# HUMAN EVOKED
# POTENTIALS
## Applications and Problems

# NATO CONFERENCE SERIES

I    Ecology
II   Systems Science
III  Human Factors
IV   Marine Sciences
V    Air—Sea Interactions
VI   Materials Science

## III HUMAN FACTORS

# HUMAN EVOKED POTENTIALS
## Applications and Problems

Edited by
**Dietrich Lehmann**
*University Hospital*
*Zurich, Switzerland*

and
**Enoch Callaway**
*University of California*
*San Francisco, California*

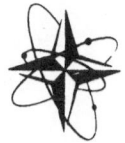

Published in coordination with NATO Scientific Affairs Division by
**PLENUM PRESS · NEW YORK AND LONDON**

Library of Congress Cataloging in Publication Data

Nato Conference on Event-Related Potentials in Man, Constance, 1978.
  Human evoked potentials.

  (NATO conference series: III, Human factors; v. 9)
  Includes index.
  1 Brain—Diseases—Diagnosis—Congresses. 2. Evoked potentials (Electrophysiology)
—Congresses. 3. Brain—Localization of functions—Congresses. 4. Sensory stimulation
—Congresses. 5. Neuropsychiatry—Congresses. I. Lehmann, Dietrich. II. Callaway,
Enoch. III. Nato Special Program Panel on Human Factors. IV. Title. V. Series.
[DNLM: 1. Evoked potentials—Congresses. W3 N138 v. 9 1978 / WL102.3 N105e
1978]
RC386.6.E86N37  1978                   616.8'04'754                        79-4320
ISBN-13: 978-1-4684-3485-9      e-ISBN-13: 978-1-4684-3483-5
DOI: 10.1007/978-1-4684-3483-5

Proceedings of the NATO Conference on Human Evoked Potentials held
at Konstanz, West Germany, August 25-28, 1978, and sponsored by the NATO
Special Program Panel on Human Factors

© 1979 Plenum Press, New York
Softcover reprint of the hardcover 1st edition 1979
A Division of Plenum Publishing Corporation
227 West 17th Street, New York, N.Y. 10011

PREFACE

From August 25 - 28, 1978 a conference on averaged evoked potentials was held at Konstanz, West Germany.  Research on human
evoked potentials has progressed rapidly in the past decade, and
a series of international conferences have served to maintain communication between active workers in the field.  Among the organiza-
tions that have a tradition of supporting such multi-national communication are the North Atlantic Treaty Organization Scientific
Affairs Division, the U.S. Office of Naval Research and the German
Research Society (Deutsche Forschungsgemeinschaft).  We have been
fortunate to have the support of all three.

In the early stages of planning, a committee was formed
composed of Professors Rudolph Cohen (Konstanz), Otto Creutzfeldt
(Goettingen), John Desmedt (Brussels), A.M. Halliday (London),
Anthony Remond (Paris) and Herbert Vaughan (New York).  A call for
papers was circulated as widely as possible, and this committee
carried out the difficult task of selecting a limited number of
participants from a large number of excellent abstracts.

At the same time Professor Cohen of the University of Konstanz
was generous enough to shoulder the task of playing host to the
conference.  His thoughtful arrangements contributed enormously to
the comfort of the participants.  He and his colleagues also engi-
neered an ideal ambience for sharing of ideas and observations,
while the University of Konstanz generously provided audio-visual
support.

Finally, it would be entirely appropriate for Danielle Thouvenin
to be one of the senior authors on this volume, for she not only
supervised the organization of the conference but edited and retyped
all the manuscripts.

This volume represents an attempt to make available the results
of a conference on ongoing research.  Speed of publication has been
our primary goal, and we have forgone some editorial niceties so
these papers can be made available to other working groups while
they are still current.  The topic is an interdisciplinary one, and

papers could have been classified a number of ways (methods, dis-
ciplines, major focuses, etc.). We have, however, arranged them by
senior author in alphabetical order.

Poster sessions played a large role in the sharing of new ideas
and data, and the abstracts of these poster presentations are also
in this volume.  Active participation of all who attended was perhaps the most crucial factor in the conference, and the editors wish
to thank them for their enthusiasm and their efforts.  The final
preparation of this volume has depended on the cooperation of Plenum
Press and the technical assistance of Dr. Charles Yingling.

CONTENTS

# CONTENTS

AUDITORY, SOMATOSENSORY AND VISUAL EVOKED POTENTIALS IN THE
DIAGNOSIS OF NEUROPATHOLOGY: RECORDING CONSIDERATIONS AND
NORMATIVE DATA

T. Allison, W.R. Goff and C.C. Wood

Veterans Administration Hospital, West Haven, Conn.

Yale University School of Medicine, New Haven, Conn.

Recent advances have led to an increased ability to use initial
components of the human auditory (AEP) and visual (VEP) evoked
potential as a neurophysiological probe for the detection of CNS
disorders (for reviews see e.g., Starr et al., 1978; Halliday, 1978).
These advances were quickly followed by a successful search for
subcortical portions of the somatosensory evoked potential (SEP)
which could be applied similarly to neurological problems (Matthews
et al., 1974; Cracco and Cracco, 1976; Jones, 1977; Hume and Cant,
1978). For purposes of differential diagnosis and better localization of lesions it will often be desirable to record EPs to the
three modalities of stimulation. A few studies have already appeared using combinations of EPs (e.g., Mastaglia et al., 1976; Stockard and Sharbrough, 1978). The need thus arises for a review of
the problems involved in combining AEP, SEP and VEP recording in a
test which can be carried out in a single recording session. This
paper will consider recording conditions and available normative
data in such a clinical context. In referring to electrode location
the subscripts $c$ and $i$ will denote locations contralateral and
ipsilateral to the side of stimulation. All components are labelled
by their polarity and approximate peak latency; AEP components P2-P9
correspond to waves I-VII as usually described.

Interest in subcortical AEP components is intense, and they
have been applied to various diagnostic problems. Component amplitudes vary considerably in the normal population and are not generally useful. Peak latencies in studies reporting quantitative
data are summarized in Figs. 1 and 2 and lead to these conclusions:
(1) Most of the normative data reported to date are for young
children or young adults. (2) On the right of Figs. 1 and 2, peak

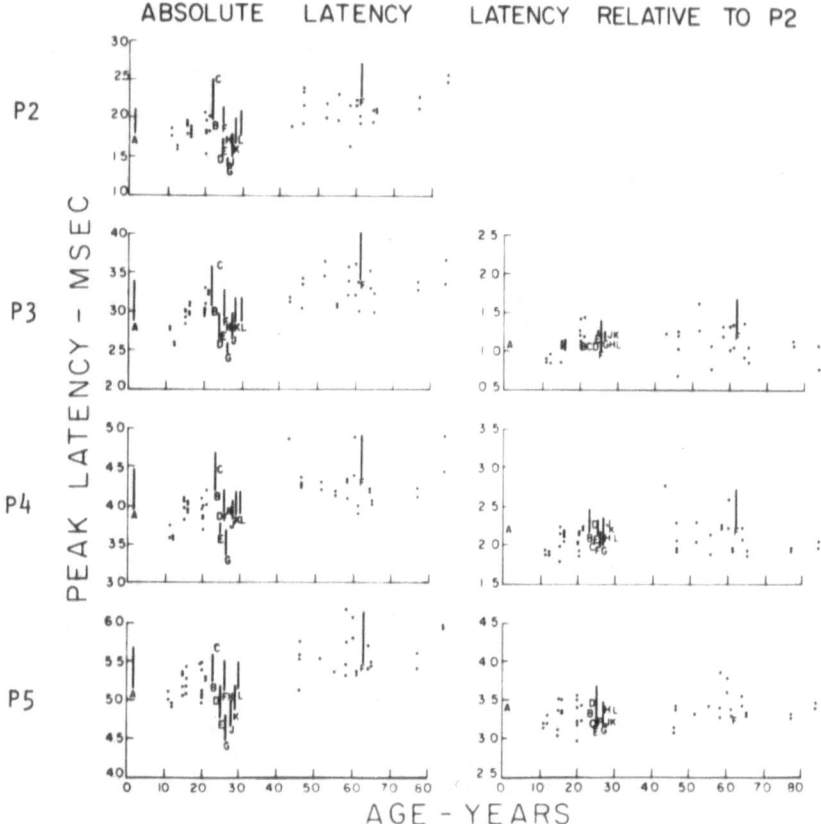

Fig. 1.  Age related changes in AEP peak latencies and latencies relative to P2.  Mean latency (letter) and +2 SD (vertical line) as determined by:  A, Salamy and McKean, 1976; B, Stockard and Rossiter, 1977; C, Goff et al., 1978; D, Picton et al., 1974; E, Gilroy and Lynn, 1978; F, Rowe, 1978; G, Gilroy et al., 1977; H, Don et al., 1976; J, Starr and Achor, 1975 (75dB HL); K, Starr and Achor (65 dB HL); L, Picton et al., 1977.  Dots are preliminary data of present study.

latencies are given relative to P2 which reflects the eighth nerve volley.  Use of the peripheral nerve benchmark against which later components are measured provides a considerable reduction in between-laboratory variability, primarily because the effects of varying stimulus intensities used by different workers are partialed out due to parallel latency-intensity functions (e.g., Starr and Achor, 1975; Huang and Buchwald, 1978).  (3) Fewer data are available for P7 and P9 which may reflect activity at the level of the medial geniculate nucleus and thalamocortical radiations, respectively (Stockard and

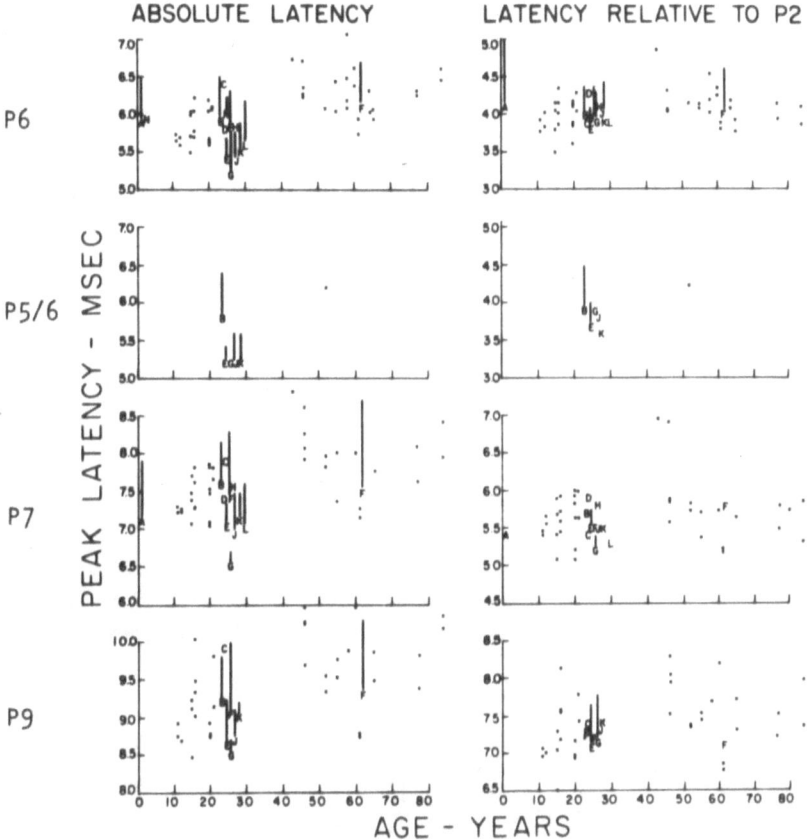

Fig. 2.   AEP component latencies.   Details as in Fig. 1.


Rossiter, 1977).   P9 is often followed by a small deflection, P12,
of unknown origin; no previous data are available.   While P7, P9 and
P12 are more variable in latency and appearance than are the earlier
components, they are usually reproducible in a given subject.   The
preliminary data summarized in Figs. 1 and 2 suggest that absolute
latencies increase with age but that latencies relative to P2 are
fairly constant.

     Recording electrode locations are reasonably consistent in
previous work.   Activity is typically recorded between Cz and an
electrode on the mastoid or earlobe ipsilateral to the ear stimulated.   Considerable variation exists in other recording parameters.
The following are representative and were used for the preliminary
data summarized in Figs 1 and 2: N = 1024 (2048 if necessary); filters at 30-3000 Hz (-3 dB points); intensity, 75 dB SL; stimulus
rate, 10 sec; recording from Cz-Ai.

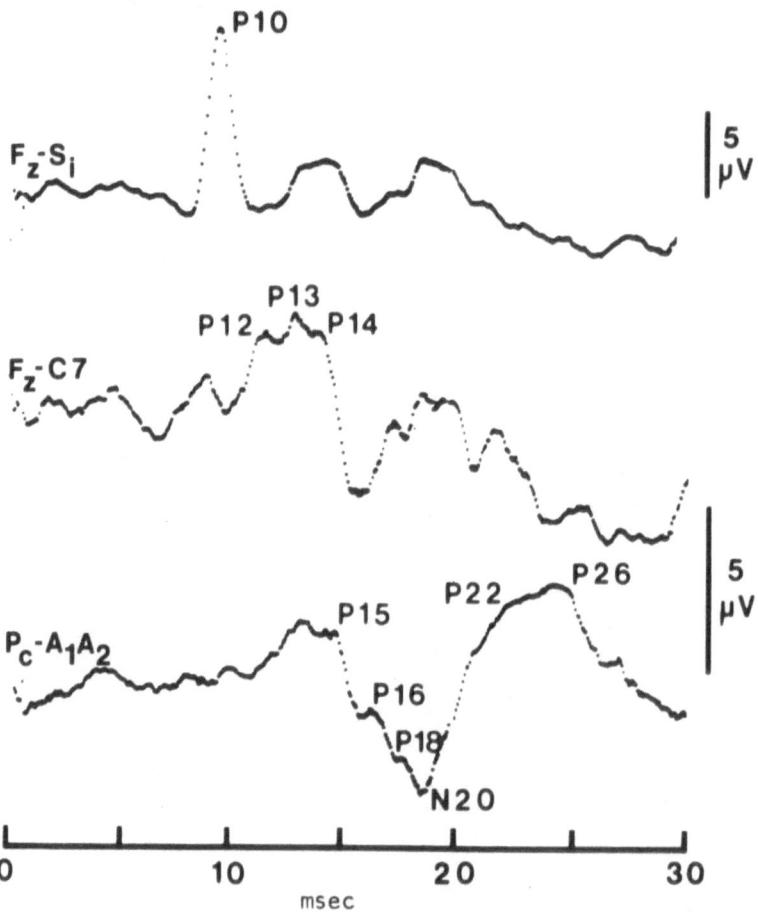

Fig. 3.  Early SEP components recorded from derivations shown;
details in text.


        Although short latency SEPs of subcortical origin have been
recorded for years (for a review see Allison et al., 1978), detailed
recording of such activity using high resolution techniques is
recent.  No consensus has been reached as to optimal recording conditions, nor is it clear that all workers are observing exactly the
same activity.  By analogy with the subcortical AEP, it should be
possible to use the subcortical SEP in evaluation of brain stem and
midbrain pathology; promising preliminary results have been reported (Mastaglia et al., 1976; Greenberg et al., 1977; Hume and Cant,
1978; Stockard and Sharbrough, 1978).

We will first describe these components obtained from our standard recording conditions, then discuss the rationale for these conditions.  The potentials are illustrated in Fig. 3 and are derived from a combination of the techniques described by Matthews et al., Cracco and Cracco, Jones and Hume and Cant.  Following the convention used for the subcortical AEP, positive at scalp leads (Fz or Pc) is recorded upward.  The top trace is the median nerve compound action potential recorded at the level of the shoulder ipsilateral (Si) to the stimulated median nerve.  The middle trace illustrates later subcortical potentials Pl2, Pl3 and Pl4.  The lower trace shows the subcortical potential Pl5 and the earliest cortical potential N20.

By analogy with the AEP, it should be useful to record a peripheral nerve benchmark with which later components can be compared.  As would be expected there is a high correlation (about .80) between the latency of these components and body height or arm length (Matthews et al.; Hume and Cant; Dorfman 1977).  Use of a peripheral nerve benchmark removes most of this source of variability in adults.  Peripheral nerve conduction velocity varies with temperature (e.g., Buchthal and Rosenfalck, 1966).  For clinical purposes it is not feasible to regulate arm temperature; use of the benchmark should remove this source of variability.  Cracco and Cracco recorded the peripheral nerve volley at the level of the brachial plexus from Erb's Point, while Jones recorded it from the clavicle.  In most subjects either of these locations yields a large, easily quantified potential.  In normal subjects we found that a location midway along the clavicle yielded a potential about one-third larger (and earlier by 0.3-0.4 msec) than that recorded from Erb's Point.  Since Pl0 is small in some older subjects and patients, the mid-clavicular placement seems preferable.

Components Pl2, Pl3 and Pl4 can be recorded either from scalp electrodes to a noncephalic reference (Cracco and Cracco), from electrodes over the cervical spine to a noncephalic reference (Jones) or from a cervical spine-midfrontal scalp derivation (Matthews et al.; Jones; Hume and Cant).  In the scalp-noncephalic derivation these components are recorded as positive potentials, whereas in cervical spine-noncephalic recordings they appear as negativities (Fig. 4A).  The origin of these potentials is not considered here (see Jones; Hume and Cant; Goff et al., 1978), but it will be useful to determine why they are recorded "locally" as negativities and rostrally as positivities.  Cracco (1973) and Allison et al., (1978) interpreted an N14 potential (an amalgam of the Pl2, Pl3 and Pl4 components as recorded here) as reflecting the cervical cord afferent volley.  If this interpretation is correct for Pl2, Pl3 and Pl4, a "killed-end equivalent" recording would satisfactorily account for the fact that these potentials are recorded from the scalp as positivities (Fig. 4B).  On the other hand, some of these

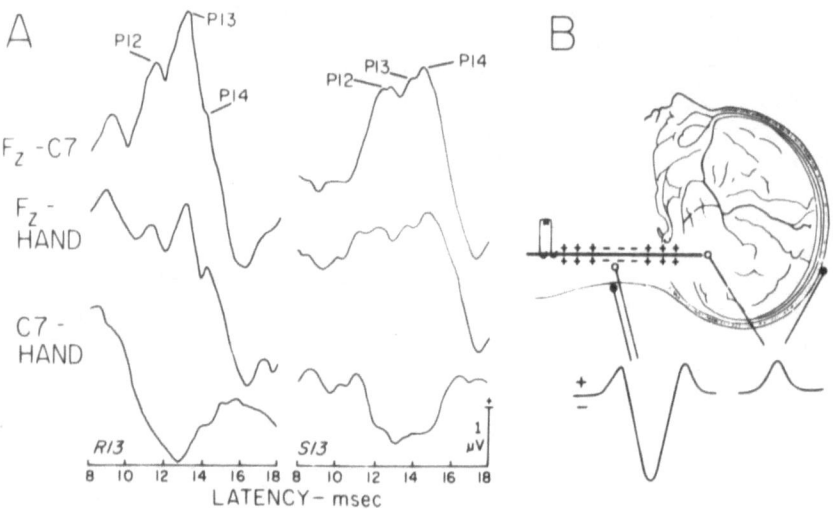

Fig. 4.  Field potential properties of SEP P12, P13 and P14.  A.
P12, P13 and P14 are recorded as positivities in the Fz-hand
derivation and as negativities in the C7-hand derivation; the Fz-C7
derivation yields their sum.  B.  Possible model to explain the
results of A.  Assume an isolated nerve preparation with recording
(open circles) and stimulating electrodes as shown.  An electrode
on the nerve will record a negativity (sink) when the region of
depolarization passes under the electrode and positive (source)
potentials just before and after.  An electrode at or beyond the
end of the nerve will record a monophasic positive source potential
("killed-end effect"; e.g., Landau, 1967).  Now imagine this nerve
to be a fiber tract (e.g., dorsal column or medial lemniscus).  As
recorded from surface electrodes (closed circles) its compound
action potential will be recorded as a negativity from the neck and
as a positivity from the scalp.

components are thought to reflect activity generated in fixed sites
(Matthews et al.; Jones; Hume and Cant); in this case it may be
assumed that local sources mainly lie rostral to the depolarizing
sinks and form a dipole field oriented in the rostral-caudal plane.
Whatever the origin of these potentials, operationally the Fz-C7
derivation introduced by Matthews et al. takes advantage of their
dipolar properties (cf. Jones) and yields an optimal recording.
Noncephalic reference derivations are more subject to stimulus, EKG
and muscle artifact and yield components of variable waveform.  P12
and P13 are robust potentials, measurable in almost all normal subjects.  P14 sometimes appears as a distinct peak (e.g., Fig. 3) but
more often appears as a shoulder or inflection on the falling phase
of P13.  When P14 is difficult to measure in the Fz-C7 derivation

it can sometimes be seen better in the Pc-AlA2 derivation (Matthews et al., Fig. 1).  As noted by Jones, P12 and P13 sometimes break up into subpeaks which can make determination of latency difficult.

In the Pc-AlA2 derivation, P13 and P14 are followed by P15 (Fig. 3).  P15 can be the largest in this sequence of potentials, or it can appear only as a shoulder.  It should be noted that the P15 potential recorded in earlier work (e.g., Allison et al., 1978) is an amalgam of the P13, P14 and P15 potentials as recorded here. N20 is generally regarded as reflecting initial activity of somato-sensory cortex.  It is large and easily measured in normal subjects. As noted by Cracco and Cracco, one or two positive deflections are often seen between P15 and N20; in Fig. 3 they are tentatively labelled P16 and P18.  When only one deflection is apparent its categorization may be difficult.  As noted by Hume and Cant, the waveform following N20 is variable in morphology.  In some cases there is a single positivity at about 25 msec, but two peaks at about 22 and 26 msec are often seen.  These are tentatively labelled P22 and P26 in Fig. 3 although in this example they are not clearly distinct.  It is likely that P22 and P26 as measured here correspond to P25 and P30 as recorded by "standard" methods (e.g., Goff et al., 1977), the difference being due primarily to differing preamplifier high frequency bandpass.

Hume and Cant studied amplitude and latency of some of these potentials as a function of stimulus intensity.  They found virtual-ly no change in latency from an intensity just above sensory thres-hold to the maximal level tolerated.  Amplitude increased only slightly from an intensity just below thumb twitch to the maximal level tolerated.  Thus an intensity near thumb twitch threshold appears to be a good compromise between response amplitude and sub-ject comfort.

Most studies not dealing specifically with the lower extremi-ties have used median nerve stimulation at the wrist as a stimulus because it is convenient, because it evokes a large SEP and because the thumb twitch so produced provides an objective measure of stimu-lus intensity.  It has been argued, however, that stimulation of a mixed nerve has the disadvantage of evoking an antidromic volley in motor fibers which might confound the recording of sensory affer-ent activity (Desmedt, 1971).  While this argument has merit, the following considerations weigh against the use of finger stimulation: (1) Jones compared early SEP components to wrist and finger stimu-lation and found that all components were smaller but identifiable to finger stimulation.  He concluded that none of the early SEP components can be wholly due to antidromic conduction in motor fibers since such fibers are not present at the base of the fingers and stimulation of the fingers was not seen to produce a direct motor response.  We have also investigated this question and reach the

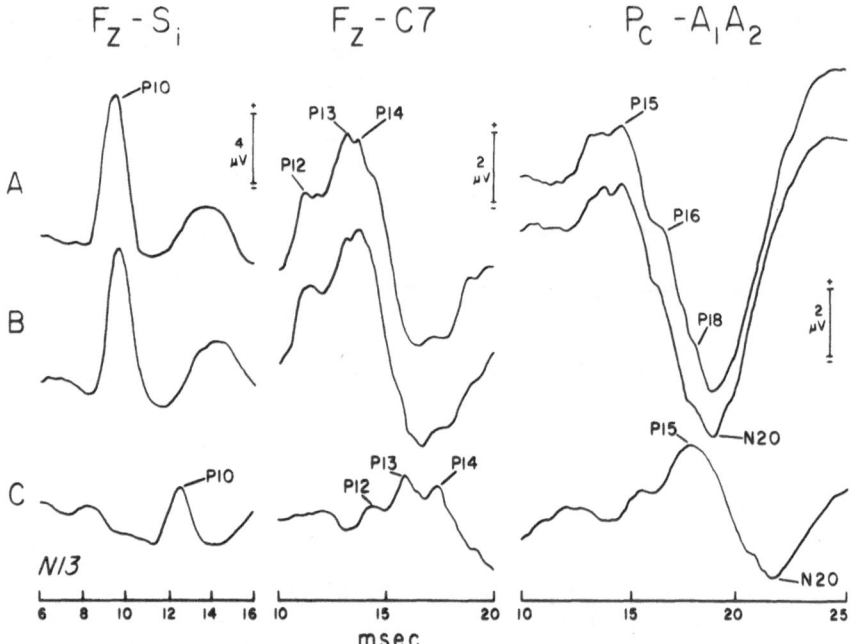

Fig. 5.  Early SEP to stimulation of median nerve at an intensity
just suprathreshold for thumb twitch (A), below thumb twitch
threshold (B) and to stimulation of first and second fingers (C).
Note similarity of waveforms in middle and top rows and presence of
all components (except P16?) to finger stimulation.

same conclusion (Fig. 5).  Note that all components are present at
a stimulus intensity below thumb twitch threshold and to stimulation
of the second and third fingers at an intensity subjectively equal
to that evoking a thumb twitch.   (2) Most patients are apprehensive
about being "shocked", and subjective estimates of stimulus intensity to finger stimulation will often be unreliable.  The small size
of the peripheral nerve volley recorded from Si to finger stimulation (Fig. 5) renders it unsatisfactory as an index of stimulus
efficacy.   (3)  Dawson (1956) first showed, and later studies (e.g.,
Rosner and Goff, 1967; Hume and Cant) have amply confirmed, that
SEP components are near their maximum amplitude at threshold for a
motor response.   (4)  Comparative studies have concluded that SEP
waveform to tactile stimuli is similar to (although smaller and later
than) the response evoked by median nerve stimulation (e.g., Nakanishi et al., 1973).  These facts argue that little or none of the
SEP is attributable to stimulation of motor nerve fibers.  In our
opinion the known advantages of using median nerve stimuli outweigh
the potential disadvantages which remain to be demonstrated.

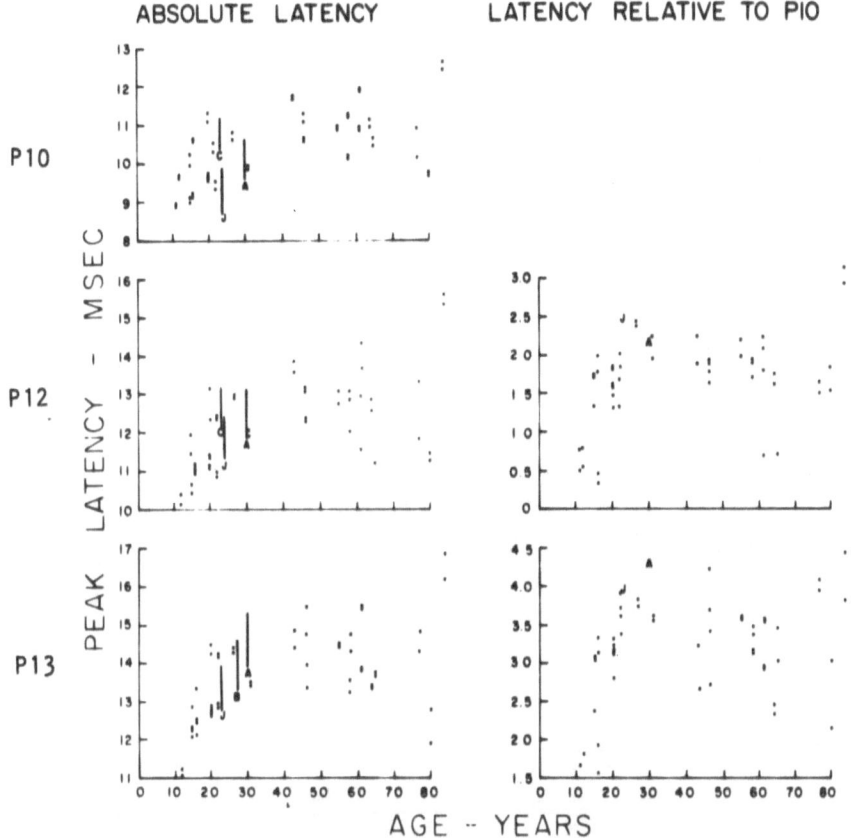

Fig. 6.  Age related changes in SEP latencies in this and previous
studies:  A, Hume and Cant, 1978; B, Matthews et al., 1974; C,
Cracco and Cracco, 1976; D, Nakanishi et al., 1973; E, Levy et al.,
1971; F, Goff et al., 1977; G, Luders, 1970; H, Laget et al., 1976;
J, Jones, 1977; L, Dorfman and Bosley, 1978; M, Aleeve and Varezhkin,
19761  Details as in Fig. 1.  Discrepancies in P10 and P10-relative
latencies result from fact that P10 latency is earlier in the Fz-C7
derivation used by Jones and Hume and Cant than in the Fz-Si derivation (Fig. 3).


        Stimulus frequencies of 1-10/sec have been used to record these
potentials.  In a pilot study we stimulated at 5 and 10/sec; waveforms and latencies were similar in both cases.  In addition to
requiring less recording time, the use of 10/sec stimuli might have
the advantage of providing more of a neurophysiological "challenge",
thus revealing abnormalities not detectable at lower rates of
stimulation (Hecox et al., 1977).  However, stimuli evoking a thumb
twitch can be unpleasant at this rate; hence we have adopted 5/sec
as a standard rate.

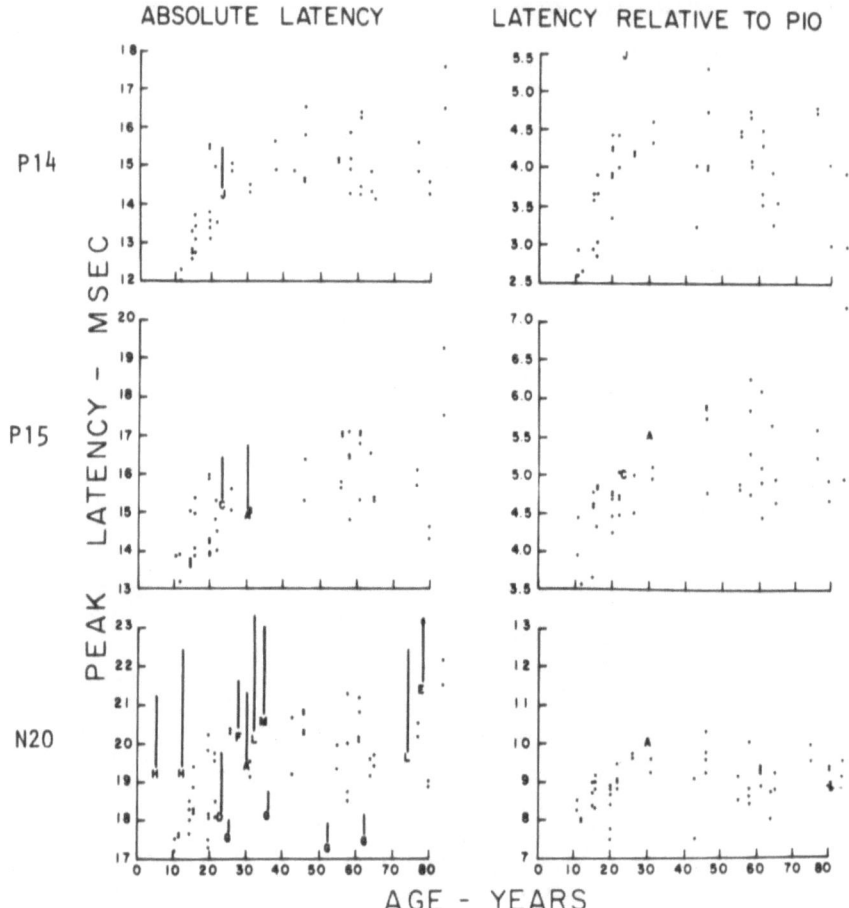

Fig. 7.  Age related SEP latency changes.  Details as in Figs. 1 and
6.

Components P15, N20, P22 and P26 are best recorded from the
scalp to an ear reference.  Some workers have recorded N20 from a
Cc lead.  However, this potential inverts in polarity across the
central sulcus and hence is small in amplitude and variable in
waveform at Cc (Goff et al., 1977).  We record P15 and later components from a Pc-A1A2 derivation.

These considerations led to adoption of the following para-
maters:  N = 512; filters at 30-3000 Hz (-3dB points); median nerve
stimulus which just produces a thumb twitch; stimulus rate, 5/sec;
three recording channels as in Fig. 3.  Preliminary data using

these conditions are summarized in Figs. 6 and 7.  It appears that
both absolute latencies and latencies relative to P10 will show
significant age related trends.  Use of these potentials in the
assessment of neuropathology has hardly begun (but see Mastaglia et
al., 1976; Small et al., 1977; Hume and Cant; Stockard and Sharbrough, 1978), and it is too early to say which will be useful.  Of
the subcortical components, P14, P16 and P18 may prove less useful
than the others because of difficulty of measurement.  P22 and P26
may reflect cortical activity occurring later than that generating
N20 and may not yield additional information.

The P100 component of the pattern reversal VEP has proved useful
in detection of optic nerve pathology of varying etiology (Halliday,
1978).  A drawback of this test is that P100 latency varies as a
function of several stimulus parameters, primarily luminance and
pattern reversal time.  Analogous to the subcortical AEP, a peripheral benchmark component which would partial out these effects
would be useful in allowing between-laboratory use of normative
data, a hazardous procedure at present (Fig. 8A).  Since the optic
nerve is itself the primary source of abnormality (assuming no retinal pathology), the ERG provides the only possible benchmark.  The
b-wave of the ERG has been recorded to pattern reversal stimuli using
a contact lens (Armington et al., 1971) but this method is not feasible for routine use.  Halliday et al. (1973) recorded a small ERG to
pattern reversal stimuli using a canthus-infraorbital derivation.
In a number of normal subjects and patients we have attempted to record the ERG from various locations near the eye but with little
success.  We agree with Halliday (personal communication) that in
this recording situation the ERG is too low in amplitude and broad
in waveform to be useful.  Unfortunately, this means that each laboratory must construct its own normative standards or adhere very
closely to the stimulating and recording conditions of a laboratory
reporting such data.

It is clear that P100 latency can increase in older persons
(e.g., Asselman et al., 1975; Hennerici et al., 1977), but the form
of the age-latency function is not clear.  The data of Keltner et
al. (in prep.) (Fig. 8B) suggest a gradual decline in latency to
about age 50 with a progressive increase thereafter, whereas Celesia
(in Starr et al., 1978) reports a progressive increase in latency
with age.  Preliminary results of the present study (Fig. 8B) do
not resolve the question.  The difference may be more apparent than
real and reflect the small sample sizes and their age distribution.
The present data were obtained using the following conditions which
are representative of those employed in previous work: N = 128
(256 if necessary); filters at 1-300 Hz (-3dB points); intensity
1760 cd/m2 (light squares), 35 cd/m2 (dark squares); squares subtend
a visual angle of 50'; entire pattern subtends 16°; reversal rate,
2/sec; electrode locations, O1 and O2 referenced to Fz.  Halliday

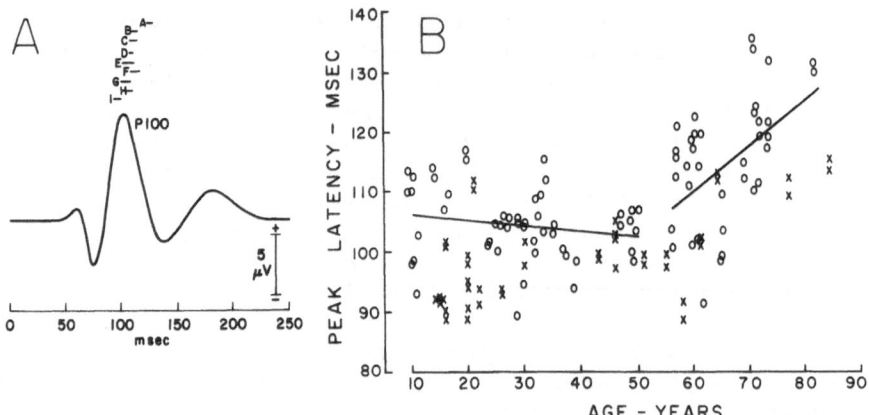

Fig. 8.  A.  Mean (letter) +2 SD (horizontal line) of VEP P100 peak
latency as determined by:  A, Halliday et al., 1973; B, Halliday
(in Goff et al., 1978); C, Shahrokhi et al., 1978; D, Zeese, 1977;
E, Celesia (in Starr et al., 1978); F, Keltner et al., in prep.; G,
preliminary results of present study; H, Hennerici et al., 1977;
I, Asselman et al., 1975.  B.  Age related changes in VEP P100.
Circles:  data of Keltner et al., in prep.  Regression lines for
10-50 and 50-80 age groups shown.  Crosses:  preliminary results of
present study.  Latency differences in the two studies are due mainly to differences in checkerboard luminance and rapidity of pattern
reversal.

prefers locations slightly rostral and lateral to O1 and O2; we find
that Halliday's placements yield a P100 whose latency is equal to
or earlier than that recorded from O1 and O2 but whose amplitude
is usually smaller.

    Using the recording conditions described above, three replica-
tions to stimulation of each ear, median nerve and eye can be obtained in approximately two hours including hook-up time.  It is,
therefore, feasible to obtain a fairly comprehensive assessment of
the functional integrity of afferent sensory pathways up to or including sensory cortex.  However, proper interpretation of such
recordings will require adequate age-related normative data which
the present preliminary results suggest will be complex.

                              SUMMARY

    The early subcortical portion of the auditory and somatosensory
evoked potentials and the P100 component of the pattern reversal
visual evoked potential are increasingly used in neurological assessment.  Review of the current state of such recordings suggests these

conclusions: 1. Recording of subcortical SEP components with high resolution techniques is recent; no consensus has emerged regarding optimal recording conditions or component origins. 2. Adequate age-related normative data for peak latencies are not available for any modality. This problem is compounded by the sensitivity of latency to stimulus parameters and recording conditions. 3. In the AEP and SEP, latency variability can be reduced by using the peripheral nerve volley as a "benchmark". 4. Preliminary results suggest that age-related latency changes are complex and must be taken into account in assessing neurological dysfunction.

REFERENCES

Aleev, L.S. and Varezhkin, J.P. Somatosensory evoked potentials of healthy people. Neurophysiol., 1976, 8, 447-454.

Allison, T., Goff, W.R., Williamson, P.D. and VanGilder, J.C. On the neural origin of early components of the human somatosensory evoked potential. In J.E. Desmedt (Ed.), Progress in Clinical Neurophysiology, Vol. 7, Basel: Karger, 1978.

Armington, J.C., Corwin, T.R. and Marsetta, R. Simultaneously recorded retinal and cortical responses to patterned stimuli. J. Opt. Soc. Amer., 1971, 61, 1514-1521.

Asselman, P., Chadwick, D.W. and Marsden, C.D. Visual evoked responses in the diagnosis and management of patients suspected of multiple sclerosis. Brain, 1975, 98, 261-282.

Buchthal, F. and Rosenflack, A. Evoked action potentials and conduction velocity in human sensory nerves. Brain Res., 1966, 3, 1-122.

Cracco, R.Q. Spinal evoked response: Peripheral nerve stimulation in man. Electroenceph. Clin. Neurophysiol., 1973, 35, 379-386.

Cracco, R.Q. and Cracco, J.B. Somatosensory evoked potential in man: Far field potentials. Electroenceph. Clin. Neurophysiol., 1976, 41, 460-466.

Dawson, G.D. The relative excitability and conduction velocity of sensory and motor nerve fibres in man. J. Physiol., 1956, 131, 436-451.

Desmedt, J.E. Somatosensory cerebral evoked potentials in man. In A. Remond (Ed.), Handbook of Electroencephalography and Clinical Neurophysiology, Vol. 9, Somatic Sensation, Amsterdam: Elsevier, 1971.

Don, M., Allen, A. and Starr, A.  Recovery functions of human audi-
    tory brain stem potentials to paired click stimuli., 1976 (un-
    published paper).

Dorfman, L.J.  Indirect estimation of spinal cord conduction velocity
    in man.  Electroenceph. Clin. Neurophysiol., 1977, 42, 26-34.

Dorfman, L.J. and Bosley, T.M.  Age-related changes in peripheral
    and central nerve conduction in man.  Neurol., in press.

Gilroy, J. and Lynn, G.E.  Computerized tomography and auditory
    evoked potentials.  Arch. Neurol., 1978, 35, 143-147.

Gilroy, J., Lynn, G.E., Ristow, G.E. and Pellerin, R.J.  Auditory
    evoked brain stem potentials in a case of "locked-in" syndrome.
    Arch. Neurol., 1977, 34, 492-495.

Goff, W.R., Allison, T., Lyons, W., Fisher, T.C. and Conte, R.
    Origins of short latency auditory evoked potentials in man.
    In J.E. Desmedt (Ed.), Progress in Clinical Neurophysiology,
    Vol. 2, Basel: Karger, 1977.

Goff, W.R., Allison, T. and Vaughan, H.G., Jr.  The functional
    neuroanatomy of event related potentials.  In E. Callaway, P.
    Tueting and S. Koslow (Eds.), Event Related Brain Potentials
    in Man, New York: Academic Press, in press.

Greenberg, R.P., Mayer, D.J., Becker, D.P. and Miller, J.D.  Eval-
    uation of brain function in severe human head trauma with
    multimodality evoked potentials.  Part 1:  Evoked brain injury
    potentials, methods and analysis.  J. Neurosurg., 1977, 47,
    150-162.

Halliday, A.M.  Clinical applications of evoked potentials.  In
    W.B. Matthews and G.H. Glaser (Eds.)  Recent Advances in
    Clinical Neurology, Livingstone: Chruchill, in press.

Halliday, A.M., McDonald W.I. and Mushin, J.  Delayed pattern evoked
    responses in optic neuritis in relation to visual acuity.  Trans.
    Ophthalmol. Soc. U.K., 1973, 93, 315-324.

Hecox, K., Cone, B. and Cooper, P.  Principles of stimulus selection
    in evoked response studies.  In J.I. Martin (Ed.), Proceedings
    of the San Diego Biomedical Symposium, Vol. 16, New York:
    Academic Press, 1977.

Hennerici, M., Wenzel, D. and Freund, H.-J.  The comparison of small
    size rectangle and checkerboard stimulation for the evaluation
    of delayed visual evoked responses in patients suspected of

multiple sclerosis.  Brain, 1977, 100, 119-136.

Huang, C.-M. and Buchwald, J.S.  Factors that affect the amplitudes
    and latencies of the vertex short latency acoustic responses
    in the cat.  Electroenceph. Clin. Neurophysiol., 1978, 44,
    179-186.

Hume, A.L. and Cant, B.R.  Conduction time in central somatosensory
    pathways in man.  Electroenceph. Clin. Neurophysiol., in press.

Jones, S.J.  Short latency potentials recorded from the neck and
    scalp following median nerve stimulation in man.  Electro-
    enceph. Clin. Neurophysiol., 1977, 43, 853-863.

Laget, P., Raimbault, J. D'Allest, A.M., Flores-Guevara, R., Mari-
    ani, J. and Thieriot-Prevost, G.  La maturation des potentiels
    evoques somesthesiques (PES) chez l'homme.  Electroenceph.
    Clin. Neurophysiol., 1976, 40, 499-515.

Landau, W.M.  Evoked potentials.  In G.C. Quarton, T. Melnechuk
    and F.O. Schmitt (Eds.), The Neurosciences. A Study Program,
    New York: Rockefeller University Press, 1967.

Levy, R., Isaacs, A. and Behrman, J.  Neurophysiological correlates
    of senile dementia: II. The somatosensory evoked response.
    Psychol. Med., 1971, 1, 159-165.

Luders, H.  The effects of aging on the waveform of the somatosensory
    cortical evoked potential.  Electroenceph. Clin. Neurophysiol.,
    1970, 29, 450-460.

Mastaglia, F.L., Black, J.L. and Collins, D.W.K.  Visual and spinal
    evoked potentials in diagnosis of multiple sclerosis.  Brit.
    Med. J., 1976, 2, 732.

Matthews, W.B., Beauchamp, M. and Small, D.G.  Cervical somatosensory
    evoked responses in man.  Nature, 1974, 252, 230-232.

Nakanishi, T., Takita, K. and Toyokura, Y.  Somatosensory evoked
    responses in tactile tap in man.  Electroenceph. Clin. Neuro-
    physiol., 1973, 34, 1-6.

Picton, T.W., Hillyard, S.A., Krausz, H.I. and Galambos, R.  Human
    auditory evoked potentials.  I. Evaluation of components.
    Electroenceph. Clin. Neurophysiol., 1974, 36, 179-190.

Picton, T.W., Woods, D.L., Baribeau-Braun, J. and Healy, T.M.G.
    Evoked potential audiometry.  J. Otolaryngol., 1977, 6, 90-119.

Rosner, B.S. and Goff, W.R.  Electrical responses of the nervous
    system and subjective scales of intensity.  In W.D. Neff (Ed.)
    Contributions to Sensory Physiology, Vol 2, New York: Academic
    Press, 1967.

Rowe, M.J. III.  Normal variability of the brain stem auditory evoked
    response in young and old adult subjects.  Electroenceph. Clin.
    Neurophysiol., 1978, 44, 459-470.

Salamy, A. and McKean, C.M.  Postnatal development of human brain
    stem potentials during the first year of life.  Electroenceph.
    Clin. Neurophysiol., 1976, 40, 418-426.

Shahrokhi, F., Chiappa, K.H. and Young, R.R.  Pattern shift visual
    evoked responses.  Arch. Neurol., 1978, 35, 65-71.

Small, D.G., Beauchamp. M. and Matthews, W.B.  Spinal evoked poten-
    tials in multiple sclerosis.  Electroenceph. Clin. Neurophysiol.,
    1977, 42, 141.

Starr, A. and Achor, L.J.  Auditory brain stem responses in neuro-
    logical disease.  Arch. Neurol., 1975, 32, 761-768.

Starr, A., Sohmer, H. and Celesia, G.G.  Some applications of evoked
    potentials to patients with neurological and sensory impairment.
    In E. Callaway, P. Tueting and S. Koslow (Eds.), Event Related
    Brain Potentials in Man, New York: Academic Press, in press.

Stockard, J.J. and Rossiter, V.S.  Clinical and pathologic corre-
    lates of brain stem auditory response abnormalities.  Neurol.,
    1977, 27, 316-325.

Stockard, J.J. and Sharbrough, F.W.  Unique contributions of short
    latency sensory evoked potentials to neurologic diagnoses.  In
    J.E. Desmedt (Ed.), Progress Clinical Neurophysiology, Vol. 7,
    Basel: Karger, in press.

Zeese, J.A.  Pattern visual evoked responses in multiple sclerosis.
    Arch. Neurol., 1977, 34, 314-316.

# ADAPTATION EFFECTS IN THE TRANSIENT VISUAL EVOKED POTENTIAL

C. Barber and N.R. Galloway

Departments of Medical Physics and Ophthalmology

Queen's Medical Centre, Nottingham

## INTRODUCTION

Implicit in the measurement of the averaged transient visual evoked potential (VEP) is the assumption that the visual system returns to a state of rest between stimuli. A signal enhancement technique such as averaging should display the signal which is the technique itself. Hence the temporal characteristics (stimulus duration and presentation rate) of the stimulus regime should be such that the above assumption is valid, or the averaging procedure may itself alter that which it seeks to measure. A lower limit to the rate of stimulation is effectively set by the stationarity of the background EEG (Cohen and Sances, 1977), and by the difficulty of maintaining a constant psychological state over periods of more than a few seconds. The upper limit is set by the transition to a steady state VEP, when the individual components become indistinguishable. Between these limits there is considerable scope for variation. The aim of this study is to investigate the dependence of the averaged transient VEP upon temporal stimulus parameters, with particular reference to the effects of adaptation upon the components of the pattern VEP.

Pattern adaptation was demonstrated by Gilinsky (1968) who showed that pre-exposure to a patterned light flash raised the psychological threshold for perception of a visual display of the same pattern form (but not others). That the VEP could be affected was shown by Blakemore and Campbell (1969) who used prestimulus adaptation to a pattern to produce a general reduction in the amplitude of the VEP, the amount of reduction depending upon the length of time for which the adapting pattern was presented. James and Jef-

freys (1975) investigated the effect of pattern pre-exposure on the
components of the pattern onset VEP and commented that these effects
could be observed in a conventional averaging run unless the stimulus
duration is a small fraction of the interstimulus interval.  Subsequently Jeffreys (1977) showed how variations in stimulus duration
and interstimulus interval could affect the VEP waveform, and
MacKay (1977) demonstrated that adaptation effects could be observed
even if the pre-exposed pattern was formed by contrasting textures.
Long stimulus sequences might be expected to accentuate any adaptation effects, and a number of authors have reported results of such
statistics.

## METHODS

Four subjects between 26 and 43 years of age participated in
these experiments, three males and one female, two right-handed and
two left-handed.  All had normal visual acuities and visual fields
and all were experienced observers.

The visual stimulus is a television based system, similar in
many respects to that described by Arden et al. (1977).  Two differences are worthy of note.  The pattern generator has crystal-
controlled synchronization giving a frame rate slightly different
from the mains and thus permitting frame-locked stimulus presentation without mains-locked artifacts.  Secondly, it is used with a
projection television (Advent Videobeam).  In this study a black
and white checkerboard pattern was used throughout with check sizes
subtending either 15', 30' or 60' of arc at the subject.  The screen
itself subtended angles of $26^{o}$ (horizontal) and $20^{o}$ (vertical).  A
fixation spot produced by slightly incrementing the pattern luminance at the appropriate point was positioned at the screen center.
The luminance of the bright squares was 10 cd m$^{-2}$ and that of the
dark squares 3.1 cd m$^{-2}$  For pattern onset VEPs the background
(i.e., interstimulus) luminance was adjusted so that the integrated
illuminance remained constant for both pattern and blank display.
For flashed pattern VEPs the screen was dark (0.1 cd m$^{-2}$) between
stimulus presentations.  For pattern reversal VEPs the luminance
values of adjacent checks were interchanged at the stimulus
frequency.

A silver/silver chloride electrode was used, positioned 2.5
cm above the inion on the midline and referenced to a similar
electrode placed midfrontally (as Michael and Halliday, 1971).
Earlobes were grounded.  The bandwidth of the (Medelec Van Gogh)
amplifier was 0.1 - 35 Hz, and the signals were averaged on a
Nicolet MED-80 minicomputer using a simple amplitude criterion for
artifact rejection.  Raw data was also recorded on magnetic tape.

For experiments involving variation of either stimulus duration or interstimulus interval an average of 64 VEPs was taken. The
various different values of independent variable were presented to
the subject over a number of sessions in a balanced square design
as appropriate.  The procedure was replicated for each stimulus mode
and, where used, for each different check size.  For experiments
involving long term adaptation a run of 600 stimulus presentations
was used; each presentation mode and, where applicable, check size
was presented to each subject on three separate occasions.  Subjects
were seated in a dimly illuminated room (illuminance at the subject
equal to the stimulus illuminance used) and allowed to adapt to this
level for a period of ten minutes in order for the effect of dark
adaptation upon the VEP to become stable (Klingaman, 1976).  Subjects
were instructed to count the number of stimulus presentations in an
attempt to maintain a constant level of attention.  Binocular
stimulation was used throughout.


## RESULTS

For pattern onset and flashed pattern VEPs three peaks are
always clearly visible:  a positive peak at 100-120 msec latency, a
negative peak at 130-150 msec and a second positive peak at 200-220
msec.  They are taken to be components I, II and III as described by
Jeffreys (1972), Lesevre and Remond (1972) and Spekreijse et al.
(1973).  Differences in latency are assumed to be due to differences
in luminance and contrast of the patterns used by different authors.
It is expected that the latencies in this study will be relatively
long since, although a high contrast pattern is used, the luminance
is relatively low.  For pattern reversal responses a single positive
peak at approximately 100 msec latency is predominant, although in
some subjects negative peaks on either side of it, and even a second
positive peak at around 200 msec latency are seen with varying
degrees of clarity.  The 100 msec peak, as described by Halliday and
Michael (1970) is used as the measure in this study. If it is assumed
that these components may represent distinct cortical processes, then
it is essential to measure their amplitudes independently; peak-to-
peak measures will always confound the properties of two components.
It is thus necessary to define a suitable baseline, and in this
work it was taken to be the mean value of VEP recorded in the first
40 msec after stimulus presentation.  The notations CI, CII and CIII
will be used hereafter to apply to the positive 100-120 msec, negative 130-150 msec and positive 200-220 msec peaks, respectively, as
measured from this baseline.  P100 will be used for the predominant
peak in the reversal VEPs.


## Experiment (i)

The effect of different stimulus duration upon component

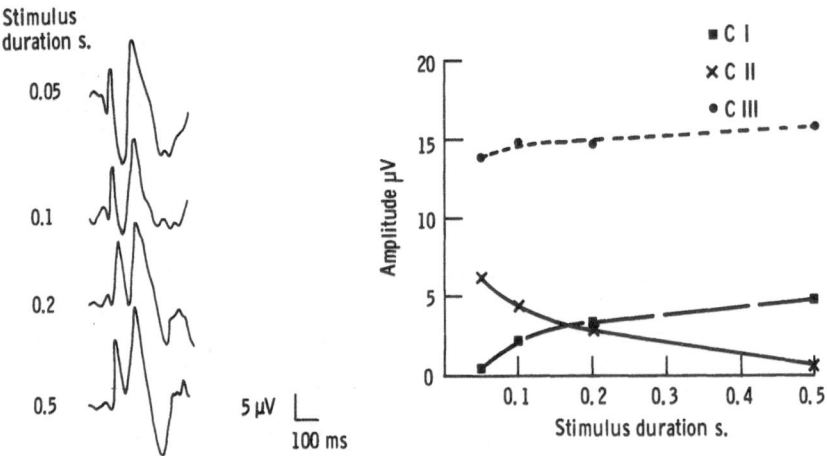

Fig. 1. The effect of stimulus duration. The left half-figure
shows (single subject) flashed pattern VEPs for stimulus durations
of 50, 100, 200 and 500 msec with a constant interstimulus interval
of 500 msec. Positivity is up. The right half-figure shows component amplitude as a function of duration (mean across subjects and
sessions). 15' checks were used.

amplitudes was investigated for a fixed interstimulus interval of
500 msec using flashed pattern presentation of a 15' check.

     The VEPs obtained (Fig. 1) show an increase in the amplitude of
CI and a clear decrease in the amplitude of CII, with increasing
stimulus duration; changes in CIII are less marked. A description
of the behavior of CI is possible using the concept of "residual
contrast" which is present at stimulus onset due to the incomplete
disappearance of contrast representation from the previous stimulus
presentation. Such a mechanism was proposed by Spekreijse et al.
(1973). They also demonstrated that the VEP to an increase in
standing contrast may be treated as a pattern onset VEP with its
starting point part way up the amplitude vs contrast curve,
providing the standing contrast does not produce appreciable
adaptation. Since the component amplitude reaches zero whilst there
is still some contrast present, it is possible for a small standing
contrast to produce an increase in amplitude. Hence it could be
postulated that for CI there is a small residual contrast, the
magnitude of which increases with stimulus duration but remains subthreshold under the conditions of the experiment. The behavior of
CII is indicative of adaptation with an integrative adaptation
process. Although the data are few, regression analysis provides
a good fit to an exponential relationship (correlation coefficient
> 0.99) with an adaptation time constant of approximately 200 msec.
CIII shows an insignificant amplitude increase with duration

increase, which could be interpreted as evidence of adaptation
obviating the residual contrast.


### Experiment (ii)

An alternative way of examining the same effects is to keep
the stimulus duration constant and vary the interstimulus interval.
In the first instance this was carried out using a flashed pattern
stimulus of 200 msec duration with intervals from 0.3 sec to 4.0
sec.  The duration of 200 msec was chosen so that the pattern offset response, which was clear in some subjects (but absent in
others), was sufficiently delayed with respect to the components
being measured, so as not to interfere with them.  Check sizes of
15', 30' and 60' of arc were used.

Examination of the VEPs (Fig. 2) shows a clear and steady
increase in CII with increase in interstimulus interval.  The
changes in both of the positive components are less marked.  The
relationship between check size and component amplitude is as
previously described (Barber and Galloway, 1976), with CI maximized
for large checks and CIII for small; this relationship holds over
the whole range of intervals tested.  For each component at each
check size the graph has a bifid form, suggesting the involvement
of more than one process.  For CI and CIII the bifid nature is much
more apparent for the larger checks.  The initial peaks in the curves
for CI may be explained by means of the residual contrast model used
previously.  If the responses to medium rate stimulation are
unsaturated, the effect of high values of residual contrast will be
to cause saturation and decrease the VEP amplitude; this condition
will apply for very short interstimulus intervals.  As the interval
is increased the amount of residual contrast will decrease, and a
point will be reached where it becomes subthreshold.  This corresponds to the initial maximum on the curve.  Thereafter, as the
residual contrast becomes further subthreshold, the component
amplitude will decrease until it reaches a steady value at the
interval for which no residual contrast remains.  The shape of the
curve for intervals in excess of this value is not in good agreement
with the model; one possible source of error may be the presence
of luminance related effects due to the flashed pattern presentation.
The more marked effect for larger checks for both CI and CIII is in
agreement with the findings of Kulikowski (1977), who has shown that
the contrast threshold is higher for patterns of low spatial frequency.  The curves for CIII are similar in form to those of CI,
and the initial part, at least, could be explained in terms of
residual contrast attenuated by adaptation.  The apparent shift of
the first peak towards a shorter value of interstimulus interval
would be in agreement with this, as would the more pronounced slope
for the larger checks.  The minimal net effect for the small checks
might account for the insignificant variation in CIII in the previous

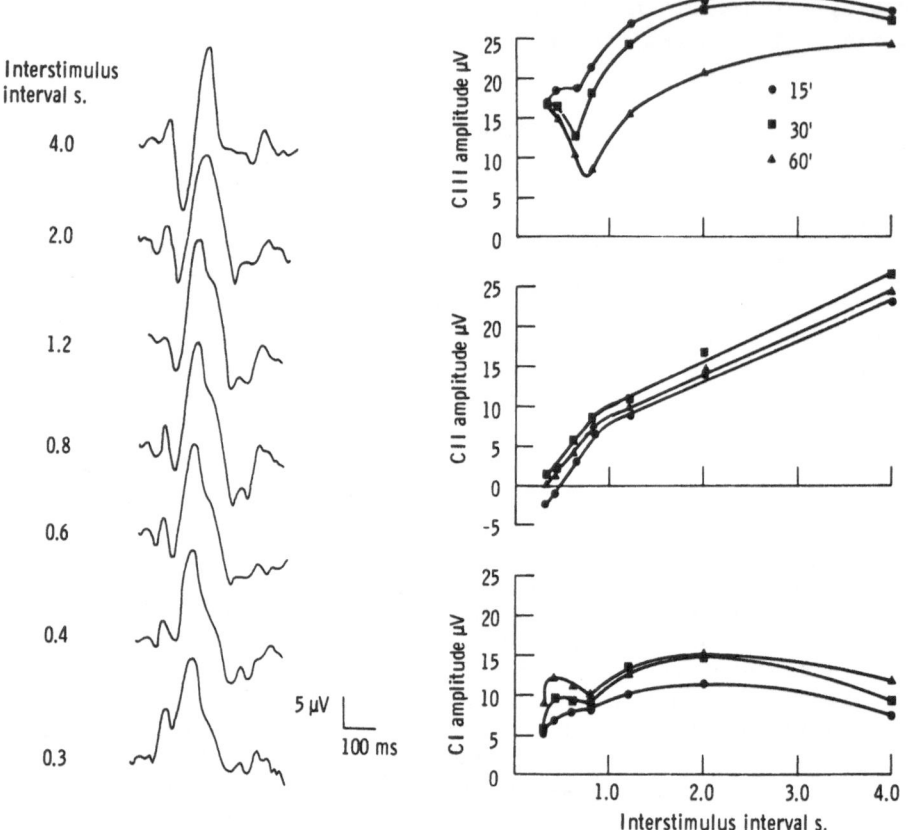

Fig. 2.   The effect of interstimulus interval.   The left half-figure
shows (single subject) VEPs to a flashed pattern of 15' checks.
Interstimulus intervals from 013 to 4.0 sec are used with a constant
duration of 200 msec.   Positivity is up.   The monotonic increase in
CII is clearly seen.   The right half-figure shows component amplitude as a function of interstimulus interval for check sizes of 15',
30' and 60'.

experiment.   The duplex linear curves obtained for CII are unusual,
but regression analysis shows a much better fit (correlation
coefficient > 0.99 for all subjects and all check sizes) than for
the exponential function which might be expected.   Having adapted
during the stimulus presentation, CII appears to undergo linear
recovery, with accelerated recovery in the residual contrast period.
The parallel curves indicate that the effect is independent of check
size.   Again, the involvement of luminance effects is a possibility.

       The experiment was repeated for pure pattern onset responses
and the opportunity taken to increase the range of interstimulus

intervals in order to try to determine the interval at which CII
levels off.  The stimulus duration was increased to 500 msec so that
the response recorded was pure pattern onset.  In other respects the
procedure was identical to that used for the previous part of this
experiment except that only one check size (30') was used.

The results (Fig. 3) show that for CI there is definitely a
luminance contribution.  With this removed, the residual adaptation
model describes the curve well.  For short interstimulus intervals
it also describes the curve for CIII, but for the longer intervals
the amplitude of this component begins to decrease.  Examination of
our VEPs suggests that CIII may be composed of two peaks which are
not resolved at normal intervals, but which are visible for a very
long interval.  Hence the peak normally measured may be a summation
of two peaks.  The length of time for which residual contrast per-
sists shows an increase compared with the flashed pattern curves.
This is due to the increase in stimulus duration from 200 msec to
500 msec, and the size of increase is in good agreement with the
200 msec adaptation time constant derived earlier.  The curve for
CII is unchanged; furthermore, the rate of increase in amplitude is
unchanged, even for intervals as long as 9 msec.

In all the work described thus far, stimulus presentation has
been regular, and there remains the possibility that this regularity
itself influences the VEP.  The experiment was, therefore, repeated
using a series of random interstimulus intervals, each with a mean
value equal to one of the values of intervals used previously and a
range of ± 50% of this value.  The results show a similar relationship for the positive component as has been obtained previously.
For CII, however, whilst there is still a clear increase in amplitude with interval, the bifid form obtained for regular presentation
is not discernable.  Clearly, regularity has an effect, though it

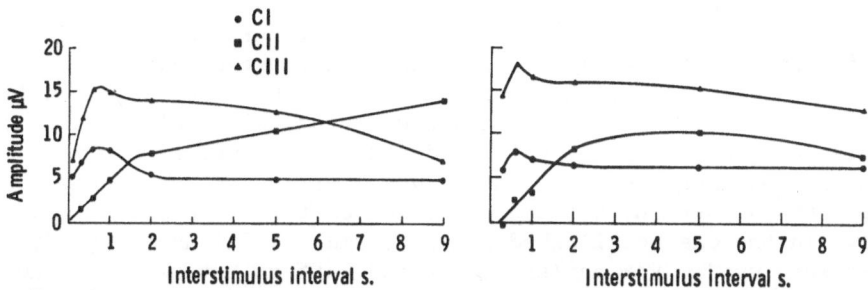

Fig. 3.  Component amplitude as a function of interstimulus interval
for pattern onset VEPs (mean across subjects and session).  The left
hand graph refers to a regular stimulus sequence.  The curves for CI
and CIII are modified compared with those for flashed pattern VEPs,
but that for CII is unchanged.  The use of an "interval indicator"
(right hand graph) modifies the behavior of CII for long interstimulus intervals.

is not clear whether this is due to physiological or psychological
factors; controlling temporal uncertainty by means of an "interval
indicator" modifies the latter part of the CII curve but nothing else.

The basic experiment was also carried out using regular stimulus periods for pattern reversal responses. In this case the P100
component was measured, being the only component recognizable in all
cases. The largest response was obtained from a subject from whom
we have consistently been unable to obtain an offset VEP. This
suggests that reversal VEPs, obtained by a television stimulus, may
be similar to those described by Jeffreys (1977) for tachistoscope
presentation as opposed to those obtained by pattern movement. The
dependence of P100 on interstimulus interval was slight and varied
from subject to subject. In some there was a slight increase in
amplitude with increase in period; in others a slight decrease.
Overall, no adaptation effects were observed for reversal VEPs. It
is not possible to tell from this experiment whether pattern reversal
fails to stimulate those components which are subject to adaptation
or whether the constant presence of the pattern simply adapts them
out.

## Experiment (iii)

Whereas the previous experiments have been concerned with
processes occurring with individual stimulus presentations and
interstimulus intervals, the final experiment is aimed at demonstrating the effects of these processes as observed over large
numbers of stimulus presentations. There are two reasons for doing
this. One is that any small effects may thereby become more
apparent. The other is to test the predictions of the model derived
for the adaptation and recovery of CII. A system with exponential
adaptation and linear recovery characteristics gives a value for the
amplitude of the VEP to the nth stimulus which converges quite
rapidly to a steady value as n increases from zero and thus predicts
a rapid decrease in amplitude followed by a constant amplitude VEP.
The actual rate of convergence in any given set of conditions will
depend upon the values of the parameters used; with values obtained
in this study a steady value is predicted after approximately five
stimuli. Long sequence experiments were carried out on each subject
using flashed pattern, pattern onset and pattern reversal stimulus
modes. In the case of flashed pattern, small (15') and large (60')
checks were used. For pattern onset and pattern reversal, medium
(30') checks were used. The VEPs were evaluated simply by averaging
contiguous blocks and producing plots of amplitude vs block number.
In the first instance 32 VEPs were averaged per block.

The results for each of the different components and stimulus
presentation modes are shown in Fig. 4, except that the graphs for
pattern onset and flashed pattern presentation are very similar and

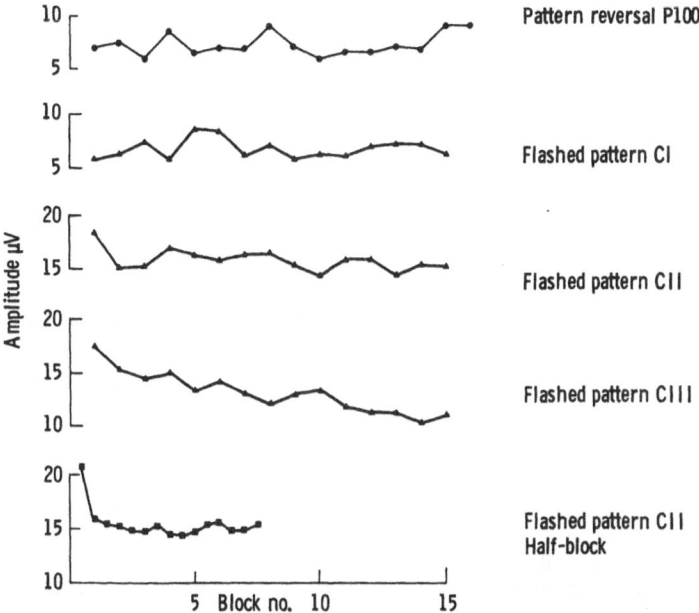

Fig. 4.   Variation in component amplitude during a long stimulus sequence for pattern reversal and flashed pattern VEPs.   Each contiguous block contains 32 VEPs.   For the last graph there are 16 VEPs per block, and these have been plotted as "half blocks" to preserve the time scale for the figure.

are not shown separately.   For reversal VEPs the P100 component remains unchanged over the long sequence.   For pattern onset and flashed pattern VEPs CI shows no overall change in amplitude, and this is independent of check size.   CII shows a gradual decrease in amplitude which is described reasonably well by an exponential function (correlation coefficient 0.96).   The rhythmical super-imposed fluctuations were more marked for pattern onset VEPs and increased in amplitude with time; they may be due to variations in attention.   CII shows a sharp initial drop and then remains essentially constant.   This is clearly visible for each check size for each subject.   A block size of 32 is a rather coarse measure, and so one set of data was recalculated for blocks of sixteen (smaller blocks than this give inadequate signal enhancement).   The initial amplitude drop and subsequent stabilization become more apparent.

DISCUSSION

The main findings from this work are that the amplitude of each component of the averaged VEP is affected to some extent by the temporal properties of the stimulus regime; since they are differ-

entially affected, changes in waveform are produced.  The behavior
of CI may be explained in terms of saturation induced by residual
contrast; CI does not appear to be subject to adaptation at all.
CIII adapts slowly, and the effects of this are visible only after
a fairly large number of stimulus presentations.  The behavior of
CII is quite different: it adapts quickly and reaches a stable, and
considerably reduced, amplitude in a small number of presentations.
These findings are in general agreement with those of James and
Jeffreys (1975) but differ in the degree of attenuation found in
CIII.  This may be due to the length of pre-exposure used; a long
pre-exposure would increase the adaptation of CIII relative to CII.
An alternative explanation is suggested by Jeffreys' data (1977)
from which it appears that CIII amplitude is relatively constant
except for a single condition (100% contrast, 25 msec duration),
which may be anomolous.

A number of other studies have produced results which are
compatible with the residual contrast model, although comparisons
of data can only be made with caution as most previous work has been
carried out on flash VEPs, often with different electrode placements
and invariably with peak to peak measures of amplitude.  Differences
between vertex and occipital VEPs were pointed out by Lehtonen (1973),
particulary for CII (his N3).  He also noted that this component
increased in amplitude in the presence of stimulus contour.  In fact,
the amount of contour used - simply the rectangular boundary of the
stimulus screen - was very small and approximates to the blank flash
stimulus used in the present study.  This does emphasize the point
that, although the difficulties of producing a pattern VEP uncontami-
nated by luminance components are well known it is also difficult
to produce a luminance VEP free of pattern components.  Hence
many supposedly flash VEPs do contain recognizable contour components, in some cases enough to permit comparisons with pattern VEPs
to be made.  An initial peak similar to that ascribed to residual
contrast in the data presented here is present in the data of Mecacci
and Spinelli (1976) who measured VEP amplitude (steady state,
sinusoidal grating, reversal VEP) as a function of recovery time
after adaptation to a similar high contrast pattern.  Residual
contrast may also be involved in the enchancement of VEP by pre-
exposure to conditioning (adapting) lights, which was described by
Kitajima et al. (1975).  Although their data relates to flash VEPs
a component corresponding to CII is clearly visible and markedly
affected by adaptation.  An effect due to stimulus regularity is
indicated, but its origins are not resolved.  The effects of
attention and expectation on EP amplitudes are well documented
(e.g., Squires et al., 1976), and in this study CII amplitude for
long interstimulus intervals was modified by controlling temporal
uncertainty.  However, psychological variables seem unlikely to be
involved for the early parts of the graphs.  The value of interstimulus interval at which the slopes change is not correlated with
any subjective temporal performance criteria such as an instanta-

neous/durable transition   (Serviere et al., 1977), optimum interval
estimation (Woodrow, 1934) or loss of sense of rhythm (Fraise, 1956),
whilst it is increased by an increase in previous adaptation time.
Hence a physiological explanation is indicated.  If the contention
of Basar et al. (1975), that EPs mostly result from frequency
stabilization of spontaneous activity, triggered by stimulation,
is correct, then this may reflect the different effectiveness of
regular as opposed to irregular stimulation in frequency stabilization.  The findings from the long stimulus sequences confirm the
predictions of component behavior derived from the data of the
short term experiments, and other authors have demonstrated similar
results (for example, Armington, 1964; Laurian and Gaillard, 1976;
Shipley and Hyson, 1977).  Shipley and Hyson discuss the shape of
the attenuation curve (for various modalities) and suggest that it
becomes more nearly a duplex function as stimulus rate is increased.
Our results show that for pattern VEPs the initial decrease will be
steeper for shorter interstimulus intervals accentuating the break
between the CII-dominated and CIII-dominated parts of a curve of
peak-to-peak amplitude.  This is in agreement with their suggestion.

These results show what is well known to anyone who has
watched VEPs being averaged: the first response is invariably much
larger than subsequent ones, and the conclusions to be drawn are of
practical significance.  Attempts to choose temporal stimulus
parameters, such that the measurement procedure itself produces no
adaptation effects on the VEP, are likely to be unsuccessful.
Generally CI will exhibit no adaptation effect, and CIII little.
CII, on the other hand, will be subject to rapid initial adaptation,
and the use of a very long interstimulus interval to avoid this
will increase the likelihood of psychological variations, to which
this component is also shown to be subject.  A practical procedure
would be simply to discard the VEPs to the first six or so stimuli.
In this way a stably adapted VEP will be obtained.

## SUMMARY

The effect of adaptation-type processes upon the waveform of
the transient visual evoked potential (VEP) was investigated in
normal subjects using flashed pattern, pattern onset and pattern
reversal stimuli.  A checkerboard pattern was used with check sizes
of, variously, 15', 30' or 60' of arc.  Changes in amplitude of the
individual components of the VEP were measured as a function of
stimulus duration and interstimulus interval (flashed pattern and
pattern onset) or stimulus period (pattern reversal).  For pattern
onset VEPs both regular and random interstimulus intervals were
used.  Each component was shown to have some dependence upon temporal
stimulus parameters, although a marked adaptation effect occurred
for only one.  The variation in component amplitude as a function
of interstimulus interval had, in each case, a bifid form, indicat-

ing the involvement of more than one physiological process.  There
was also some dependence upon check size.  The findings were used
to describe the behavior of component amplitude in an averaging run,
and the validity of this description was tested by investigating
variations occurring during a long stimulus sequence.

## REFERENCES

Arden, G.B., Faulkner, D.J. and Mair, C.  A versatile television
    pattern generator for visual evoked potentials.  In J.E.
    Desmedt (Ed.)  Visual Evoked Potentials in Man:  New Develop-
    ments, Oxford: Clarendon Press, 1977.

Armington, J.C.  Adaptational changes in the human electroretinogram
    and occipital responses.  Vision Res., 1964, 4, 179-192.

Barber, C. and Galloway, N.R.  A pattern stimulus for optimal res-
    ponse from the retina.  Doc. Ophthal., 1976, 10, 77-86.

Basar, E., Gonder, A., Ozusmi, C. and Ungan, P.  Dynamics of brain
    rhythmic and evoked potentials.  Biol. Cybernetics, 1975, 20,
    137-169.

Blakemore, C. and Campbell, F.W.  On the existence of neurones in
    the human visual system selectively sensitive to the orienta-
    tion and size of retinal images.  J. Physiol., 1969, 203,
    237-260.

Cohen A.C. and Sances, A.  Stationarity of the human electroenceph-
    alogram.  Med. Biol. Eng. Comput., 1977, 15, 513-518.

Fraise, P.  Les Structures Rythmiques, Paris: Erasme, 1956.

Gilinsky, A.S.  Orientation-specific effects of patterns of
    adapting light on visual acuity.  J. Opt. Soc. Amer., 1968,
    58, 13-18.

James, C.R. and Jeffreys, D.A.  Properties of individual components
    of pattern-onset evoked potentials in man. J. Physiol., 1975,
    249, 57-58P.

Jeffreys, D.A. and Axford, J.G.  Source locations of pattern-
    specific components of human visual evoked potentials.  Exp.
    Brain Res., 1972, 16 1-40.

Jeffreys, D.A.  The physiological significance of pattern visual
    evoked potentials.  In J.E. Desmedt (Ed.), Visual Evoked
    Potentials in Man: New Developments.  Oxford: Clarendon Press,
    1977.

Kitajima, S., Morotomi, T. and Kanoh, M.   Enhancement of averaged
     evoked responses to brief flashes after offset of pre-exposed
     light stimulation:  A critical moment.  Vision Res., 1975, 15,
     1213-1216.

Klingaman, R.L.   The human visual evoked cortical potential and
     dark adaptation.  Vision Res., 1976, 16, 1471-1477.

Kulikowski, J.   Visual evoked potentials as a measure of visibility.
     In J.E. Desmedt (Ed.), Visual Evoked Potentials in Man:  New
     Developments, Oxford: Clarendon Press,1977.

Laurian, S. and Gaillard, J.-M.   Habituation of visually evoked
     responses in man:  A study of its time course.  Neuropsycho-
     biol., 1976, 2, 297-306.

Lehtonen, J.B.   Functional differentiation between late components
     of visual evoked potentials recorded at occiput and vertex:
     Effect of stimulus interval and contour.  Electroenceph. Clin.
     Neurophysiol., 1973, 35, 75-82.

Lesevre, N. and Remond, A.   Potentials evoques par l'apparition
     de patterns:  Effets de la dimension du pattern et de la
     densite des contrasts.  Electroenceph. Clin. Neurophysiol,
     1972, 32, 593-604.

MacKay, D.M.   Adaptation of evoked potentials by patterns of
     texture-contrast.  Exp. Brain Res., 1977, 29, 149-153.

Mecacci, L. and Spinelli, D.   The effects of spatial frequency
     adaptation on human evoked potentials.  Vision Res., 1976,
     16, 477-479.

Michael, W.F. and Halliday, A.M.   Differences between the occipital
     distribution of upper and lower pattern-evoked responses in
     man.  Brain Res., 1971, 32 311-324.

Serviere, J., Miceli, D. and Galifret, Y.   Electrophysiological
     correlates of the visual perception of "instantaneous" and
     "durable".  Vision Res., 1977, 17, 65-69.

Shipley, T. and Hyson M.   Amplitude decrements in brain potentials
     in man evoked by repetitive auditory, visual and intersensory
     stimulation.  Sensory Processes, 1977, 1, 338-353.

Spekreijse, H., van der Tweel, L.H. ad Zuidema, Th.   Contrast
     evoked responses in man.  Vision Res., 1973, 13, 1577-1601.

Squires, K.C., Wickens, C., Squires, N.K. and Donchin, E.   The
     effect of stimulus sequence on the waveform of the cortical

event-related potential.  Science, 1976, 193, 1142-1146.

Woodrow, H.  The temporal indifference interval determined by the
    method of mean error.  J. Exp. Psychol., 1934, 17, 167-188.

# LINGUISTIC MEANING-RELATED DIFFERENCES IN ERP SCALP TOPOGRAPHY

Warren S. Brown and Dietrich Lehmann

Department of Psychiatry, University of California,
Los Angeles, Calif. 90024 and Department of Neurology,
University Hospital, Zurich, Switzerland

Certain aspects of language have been hypothesized to be processed in different cortical areas or, at least, by different neural
elements. The most obvious example is the classical differentiation
of the speech disorders associated with frontal or temporal-parietal
lesions of the dominant hemisphere, i.e. expressive versus receptive
language disorders. More specific disturbances have been reported
which showed impairment of word finding predominantly concerning
nouns in some patients and verbs in other patients (Kleist, 1934;
Brown, 1972). Nouns and grammatical words have been reported to be
differentially affected by anterior and posterior lesions in patients
with anomia (Brown, 1972).

Recent research (Brown et al., 1973; 1976, in preparation;
Marsh and Brown, 1977) has shown that different contextual meanings
of homophone words evoke waveform differences in scalp recorded
event related potentials (ERPs). For example, responses to the
word /'led/ in the ambiguous phrase "it was /'led/" differed reliably depending on whether subjects had been instructed to perceive
the stimulus word as "led" or "lead". Principal component analysis
of the data from this experiment showed that individual components
of the evoked responses exhibit maximal differences between word
meanings at different electrode sites (Brown et al., in prep.).
These data indicate that the evoked potential correlates of the
processing of meaning in speech are a complex interaction between
the particular ERP component, its amplitude and scalp topography.

The present paper investigates the scalp topography of responses
evoked by different meanings of homophones. In the simplest case,
the activity of different neural populations involved in processing

homophone nouns and verbs would be reflected by different locations
of maximal and minimal values of evoked scalp EEG fields.  The main
features of EEG scalp fields are simple (Lehmann, 1971; 1977;
Lehmann et al., 1978; Ragot et al., 1976).  Their principal characteristics at a moment in time can be described by the location of
the maximal and minimal field values (Lehmann, 1971; 1977).

One important advantage of the study of ERP topographies,
rather than waveforms recorded at individual electrodes, is that
the problem of the reference electrode can be avoided.  The location of the field maximal and minimal values and the gradients
within the field are not influenced by the choice of reference
electrode.  Only the average field value will be affected by the
reference.  Thus, analyses which utilize locations of extreme
field values or other aspects of the topography are unambiguous
relative to the behavior of the reference.

We chose to investigate the topographical differences evoked
by noun-verb homophones when given specific meaning by the context
of the sentence in which they occur.  In order to ensure that the
results would be generalizable to verbs and nouns in different
languages, one stimulus paradigm was English and the other Swiss-
German: "a pretty rose" and "the boatman rows"; and "e schöni
chlini Flüüge" (a pretty little fly) and "en Vogel chunnt z'flüüge"
(a bird comes flying).  The meanings of "rose" and "flüüge" in
these two pairs of sentences not only contain noun-verb syntactic
differences, but also connotative meaning differences (e.g., quiet-
active states).

The test sentences were tape recorded, and the same stimulus
word, with an associated trigger pulse on a second channel, was
spliced into the two sentences from each paradigm.  This ensured
that the homophone words in each sentence pair were exactly the
same physical stimulus.  A tape loop was used for recording
repetitive sentence presentations.

To rule out any effects caused by acoustic differences between
that portion of the test sentences which preceded the stimulus
word, a blurred but speech-like modulated tone sequence was produced, i.e., a 500 Hz tone was amplitude modulated using a rectified
and low pass filtered original test sentence.  The resulting sound
sequence was not understood by six different evaluators: upon suggestion of wordings ("e schöni chlini Flüüge" or "en Vogel chunnt
z'flüüge") either wording was judged to be equally likely.  Thus,
depending on the instructions to the subject, the identical degraded speech stimulus could elicit a noun or verb interpretation.
Hence, any differences in brain responses to the imagined meanings
must be exclusively cortical responses.

The 21 subjects were all right-handed, healthy females (age 18-35). The English sentences were presented to seven native English speaking subjects and the Swiss-German sentences, as well as the blurred sentences, to native Swiss-German speaking subjects (seven in each group).

Electrodes were attached in a transverse 3 X 4 array, centered around the vertex with 5 cm between electrodes (Fig. 1). Additional electrodes were attached on the two earlobes, the outer canthi of the eyes and in eleven subjects, above and below the left eye. EEG data from the scalp and left ear were recorded in thirteen channels against the right ear and lateral and vertical eye movements were recorded on two additional channels. A bandpass of 0.3 to 70 Hz (6 db down) was used. The A/D rate was 256 s/sec. The data for each run were averaged on line.

After electrode attachment, the subjects were comfortably seated in an electrically shielded and sound-attenuated chamber and instructed about the experiment. They were asked to listen to the sentences, and particularly to attend to the meaning of the test words in the specific sentence context. Subjects were also asked to keep their eyes closed during recordings. A loudspeaker was positioned 1.5 m behind the subject. There was a low level continuous background random noise (50-2000 Hz). The sentences had a peak intensity of 70 db at the subjects' ears. In each recording run a sentence was presented thirty times (4.6 sec cycle time for the English and 5.0 sec cycle time for the Swiss-German and degraded sentences). After a pause of 2.5 min, the next run presenting the other sentence was begun, and so on until each sentence had been used in seven runs. On each run, the subject was told via intercome to get ready for sentence presentation, and data collection was started after the first sentence.

For each subject, evoked potentials in all channels were averaged (N=30) during seven runs with each of the two stimulus sentences (seven runs with each meaning in the case of the degraded speech stimulus). The averaging procedure was started at the onset of the homophone word, using the trigger pulse on the audio presentation tape. Average evoked potentials to words in sentence context, although small, have identifiable waveforms (Fig. 2). Each of the resulting fourteen sets of twelve scalp recorded averaged evoked potentials was transformed into sequences of maps of scalp field distributions (see examples in Fig. 1) for forty analysis times in intervals of 15.6 msec between 33 and 642 msec after stimulus onset. In each field map, the location of the electrode with the maximal and minimal potential value was determined. For further data analysis, only this reference-free information on location was used.

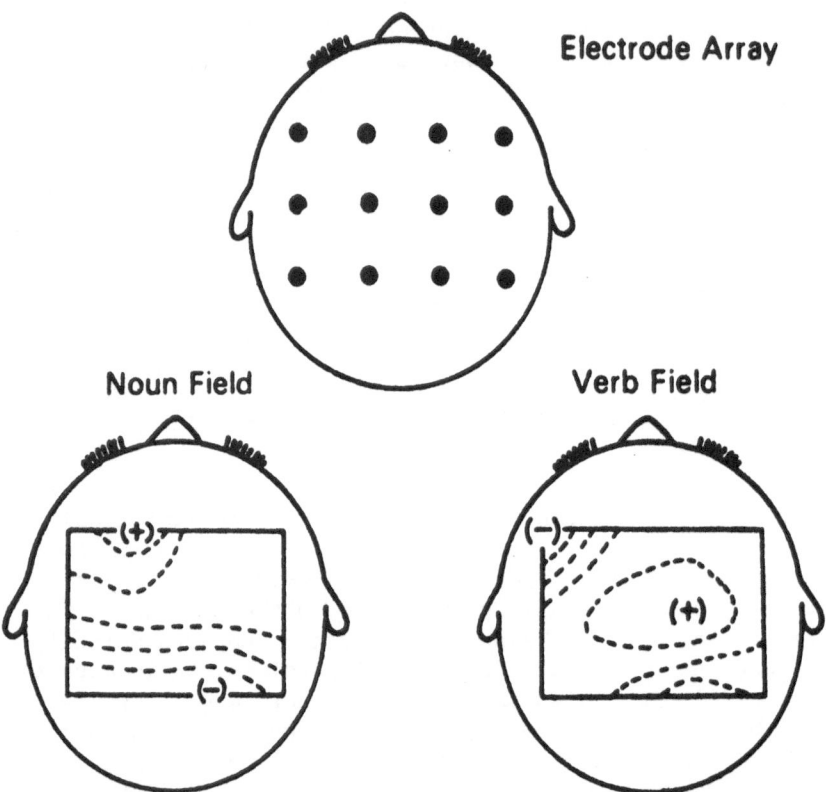

Fig. 1. Scalp electrode array (interelectrode distances of 5 cm) and sample scalp field distributions evoked by noun (left) and verb (right), 126 ms after word onset. Fields are a mean of 210 responses in one subject. Field lines are linearly interpolated between electrode positions. Note maximal and minimal field values ("+" and "-", respectively).

The median location among the seven runs in each condition was separately computed for field maxima and minima. Medians were thus computed for each subject, each condition (noun/verb), and each analysis time (196 mediams per experiment). These median field locations represent the spatial center of the cluster of maximum or minimum locations from the seven runs of each meaning condition. Since we wanted to examine the differences between noun and verb related scalp fields, the topographical relationships between noun and verb extreme value locations were plotted in a coordinate system. The position of the verb median location was plotted relative to the noun, i.e. the noun location was set at the origin. For each analysis time, in each of the three experiments, the median locations of the seven subjects were entered into separate plots for maxima

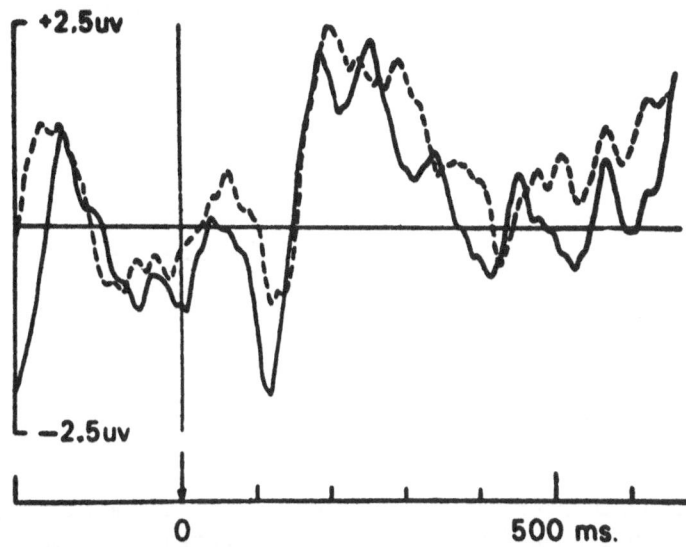

Fig. 2. Average potential waveforms evoked by "rose" (solid line) and "rows" (dotted line). Responses are a mean of seven subjects, 210 responses from each subject. Responses shown were recorded between the scalp electrode in the second row in the second column, and the right ear (as illustrated in Fig. 1). Arrow indicates the onset of the stimulus word.

and minima (see example in Fig. 3).

To summarize across subjects the relationship between locations of the extreme (maximum and minimum) values of noun and verb fields, a spatial discriminant analysis was performed. A vector was rotated through the origin of the coordinate system in order to determine the line which best divided the plot into two halves, of which one contained a maximal number of observations (see Fig. 3). The vector angle which produced the highest sum of signed ranked distances and the highest sum of signed distances of the plotted relative verb locations from the vector was determined by an iterative procedure and used as descriptor of the average field relationship across subjects. Significance of the resultant discrimination was determined by a Wilcoxon test of ranked distances.

For each group, the discriminant vector angles of all analysis times can be seen in Fig. 4. As this figure demonstrates, the three subject groups show similar results. The sum of all the entries during the entire analysis period (histograms at the bottom of each graph of Fig. 4) indicates a predominant angle of about

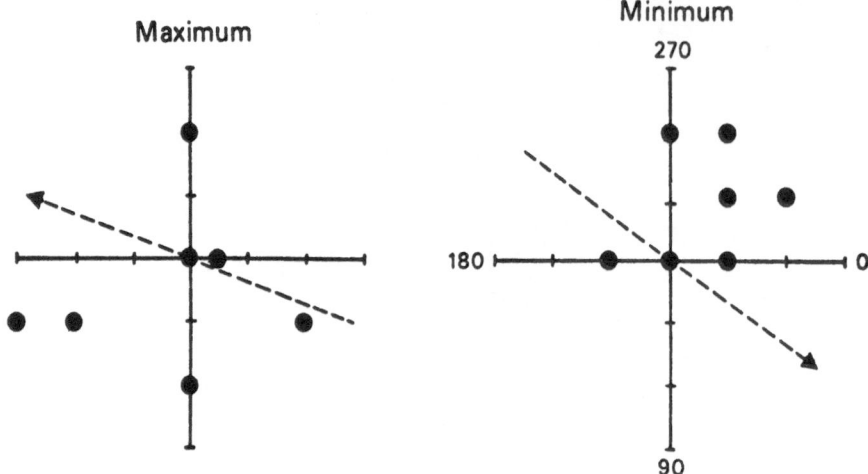

Fig. 3.  Relative positions of maximal (left) and minimal (right)
values of verb fields (dots), plotted in spatial reference to noun
field maximal and minimal values (at origin of coordinate systems).
The data are median locations of maximal and minimal values in each
of the seven subjects of one experimental group at analysis time
126 msec after word onset.  Scale markers indicate one interelectrode
distance.  Dashed line with arrow shows the discriminant angle.
Significance of the discriminations shown are p = .249 for maxima,
and p = .046 for minima (Wilcoxon tests, one tailed).  (From Brown
and Lehmann, in prep.)


180 degrees for maximal field values, and approximately 0 (or 360
degrees for minimal values, although there is considerable variance
at different analysis times.

     The 180 degree angle indicates a posterior location of the
verb maxima referred to the noun maxima, and the 360 degree angle
for minima, the opposite relationship.  Chi-square tests for nonrandomness of the histograms at the bottom of Fig. 4 were significant for all three groups for the minima (English and Swiss,
p<.001; Imagined, p<.01) and two of the three groups for the
maxima (English, p<.02; Imagined, p<.01; but Swiss, p<.10).

     If we examine changes over time by summing over only ten
analysis times across the three groups (Fig. 4, "All subjects")
and test for significant departure of the distribution from a
random distribution, it becomes evident that the locations of the
maxima are clearly separate in the two stimulus conditions in an
anterior-posterior direction (angles between 135 and 225 degrees)
during about the first 174 msec after stimulus onset, and the locations of the minima are clearly separate in the opposite direction

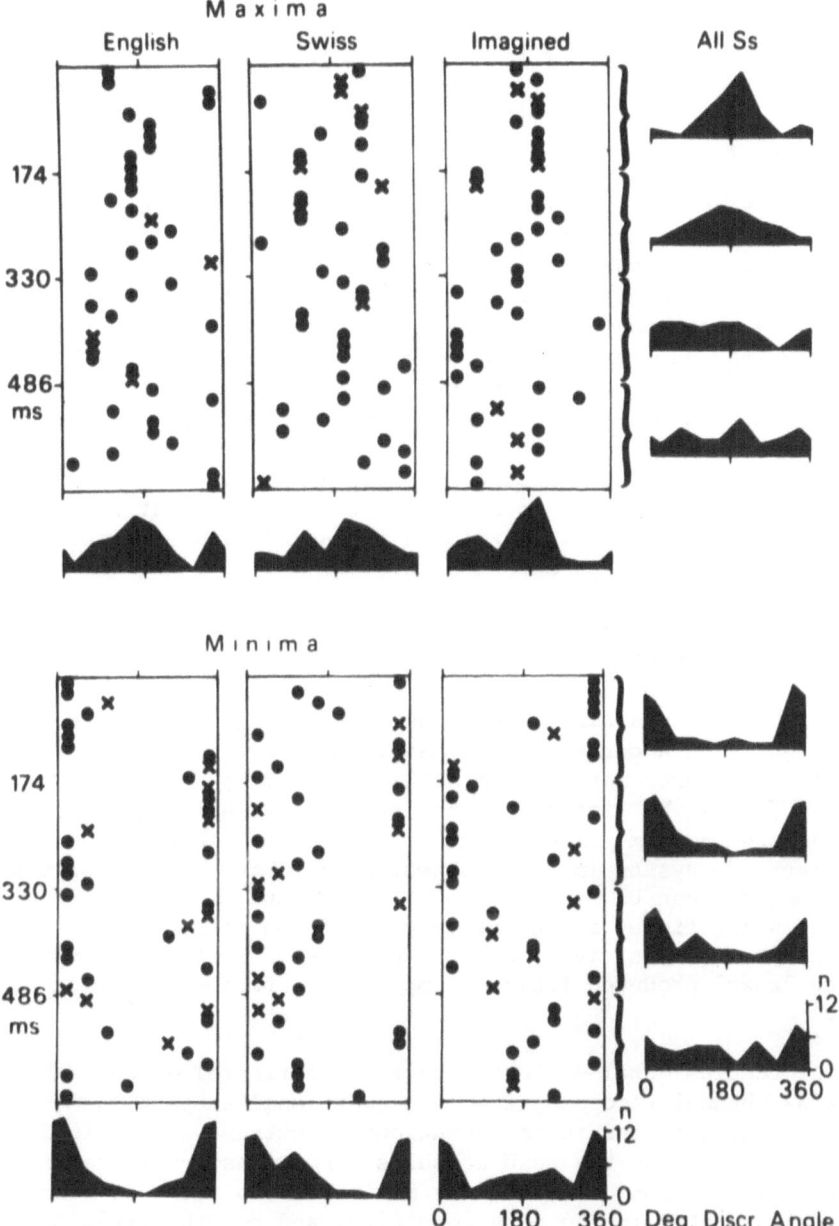

Fig. 4.  Discriminant angles between relative scalp locations of
verb and noun evoked maximal and minimal field values as a function of time (msec).  Angles with p<.06 are indicated by crosses;
p<.06, by dots.  Distribution for all forty analysis times for each
group are shown below as solid graphs, and for epochs of ten anal-
sis times over all three groups, at the right.  (From Brown and
Lehmann, in prep.)

(angles between 315 and 45 degrees) during about the first 330 msec, after which the clear preference of the discriminant angles begins to fade. Chi-square tests for nonrandomness of these distributions were significant for the first epoch of the maxima (p<.001) and first three epochs of the minima (p<.001, p<.001 and p<.02, respectively).

One may suspect vertical eye movements as a possible source of anterior-posterior displacements of extreme scalp field values. The literature, to our knowledge, does not report on vertical eye movements being related to the perception of different word meanings. However, we recorded vertical eye movements from electrodes above and below the eye with the same amplifier settings as the evoked potential data from eleven subjects (three in the English, four in the Swiss-German and four in the Imagined sentence paradigm). The eye movement recordings were averaged over all noun presentations and over all verb presentations for each subject. Comparison of these traces demonstrated no significant differences at any of the forty analysis times, which excludes a possible role of presentation related eye movements in our results.

To more precisely observe the topography of ERPs to the noun and verb meanings of homophones, an additional subject was run while recording from 37 channels simultaneously. Electrodes were placed in a 7 X 7 matrix centered on the vertex, with the three electrodes at each corner of the matrix missing. Interelectrode distance was approximately 3 cm. This subject was a native English speaking female who listened to the English stimuli. All procedures were the same as those described above. That the data from a 37 electrode system in this subject confirm the results of the other subjects can be seen in Fig. 5. The noun meaning "rose" produced scalp fields in the early part of the response epoch which have an anterior positivity and posterior negativity. The verb meaning "rows" produced fields of opposite anterior-posterior slope.

The results obtained in the three experimental groups, as well as the 37 channel recording from the additional subject, demonstrate consistent differences in the locations of extreme scalp field values between the noun and the verb stimulus conditions. For the first 175 msec after stimulus onset, the maximal field value is more anteriorly located in the noun condition, and for the first 330 msec after stimulus onset, the minimal field value is more posteriorly located in the noun condition than in the verb condition. Apparently, the functional neural elements whose activity constitutes the evoked brain response to the stimulus word are not identical in our two stimulus conditions: a critical subpopulation is different for nouns and verbs. This may mean different locations or different orientations of the active elements.

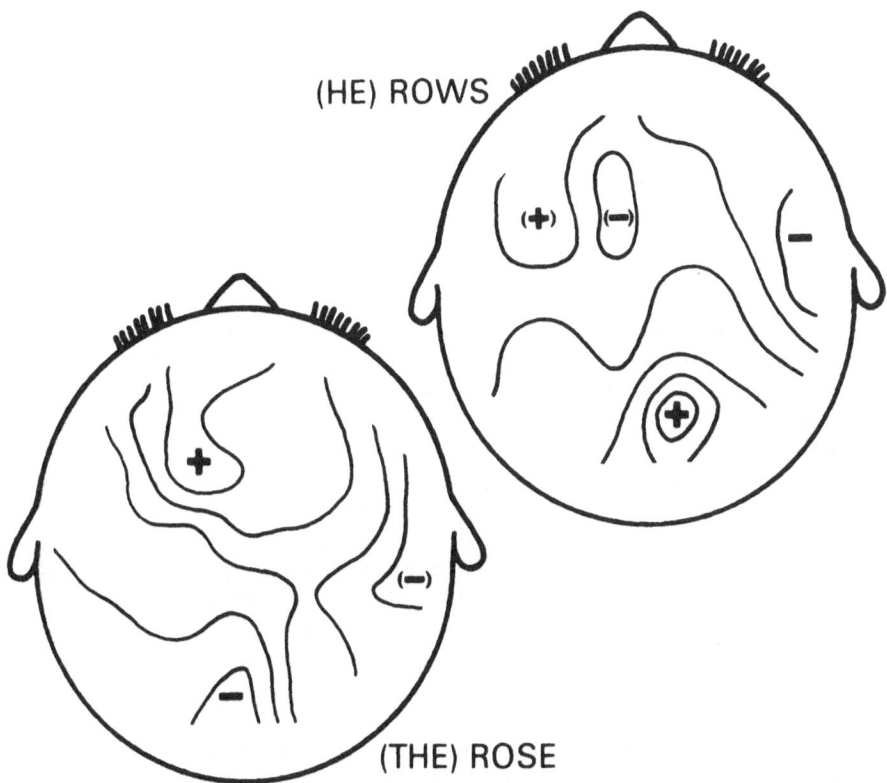

Fig. 5. Topographic maps of average (N=210 scalp fields recorded from a 37 electrode array in one subject while perceiving the English word /roz/ as a noun (labeled "the rose") and as a verb (labeled "he rows"). Field latency is 48 msec after onset of the word /roz/. Isopotential lines are linearly interpolated every 0.5 μv. (From Brown and Lehmann, in prep.).

It appears that it is not the decoding process of the physical stimulus which is manifested in the evoked EEG activity, since the degraded speech sequence evoked results which, depending on the instructions to the subject, were comparable to those from under-standable sentences. Rather, it is the syntactic or connotative meaning which is reflected by the evoked potential topography. Thus, different internally generated meanings are associated with evoked potential characteristics which are similar to those pro-duced by the same meanings when they result from the decoding of speech information.

The topographical differences which we have demonstrated are constant over two different languages, using different specific sentence meaning and different stimulus word meanings. They are

also constant over at least two different sets of phonetic representations.  The most obvious common difference of meaning between, the two sentences in the three experiments is the verb-noun
syntactic difference.  However, other more general connotative
features may be implied by the particular nouns and verbs which
we used (i.e., passive/active, contemplative/strenuous, etc.).  We
note at any rate that it is language information which evoked the
responses, whatever later stages of brain processing may be involved.

     Other reports have shown that the internal presence of specific
information or mental classification of stimulus content determined
evoked waveforms independent of the nature of the physical stimulus.
Using nonlinguistic paradigms, evoked potential differences related
to different internal representation of physically identical or
similar stimuli have been reported by John et al. (1967), Herrington
and Schneidau (1968) and Lehmann et al. (1977).  Evoked potential
differences produced by somewhat more directly linguistic interpretations of similar stimuli have been reported by Johnston and
Chesney (1974), Teyler et al. (1973), Grinberg and John (1977),
Brown et al. (1973,1976, in prep.), Marsh and Brown (1977).  Chapman et al. (1978) have demonstrated that averaging responses across
numerous words which share the same general semantic meaning results
in responses whose waveforms are reliably affected by connotative
meaning.  Our approach of strictly topographical comparisons is unlike the analysis used in other evoked potential studies of language
meaning.  Therefore, direct comparisons with the results reported
in the literature on meaning related language responses, are not
possible.

     The present paper uses strictly topographical data evaluation
(Lehmann, 1971, 1977; Remond, 1968) and does not examine conventional
evoked potential waveshapes (i.e., measurement of components of
evoked potential waveshapes in time).  The latter approach is used
after an a priori decision that the data be treated in each channel
separately, examining voltage differences between two recording
points as a function of time.  Accordingly, topography is a secondary consideration, usually dealt with indirectly.  Contrariwise,
our topographical analysis examines the data in all channels
simultaneously as a function of space, and the time effects are
evaluated in a second stage.  An advantage of this approach is the
avoidance of the classical problem in EEG analysis, the pre-
selection of the recording points from which measurements will be
compared.  Also, as pointed out previously, the choice of the
reference does not influence results of our topographical analysis.
The particular tactics of topography applied in this paper imply
considerable data reduction, i.e., reduction to location of maximal
and minimal field values, but the principles of analysis would not

be different if one decided to use a more fine grain analysis of
the scalp field structure, including the voltage difference between
recording points.

## SUMMARY

Three experiments were accomplished which compared the scalp
field topographies of potentials evoked by the noun and verb meanings of homophones.  Results were consistent in the three experiments.  Locations of scalp field maxima were more anterior for
nouns than verb meanings.  Field minima for noun meaning were more
posterior than verb minima.  The effect for maxima lasted throughout the first 180 msec of the response, and for minima, throughout
the first 230 msec.

## ACKNOWLEDGMENTS

This research was supported by: NIMH Research Scientist
Development Award MH00021; Swiss National Science Foundation;
Hartmann-Mueller Stiftung Zurich; Stiftung Wissenschaftliche
Forschung Zurich; EMDO Foundation Zurich.  We thank Mr. C. Matzener
for assistance in data collection and analysis and Mr. H. P. Meles
for development of computer software.

## REFERENCES

Brown, J. W.  Aphasia, Apraxia and Agnosia.  Springfield, Ill.:
    Thomas, 1972, 26-29.

Brown, W. S., Marsh, J. T. and Smith, J. C.  Contextual meaning
    effects on speech evoked potentials.  Behav. Biol., 1973, 9,
    755-761.

Brown, W. S., Marsh, J. T. and Smith, J. C.  Evoked potential wave-
    form differences produced by the perception of different
    meanings of ambiguous phrases.  Electroenceph. Clin. Neuro-
    physiol., 1976, 41, 113-123.

Brown, W. S., Marsh, J. T. and Smith, J. C.  Principal component
    analysis of ERP differences related to the meaning of an
    ambiguous word.  In prep.

Chapman, R., Bragdon, H., Chapman, J. and McCrary, J.  Semantic
    meaning of words and average evoked potentials.  In, J. Des-
    medt (Ed.) Language and Hemispheric Specialization in Man:
    Cerebral Event Related Potentials, Basel: S. Karger, 1977,
    36-47.

Grinberg and John, E. R.   Unpublished work described in R. W.
     Thatcher and E. R. John.  Functional Neuroscience: Vol. I
     Foundations of Cognitive Processes, New Jersey: Lawrence
     Earlbaum Assoc., 1977, p. 261.

Herrington, R. N. and Schneidau, P.   The effects of imagery on
     the visual evoked response.  Experientia, 1968, 24, 1136-
     1137.

John, E.R., Herrington, P.N. and Sutton, S   Effects of visual
     form on the evoked response.  Science, 1967, 155, 1439-1442.

Johnston, V. and Chesney, G.   Electrophysiological correlates of
     meaning.  Science, 1974, 186, 944-946.

Kleist, K.  Gehirnpathologie, Leipzig: Barth, 1934, 801.

Lehmann, D.   The EEG as scalp field distribution.  In, A. Remond
     (Ed.), EEG Informatics: A Didactic Review of Methods and
     Applications of EEG, Amsterdam: Elsevier, 1977, 365-384.

Lehmann, D.   Multichannel topography of human alpha EEG fields.
     Electroenceph. Clin. Neurophysiol., 1971, 31, 439-449.

Lehmann, D., Meles, H. P. and Mir, E.   Average multichannel EEG
     potential fields evoked from upper and lower hemiretina:
     Latency differences.  Electroenceph. Clin. Neurophysiol.,
     1977, 43, 725-731.

Lehmann, D., Koukkou, M. and Dittrich, A.   Pattern evoked average
     EEG potentials and dichoptic visual percepts.  Perception,
     1977, 6, 77-84.

Marsh, J. T. and Brown, W. S.   Evoked potential correlates of
     meaning in the perception of language.  In, J. Desmedt (Ed.)
     Language and Hemispheric Specialization in Man: Cerebral
     Event Related Potentials, Basel: Karger, 1977, 60-72.

Ragot, R., Cecchini, A. and Remond, A.   Les possibilities de la
     saisie topographique et du traitment cartographique des
     signaux EEG.  Rev. EEG Neurophysiol., 1976, 6, 278-284.

Remond, A.   The importance of topographic data in EEG phenomena,
     and an electrical model to reproduce them.  Electroenceph.
     Clin. Neurophysiol., 1968, Suppl. 27, 29-49.

Teyler, T., Harrison, T., Roemer, R. and Thompson, R.   Human scalp
     recorded evoked potential correlates of linguistic stimuli.
     Psychonom. Soc. Bull., 1973, 1, 333-334.

APPLICATION OF SOMATOSENSORY EVENT RELATED POTENTIALS TO

EXPERIMENTAL PAIN AND THE PHARMACOLOGY OF ANALGESIA

Monte S. Buchsbaum and Glenn C. Davis

National Institute of Mental Health, Biological

Psychiatry Branch, Bethesda, Maryland

## INTRODUCTION

There is increasing evidence that many neurotransmitter systems may be involved in pain appreciation including cholinergic agents, endorphins, biogenic amines and others (Mayer and Price, 1976). This suggests that there are multiple mediators of pain appreciation, each involving a possibly distinct neural pathway. Event related potentials may offer a means of separating distinct pain modulation processes in pharmacological experiments in man.

The average evoked potential (EP) to electric shocks has been used in a number of psychophysiological studies of psychogenic pain (Mushin and Levy, 1974), pain predictability (Lykken et al., 1972), hysterical anesthesia (Moldofsky and England, 1975; Levy and Mushin, 1973) and cutaneous stimulation (Satran and Goldstein, 1973).

We have previously reported that individuals who appear relatively pain tolerant (on the basis of signal detection analysis of their subjective pain ratings) show somatosensory EPs which increase in amplitude less rapidly with increasing stimulus intensity than those of relatively pain intolerant subjects (Buchsbaum, 1975). Audioanalgesia was also associated with a reduction in the amplitude/intensity slope of the EP (Lavine et al., 1976). We have also reported that naloxone, a narcotic antagonist which reverses the effects of opiates and endorphins, alters pain sensitivity and EPs when administered alone to normal subjects, suggesting a physiological role for endorphins in pain regulation (Buchsbaum et al., 1977). In these studies, the positive component at 100 msec (P100) and the following negative component (N120) were the most consistently affected, especially when recorded at C4 with contralateral stimulation.

In approaching other pharmacological interventions, including lithium, physostigmine and choline chloride where analgesia effects might possibly arise from a variety of mechanisms, we hoped that EP results might be especially valuable. By revealing distinctively different patterns of components and different topographic distribution, similarity of mechanisms might be identified.

In order to help clarify analgesic effects, experiments with a classic analgesic seemed crucial. Aspirin was chosen because of its safety and widely recognized efficacy. Taking the largest and most reliable aspirin effect as a criterion, different techniques of EP processing and peak measurement could also be compared for utility.

## METHODS

### Subjects

Forty-seven normal adult volunteers participated, fifteen (six men and nine women) in a test-retest reliability study and thirty-two (sixteen men and sixteen women) in a double-blind crossover study of aspirin.

### Experimental Protocol

All subjects participated in an identical first session. This consisted of a psychophysical pain rating procedure followed by somatosensory evoked potential (EP) recording. No drug or placebo was given. Subjects were scheduled at their convenience between 8:00 a.m. and 4:00 p.m. Stimuli were administered and both psychophysical ratings and electroencephalographic responses recorded by an on-line computer.

Test-retest. For the test-retest analysis, this session was repeated on a second occasion, usually one to two weeks later.

Aspirin. For the drug trial, two additional sessions like the first were utilized. Subjects received either 1 gram aspirin or placebo orally in a randomized, counterbalanced design and then waited 60 min before beginning the psychophysical/EP session. Aspirin and placebo were administered in identical pink capsules from coded containers and analyses, including peak identification and statistics, were done before decoding the treatment.

Stimuli. Electrical stimulation was provided by a concentric electrode (Tursky) connected to an on-line computer controlled con-

stant current stimulator and placed on the dorsal of the left forearm.  Each stimulus was a 1 msec biphasic pulse.  Skin preparation
and stimulation techniques are described in Lavine et al. (1976).

   Somatosensory EP procedure.  Four stimulus levels (2, 9, 16
and 23 mA were presented sixty-four times each at 1 sec intervals
in a random order constrained so that each stimulus intensity was
preceded by each of the others and itself an equal number of times.
EEG was recorded from vertex (Cz-right ear) and somatosensory cortex (C4-right ear), amplified and filtered (flat bandpass 1--40 Hz;
down 3 dB at 0.3 Hz and 42 dB at 60 Hz).  EEG was sampled at 250 Hz
for 500 msec, and responses to each intensity were averaged on-line.

   Psychophysical shock procedure.  Subjects received three shocks
at each milliamperage increment from 1 to 31 mA for a total of
ninety-three shocks in a random sequence at 2.5-s intervals.  Subjects rated each shock in one of four categories: noticeable, distinct, unpleasant or very unpleasant.  Signal detection analysis
yielded two pain measures: a nonparametric analog of response criterion and a sensitivity level (Sitaram et al., 1977).  The sensitivity measure has been associated with pharmacological analgesia
(Chapman et al., 1973) and response criterion has been related to
suggestion effects (Clark and Goodman, 1974).

   EP measurement.  The largest and most commonly occurring components in the EP configuration for both Cz and C4 leads are a
sequence of positive negative and positive deflections at about 100,
120 and 200 msec (termed P100, N120 and P200).  These components
were identified by visual inspection by a person blind to drug
status, and the latency from the stimulus was recorded.  Peaks were
chosen to be 1) as consistent as possible in latency across the
four intensities and two sessions and 2) to be within 25 msec of
the 100, 120 and 200 msec anchor points.  Amplitude of the components was measured in two ways.  First, the height in microvolts
from a 32 prestimulus baseline was determined.  Second, an area integration technique not dependent on visual identification peaks
was used.  EPs were divided into three time bands centered on P100
(76-112 msec), N140 (116-152 msec) and P200 (168-248 msec).  EP
amplitude was measured by calculating the area within the band.
This was done by first removing the mean of the entire epoch from
32 msec prestimulus to 480 msec poststimulus and then calculating
the mean of the absolute values of the EP time values for each time
band.  The amplitude/intensity slope was calculated by least
squares regression using the four EP amplitudes in microvolts and
the logs of the stimulus intensities in milliamperes.

   EP data were then analyzed by using paired t-tests and by using
two- and three-way ANOVA with repeated measures and trend analysis
for the intensity dimension.  For test-retest correlations and pre-

dicted analgesia effects where the statistical hypothesis is una-
voidably unidirectional, one-tailed tests are used.


## RESULTS

### Test-Retest Reliability of EP

Test-retest reliabilities were calculated for both mean amplitude (across four intensities) and for the amplitude/intensity
slope (Table 1).  Both showed reasonable consistency over time;
area measurements of amplitude appeared clearly superior to the
baseline-to-peak technique, as we have observed elsewhere for visual
EPs (Buchsbaum, 1976).


### Effect of Aspirin on Psychophysical Ratings

Consistent with the expected analgesic effect, aspirin increased the error rate (a nonparametric analog of d') for the
distinct/unpleasant dichotomy from 7.3 on placebo to 9.5 (paired
t = 2.69, p < 0.01, one-tailed).  Psychophysical results will be
reported in detail at a later date.


### Effect of Aspirin on Somatosensory EPs

Aspirin diminished the EP amplitude, especially for high intensity stimuli and for the N120 component (Fig. 1, left).  This
was confirmed statistically by paired t-tests on the amplitude/in-
tensity slope measures (t = 2.86, p < 0.005) by two-way ANOVA with
drug treatment and stimulus intensity as repeated measures for area
measures Cz-N120 (F = 7.97, p < 0.01; 1,30 d.f., linear trend analysis) and for C4-N120 (F = 5.62, p < 0.25, quadratic trend analysis)
and peak measures for C4-N120 (F = 4.92, p < 0.005, quadratic trend
analysis).  Baseline-to-peak measure P100 also showed a main effect
of aspirin (F = 5.54, p < 0.05).  Area measurements showed that
individual differences in the effects of aspirin were similar for
both N120 and P200 (Table II), when amplitudes of EPs for the highest stimulus intensity were used.


### Removal of Low Frequency Components

Both baseline-to-peak and area integration techniques could
have their measurements distorted by sustained potentials, CNV or
large P300 components which could affect baselines.  Effects actually due to these slow components might hypothetically be attributed
to earlier components such as P100 or N120.  Late slow components
appear minimal in the passive paradigm used here (Fig. 3), and base-

TABLE I

Test-Retest Reliability of EP Components

| | | Technique | | | |
| | | Area | | Baseline-to-peak | |
| Lead | Peak | Mean | Scope | Mean | Slope |
|------|------|------|-------|------|-------|
| | P100 | .50* | .43* | .56* | .06 |
| Cz | N120 | .70* | .67* | .75* | .17 |
| | P200 | .85* | .89* | .77* | .74* |
| | P100 | .05 | .46* | .57* | .47* |
| C4 | N120 | .53* | .62* | .39 | .21 |
| | P200 | .92* | .87* | .62* | .65* |

* $p < 0.05$, one-tailed

Mean is calculated from amplitude at the four stimulus intensities; amplitude/intensity slope is calculated as described in text.

TABLE II

Correlation Between Area and Baseline-to-Peak Measure
Effects of Aspirin

| Amplitude of highest intensity EP | Lead | |
| | Cz | C4 |
|-----------------------------------|------|------|
| P100 | -.38 | -.19 |
| N120 | .34* | .62** |
| P200 | .47** | .68** |

*  $p < 0.05$, one-tailed
** $p < 0.0025$, one-tailed

Change scores for placebo minus aspirin were calculated for each peak and lead in the two measurement systems.

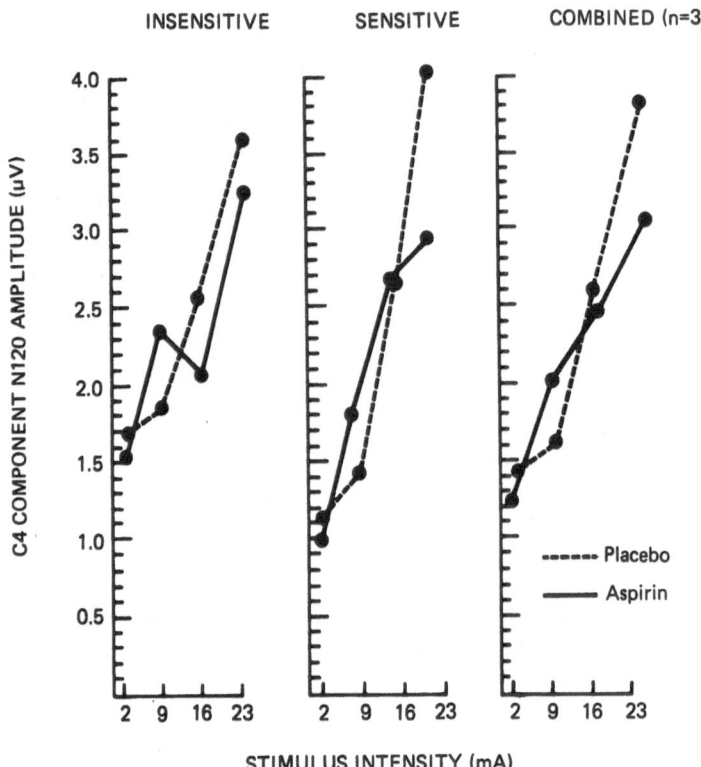

Fig. 1. Mean evoked potential amplitude in µV for negative peak
N120 at four stimulus intensities for pain sensitive (N = 15), pain
insensitive (N = 17) and total groups (N = 32). Solid lines are
aspirin, and dotted lines are placebo. EP differences at highest
intensity are consistent in the two subgroups. Drug X intensity
interactions were confirmed by ANOVA statistically, but group X drug
X intensity interactions were not significant. Note that sensitive
individuals on placebo have greater amplitude/intensity slopes (augmenting) than pain insensitive individuals.

line shifts due to the intensity of the preceding stimulus cannot
systematically influence stimulus intensity effects because of the
stimulus intensity randomization used. Nevertheless, for a rigorous
test all EPs were filtered using a high pass autoregressive filter
(Coppola, in press) with a filter constant of 0.93 yielding a 50%
amplitude value of 2.5 Hz (Fig. 2). This filtering only minimally
altered aspirin effects; for area measurement of Cz-N120, the F-

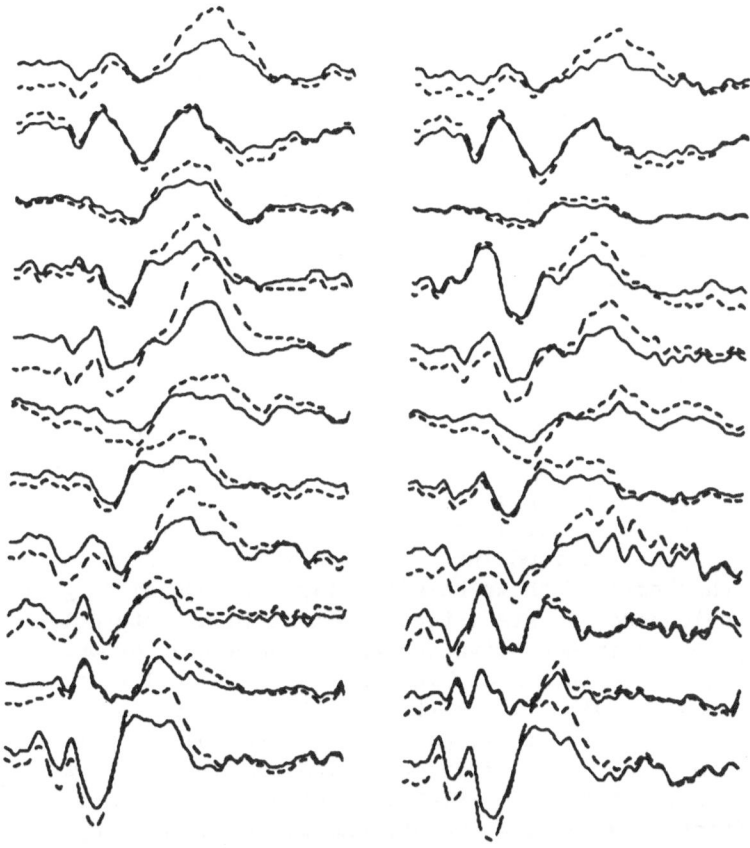

Fig. 2.  Effect of high pass autoregressive filter on EP waveform.
EPs for 23 mA stimulus, Cz lead on the left and C4 on the right, for
the eleven subjects with typical EPs in Fig. 3.  Curves before filtering (dotted) and after removal of low frequencies (solid) are
illustrated.  Note that while P200 is somewhat attenuated, early
components are minimally affected.  No P300 is evident in these
subjects.

ratio for the drug x intensity effect increased from 7.97 to 11.7.
P100 peak-to-trough effects were also enhanced.  C4-N120 F-ratio
values were somewhat diminished, but the aspirin-placebo t-tests
on the amplitude of the highest intensity EP remained statistically
significant.  Thus not only did low frequency components not appear
to be the source of the EP changes, but their removal was mildly
advantageous for the vertex EP.

Psychophysical and EP Correlations

Individuals who responded to aspirin by showing an analgesic effect on the psychophysical procedure (error rate increase) tended to show analgesia on the EP measure, the C4-N120 amplitude/intensity slope.  The correlation between the placebo minus aspirin change scores for the C4-N120 amplitude/intensity slope and distinct/un-pleasant error rates was 0.382 (p < 0.05) for the twenty-five individuals with complete psychophysical range data.  The baseline-to-peak mean P100 measure correlation was 0.481 (p < 0.01).

Individual Variation in Pain Sensitivity and Aspirin Effect

In our studies of naloxone (Buchsbaum et al., 1977) individuals who were particulary pain insensitive on the baseline day were especially likely to show naloxone-induced hyperalgesia.  Using the same pain sensitivity level used in the naloxone study as a criterion, subjects were divided into pain sensitive and pain insensitive groups on the basis of their baseline day psychophysical pain ratings.  In this study no statistically significant interaction effects were seen, both pain sensitive and pain insensitive groups sharing aspirin-induced diminution of high intensity EP amplitude.  Note that as we have previously reported, pain sensitive individuals had higher amplitude/intensity slopes (augmenters) on the placebo day than did pain insensitive individuals (reducers).  This was statistically confirmed for the C4-N140 intensity function (group by intensity effect, F = 4.76, p < 0.05) and was present as a trend for Cz-P100 and C4-P100.

Individual Differences in EP Configuration

Within the thirty-two individuals there was variation in the appearance of the EP even on placebo.  Some individuals showed a typical triphasic vertex EP, similar to visual EPs, with a positive peak at 80-110 msec followed by a clear negative-positive sequence at 120 and 220 msec.  A second group showed an earlier positive component usually at 40-60 msec, an earlier negative at 70-80 msec and a typical latency positive at 220 msec.  A third group showed variable or absent P100, most frequently dropping out at the highest intensity.  The three groups, sorted on their placebo EPs, are illustrated in Fig. 3.  Note that the early and variable groups showed considerable consistency in waveform from session to session, mitigating against recording artifacts being the source of the distortion or loss of P100.  The typical group showed the greatest aspirin effect, the P100-N140 complex almost disappearing in some cases. Ten of the eleven individuals with typical EPs showed area amplitude/intensity slope reduction for C4-N120 with aspirin and ten of the eleven also showed diminished baseline-to-peak P100 amplitudes.

**P100 range  73-113 ms**          **0-60 ms**          **varys or absent**

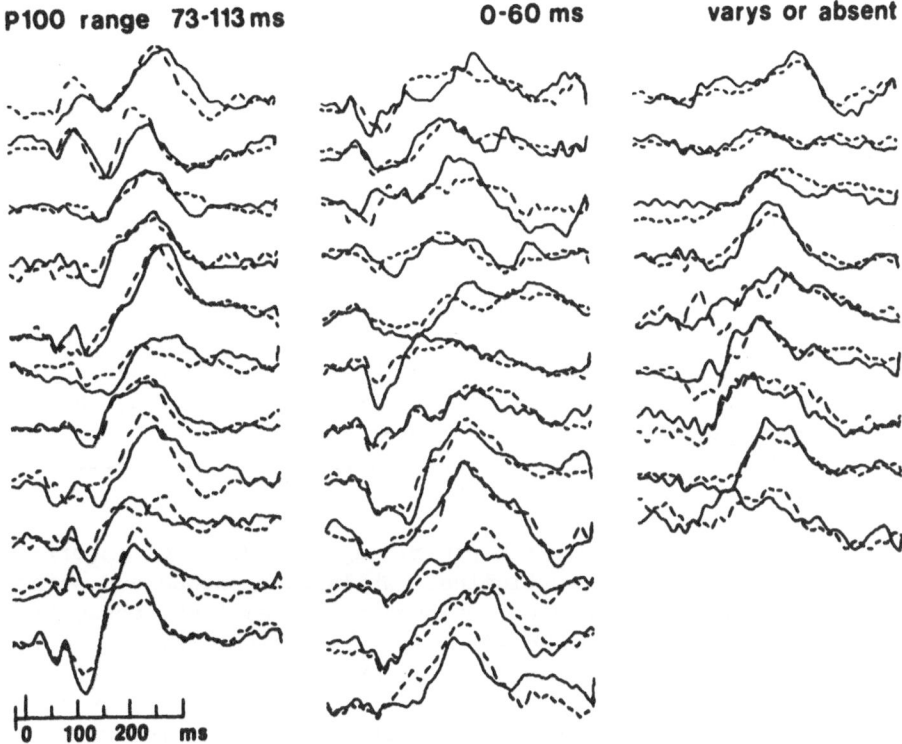

Fig. 3.  Grouping subjects by P100 configuration and latency.  EPs
for 23 mA stimulus, Cz lead are shown, positive up, for all thirty-
two subjects on placebo (solid line) and aspirin (dotted line).
Left:  subjects selected for clearest P100 at all stimulus intensities in the usual (73-113 msec) range while on placebo.  Note aspirin
diminution of P100 and N120 components.  Middle:  subjects with a
very early positive component and no 100 msec positivity.  Right:
subjects who showed variable or absent early components making assessment of stimulus intensity curves difficult.

This is seen statistically in the F-ratios for area C4-N210 for the
typical, early and variable groups which are 10.45, 3.35 and 4.16,
respectively (drug-by-intensity interaction linear trend effect).
Peak identification was helpful, and the baseline-to-peak Cz-P100
measure yielded F-ratios of 7.97, 7.56 and 4.77 (drug effect).  Thus
it appears that the early group may indeed have physiologically similar activity at a shorter latency.  Both the typical and early groups
had larger baseline-to-peak P100 amplitude at C4 than at Cz, consistent with the topographic findings of Goff et al. (1977).

DISCUSSION

In this study somatosensory EP amplitude and amplitude/inten-
sity slopes parallel psychophysical rating changes with aspirin,
both techniques confirming aspirin analgesia.  The statistical
strengths of the two techniques, as measured by the paired 't' values comparing aspirin and placebo were similar, being 2.69 for the
nonparametric analog of d' and 2.86 for the area Cz-N120 amplitude/
intensity slope.

Individual differences in analgesic effects of aspirin were
reflected in significant correlations between the magnitude of the
changes associated with aspirin in psychophysical and EP measures.
Variability in the analgesia effect of aspirin was reduced by choos-
ing individuals with typical triphasic EPs, and more consistent
effects were observed than those achieved with the psychophysical
measure used.

The analgesia associated with aspirin appears distinct in origin from that found with physostigmine.  While both showed a distinct/
unpleasant error rate increase on the psychophysical task, physostigmine showed exclusively P100 and P200 effects, whereas for aspirin,
like naloxone, the C4-N120 effect predominated.  We have suggested
(Sitaram et al., 1976) that physostigmine analgesia effects may be
mediated by arousal mechanisms. In contrast, the association of P100
and N120 reducing seen with aspirin analgesia and with audio analgesia seems more related to trait differences in pain sensitivity.
As we have earlier noted, augmenting P100 or N120 amplitude/inten-
sity slopes are related to pain sensitivity on placebo or baseline
sessions (Buchsbaum, 1975; Buchsbaum et al., 1977).  Additionally,
naloxone, a drug which showed no total group effect on the psychophysical measure, produced augmenting on the N120 component in pain
tolerant individuals, suggesting that individual differences in endogenous opiates might be reflected in the P100-N120 complex (Buchsbaum et al., 1977).  The grouping observed here of aspirin effects
with endogenous opiate effects is intriguing.  Further development
of EP techniques with measurement of primary P30 and P50 components,
and testing of a greater range of analgesics and neurotransmitter
strategies as well, may be helpful in increasing the neurophysio-
logical/neurochemical correlations.

It is noteworthy that physostigmine and aspirin were indistinguishable analgesics on the psychophysical task, and no significant
group effect appeared with naloxone; yet EP results differentiated
the first two agents and revealed individual differences in response
for the third.  This greater specificity of the EP measures, combined with its reliability, suggests the utility of somatosensory
EP recordings in psychopharmacological investigations.

## SUMMARY

Forty-seven normal subjects were tested on psychophysical and somatosensory evoked potential pain procedures during double-blind placebo controlled trials of aspirin.  Two runs of electrical stimuli were presented to each subject's forearm using the Tursky electrode; 1) ninety-three shocks of random intensities were judged noticeable, distinct, unpleasant and very unpleasant and 2) four intensities of stimuli were used to record ERPs from vertex and C4 leads.  Psychophysical pain sensitivity was assessed by nonparametric signal detection analysis.  ERP component latencies were identified visually in the ERPs, and amplitude was measured both from a prestimulus baseline and peak-to-trough; area integration measures were also obtained for comparison.  Both ERP and psychophysical pain ratings showed stable individual differences; test-retest correlations for occasions two weeks apart ranged from $r = 0.5$ for psychophysical tasks to $r = 0.7 - 0.9$ for amplitude and amplitude/intensity slopes.  N120 components recorded from both C4 and vertex were especially sensitive to aspirin analgesia, significantly diminishing in amplitude and shortening in latency especially at higher intensities.  Pain ratings also showed analgesia for the sensitivity measure (d' analog).  Comparing aspirin results with previous data on naloxone, the N120 component was most consistently influenced by pharmacological analgesia;  both P100 and P200 were also affected by time of day and individual differences in pain sensitivity.  Taken together, these results indicate the practical utility of ERP methodology in neurobiological pain research.

## REFERENCES

Buchsbaum, M.S., Davis, G.C. and Bunney, W.E., Jr.  Naloxone alters pain perception and somatosensory evoked potentials in normal subjects.  Nature, 1977, 270, 620-622.

Buchsbaum, M.S.  Self-regulation of stimulus intensity:  Augmenting/ reducing and the average evoked response.  In G.E. Schwartz and D. Shapiro (Eds.), Consciousness and Self-Regulation, New York: Plenum Press, 1976.

Buchsbaum, M.S.  Average evoked response augmenting/reducing in schizophrenia and affective disorders.  In D.X. Freedman (Ed.), The Biology of the Major Psychoses, A Comparative Analysis, New York: Raven Press, 1975.

Chapman, C. R., Murphy, T.M. and Butler, S.  Analgesic strength of 33 percent nitrous oxide: A signal detection theory evaluation. Science, 1973, 179, 1246-1248.

Clark, W.C. and Goodman, J.  Effects of suggestion on d' and cx for pain detection and pain tolerance.  J. Abnorm. Psychol., 1974, 83, 364-372.

Coppola, R.  Isolating low frequency activity in EEG spectrum analysis.  Electroenceph. Clin. Neurophysiol., in press.

Goff, G.D., Matsumiya, Y., Allison, T. and Goff, W.R.  The scalp topography of human somatosensory and auditory evoked potentials.  Electroenceph. Clin. Neurophysiol., 1977, 42, 57-76.

Lavine, R., Buchsbaum, M.S. and Poncy, M.  Auditory analgesia: Somatosensory evoked response and subjective pain rating.  Psychophysiol., 1976, 13, 140-148.

Levy, R. and Mushin, J.  The somatosensory evoked response in patients with hysterical anaesthesia.  U. Psychosom. Res., 1973, 17, 81-84.

Lykken, D.T., Macindoe, I. and Tellegen, A.  Perception: Autonomic response to shock as a function of predictability in time and locus.  Psychophysiol., 1972, 9, 318-333.

Mayer, D.J. and Price, D.D.  Central nervous system mechanism of analgesia.  Pain, 1976, 2, 379-404.

Mushin, J. and Levy, R.  Averaged evoked response in patients with psychogenic pain.  Psychol. Med., 1974, 4, 19-27.

Satran, R. and Goldstein, M.  Pain perception: Modification of threshold of intolerance and cortical potentials by cutaneous stimulation.  Science, 1973, 180, 1201-1202.

Sitaram, N., Buchsbaum, M.S. and Gillin, J.C.  Physostigmine analgesia and somatosensory evoked responses in man.  Europ. J. Pharm., 1977, 42, 285-290.

HEMISPHERIC DIFFERENCES IN EVOKED POTENTIALS TO RELEVANT AND

IRRELEVANT VISUAL STIMULI

Robert M. Chapman and John W. McCrary

University of Rochester

Rochester, New York 14627

Since the early days of averaging evoked potentials (EPs) in man, the importance of cognitive variables, as well as stimulus variables, has been recognized (e.g., Chapman and Bragdon, 1964). Using an experimental design which involves processing number and letter stimuli, we have been studying EP effects related to a variety of cognitive operations (Chapman, 1965, 1966, 1969a, 1969b, 1973, 1974a, 1974b, 1977, in press; Chapman et al., in press (a); Chapman et al. in press (b). Most of our analyses have been for the CPZ scalp location (recorded monopolar on the midline one-third of the distance from Cz to Pz; reference was linked ear-lobes). It is of interest to study the cognitive effects at other sites, with a particular focus on the question of hemispheric differences and parietal-occipital differences.

A more complete description of the experimental design and discussion of interpretations for the present chapter is given in Chapman (1973). In that paper results are given for twelve subjects for midline electrodes located over the central-parietal (CPZ) and the occipital area (Oz), as well as control data for EOG and alpha EEG. The present experiment provides comparable data for eight subjects for laterally located electrodes over parietal (P3 and P4) and occipital (O1 and O2) areas and permits an evaluation of hemispheric differences in the information processing tasks. In general, comparable information processing effects were found in both experiments. The evaluation of location differences was facilitated by the addition of control EPs to blank flashes and the use of additional analysis procedures, featuring discriminant analyses.

Earlier work on hemispheric specialization has been critically reviewed by Donchin et al. (1977). A caveat should be noted in

considering hemispheric differences, or any brain localization
effects, from EP data.  EP effects localized at some scalp site do
not necessarily mean that the adjacent brain region is responsible
for those processes.  Because the measure is a voltage difference
in an electrical field of a conducting medium, the orientation of
the source, as well as its distance, are important.  Far field
effects have been demonstrated for early auditory potentials
(Jewett et al., 1970).  The importance of source orientation is
illustrated by scalp localizations opposite to brain hemisphere in
visual field studies (Halliday et al., 1977).  Incidentally, the
same problems exist for electrical recording within brain structures
as for scalp recording.  Given this caveat, the spatial localization interpretations given in this chapter, strictly speaking,
refer to particular scalp sites (with ear reference) and should be
extended to brain localization with great caution.

Another problem relates to the assumption that larger EP
amplitudes signify more processing. We suggest a method of analysis
here which avoids this assumption, at least in its usual simplistic
form.  The method is based on discriminant analyses which focus on
variations of EP measures which maximally discriminate particular
conditions.  This approach does not rely on sheer amplitude, but
rather seeks combinations of amplitudes, large or small, which most
systematically covary with particular sets of experimental conditions.


                          EXPERIMENTAL PROCEDURE

Two numbers and two letters were flashed individually in random
order at intervals of 3/4 sec preceded and followed by a blank flash.
The subject's task was to compare numerically the two numbers on
number-relevant runs, the letters being irrelevant to the task.  On
the other half of the runs the numbers were irrelevant, and the task
was to compare alphabetically the two letters.  By appropriately
moving a momentary two-way switch at the end of each trial, the
subject indicated whether the first or second number was larger on
number-relevant runs and similarly indicated the alphabetic order on
letter-relevant runs.  The subject had a 1.5 sec time slot following
the last flash in which to answer before the next trial started.
Correct answers produced a tone; wrong answers produced a buzz.  The
number and letters were randomly selected (1-6, A-F), and the
sequences of numbers and letters were randomized.  Nearly every
stimulus was processed appropriately by the subjects, with a performance accuracy of better than 99%.  All stimuli were flashed at the
same spatial location by a Bina-View display equipped with a Grass
strobe (flash duration < 10 msec).

The stimulus processing demanded by the task depended on a

number of factors, including whether: (i) number or letter stimuli
were task relevant, (ii) the number or letter class of stimulus
could be anticipated and (iii) the character was the first or second
relevant stimulus of the pair to be compared.  For the first relevant stimulus in each trial, the information had to be stored by the
subject until the second relevant stimulus occurred, after which
the comparison could be made.

        While the subject was performing the letter or number compari-
son tasks, electrical brain activity (EEG) was recorded from scalp
electrodes at P3, P4, O1 and O2 (referenced to linked earlobes).
Frequency bandpass was 0.3 to 70 Hz; 102 samples at each 5 msec
interval were obtained beginning 30 msec before each stimulus.  The
data were collected from eight right-handed subjects (five male,
three female) over a series of six sessions each.

        By averaging the brain activity evoked by stimuli for similar
conditions, separate averaged evoked potentials (EPs) were obtained
for sixteen information processing conditions:  relevant and irrelevant numbers and letters at four intratrial positions.  From trial
to trial the first number (or letter) stimulus occurred in intratrial positions 1, 2 or 3, while the second number (or letter)
stimulus occurred in intratrial positions 2, 3 or 4.  To simplify
interpretations certain EEG data were discarded, so the EPs for
intratrial positions 1 and 2 were based only on the first number and
letter stimuli presented within each trial, while the EPs for intratrial positions 3 and 4 were based only on the second number and
letter stimuli presented within each trial.

        Even the irrelevant stimuli in this experiment must be pro-
cessed to a certain extent to determine that they are irrelevant.
The subject cannot anticipate whether the stimulus will be a letter
or a number, and hence relevant or irrelevant, except in intratrial
position 4.  To provide a control with even less processing by
subjects, runs were added in which only blank flashes occurred.
The blank flashes were provided by the same Bina-View device and
appeared as an illuminated rectangle.  The trials for those runs
had the same temporal structure as the letter-number trials: blank
flashes at the 4 intratrial positions, preceded and followed by a
blank flash, all spaced 3/4 sec apart.

        Each run contained 102 trials, each with four intratrial posi-
tions.  Each subject was given ten number-relevant, ten letter-
relevant and four blank runs spaced over a number of sessions.
Averaging across all runs, the EPs for each subject were based on
the EEG responses to 272 to 510 stimuli.  This yielded twenty EPs
for each subject:  relevant and irrelevant numbers and letters and
blanks for each of the four intratrial positions.  For each electrode, the data set consisted of 160 EPs (20 X 8 subjects).

EP MEASURES

The EPs were measured in the manner described in Chapman (1973) in order to facilitate comparison with the midline results reported there.  For each EP, five measures were obtained:  mean amplitude over 480 msec, and 315 msec.  The most global measure was mean amplitude over 480 msec relative to a baseline obtained at 0 msec (time of stimulus; the baseline was the average of four time points before and three after the stimulus).  The amplitude at 105 msec, 225 msec and 315 msec were similarly measured relative to the same baseline at 0 msec.  These measures index the amplitude at specified points within the EPs without the necessity of identifying particular peaks.  The amplitude at 0 msec was measured relative to an arbitrary voltage level across the entire trial of four intratrial positions.  The amplitude at 0 msec indexes CNV activity.

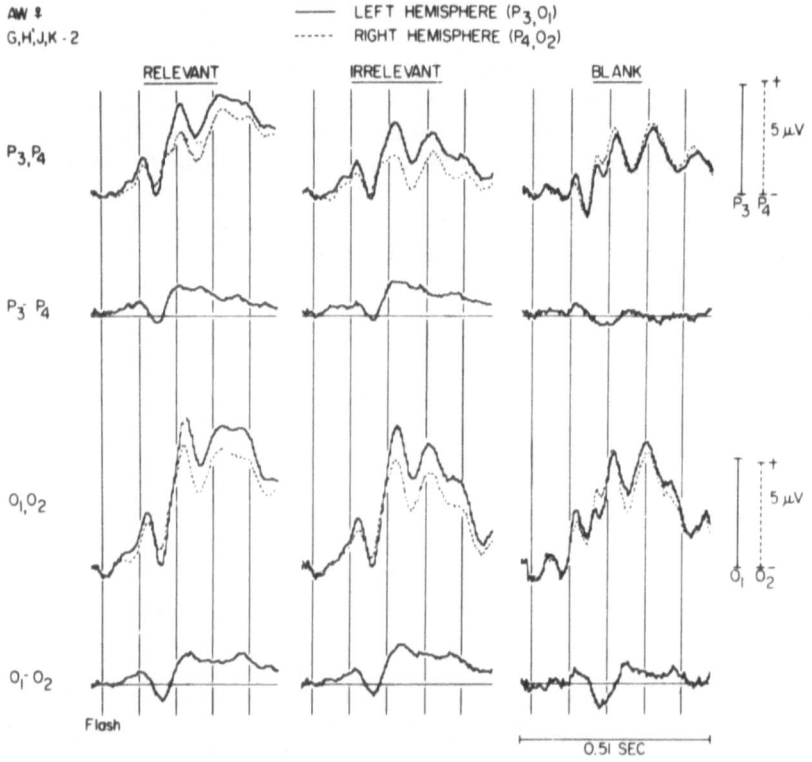

Fig. 1.  Sample evoked potentials from one subject.  Monopolar recording from left and right parietal (P3,P4) and occipital (O1, O2) scalp locations (referenced to linked earlobes).  Vertical lines 100 msec apart.

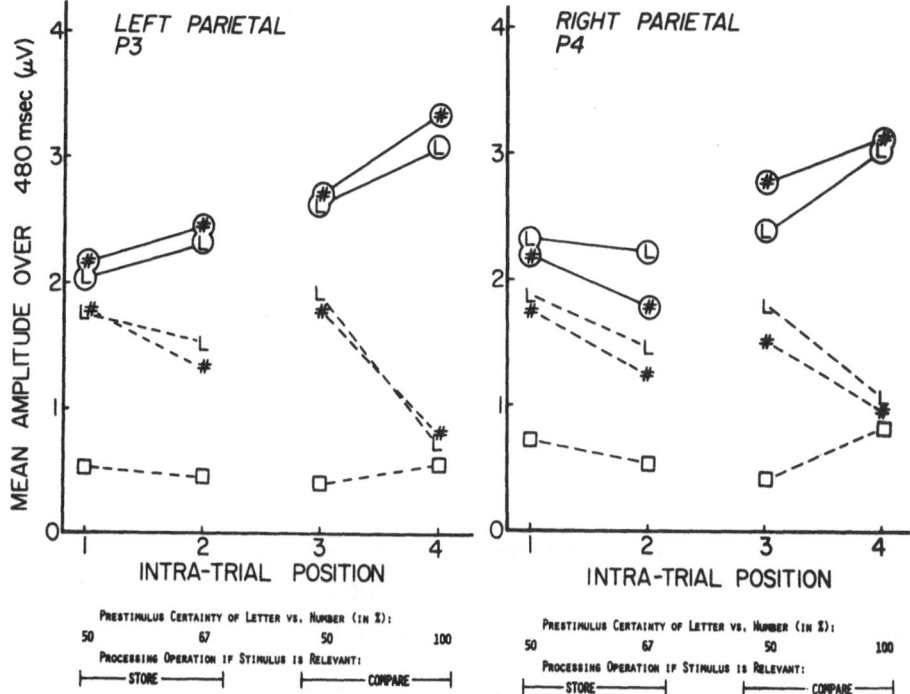

Fig. 2. Mean amplitude over 480 msec from left and right parietal electrodes for 20 experimental conditions with varying information processing demands. Number (#), letter (L) and blank (box) visual stimuli. Relevant (circled symbols and solid lines) and irrelevant (not-circled symbols and dashed lines). Information processing characteristics associated with intratrial positions are summarized below the abscissa. Data are means from eight subjects.

## RESULTS

Fig. 1 illustrates some of the EPs for one of the subjects. For this figure, the EPs were averaged across numbers and letters and intratrial positions, in order to illustrate the hemispheric differences for relevant, irrelevant and blank stimuli. In this case the EPs from the left are larger than those from the right, and this hemispheric difference is greater for relevant and irrelevant stimuli than for blank stimuli. Drawing conclusions from the data of one subject may be misleading. To assess those effects which have more generality, the data for all eight subjects have been examined as a set.

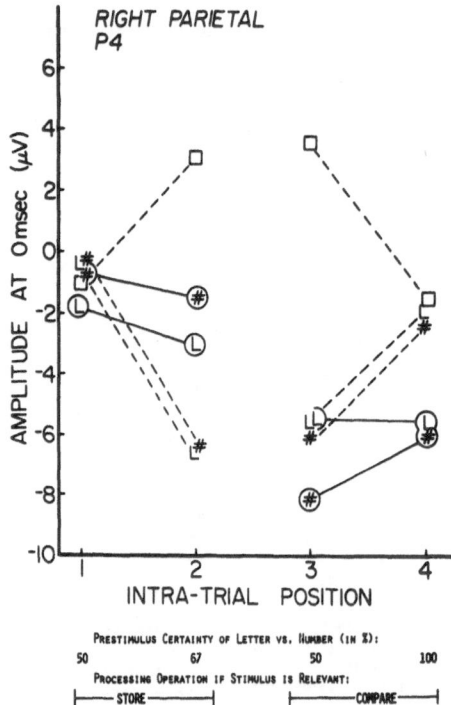

Fig. 3. Amplitude at 0 msec relative to an arbitrary voltage level
which was the same for all responses. This measure indexes CNV.
Other specification as for Fig. 2.


EP MEASURES FOR EXPERIMENTAL CONDITIONS

     The results for mean amplitude over 480 msec are quite similar
from left and right electrodes (P3 and P4 shown in Fig. 2) and are
similar to those previously obtained from midline electrodes at CPZ
and Oz (Chapman, 1973, Figs. 3.6 and 3.7). The most striking result
is the difference between relevant and irrelevant stimuli, regardless of whether numbers or letters were involved. There is also
an interaction between relevance and intratrial position. In
addition, the EPs to the blank flashes are considerably smaller than
the responses to the number and letter stimuli. However, the EPs
to the irrelevant numbers and letters in intratrial position 4,
where there is 100% prestimulus certainty of stimulus class, approach the low amplitudes obtained to the blank flash controls.

     Although there appear to be differences between the results
for P3 and P4, the similarities dominate comparisons. The results
for O1 and O2 (not shown) are also quite similar.

The amplitude at 0 msec showed a different pattern of relations to the experimental conditions (Fig. 3) which was similar to
midline data previously reported (Chapman, 1973, Fig. 3.12).  There
were essentially no differences between relevant and irrelevant
conditions at intratrial positions 1 and 3.  At these positions
there was a 50-50 chance of a letter or number occurring and,
therefore, a 50-50 chance of the stimulus being relevant or
irrelevant.  However, the prestimulus certainty of a letter or
number occurring in intratrial positions 2 and 4 was biased (67%
and 100%, respectively).  At positions 2 and 4 there was a difference in amplitude at the time of the stimulus for relevant and
irrelevant stimuli.  At intratrial position 4, where there was 100%
certainty prior to the presentation of the stimulus, the amplitude
at 0 msec was more negative when the stimulus was to be relevant
than when it was to be irrelevant.  This result is in agreement with
the CNV literature in which a negative potential is found in
anticipation of an "imperative" (relevant) stimulus.  The results
at the other electrode sites for this measure were similar (P3,
O1, O2 not shown).  Hemispheric differences were not prominent.

The other EP measures, amplitudes at 105 msec, 225 msec and
315 msec, showed major effects similar to those previously reported
for midline electrodes (Chapman, 1973).  Hemispheric differences
were not pronounced.  The measure which showed the most pronounced
hemispheric differences was the amplitude at 315 msec (Fig. 4).
The pattern of data at 315 msec suggests there may be differential
hemispheric and brain area representation of various information
processing conditions.  The most obvious of these is a differential
interaction of stimulus relevance and intratrial position with
hemisphere (F = 8.08; df = 3,21; p < .01).  The question remains
whether there is more differential representation of information
processing in one hemisphere than in the other.


HEMISPHERIC DIFFERENCES IN DISCRIMINANT ANALYSIS

One way to assess whether responses from one area or another
are more involved in various functions is by the use of discriminant analyses.  If measures of responses from two (or more) brain
areas are used to discriminate two (or more) experimental conditions,
which measures do the best job?

Do EPs from the left (P3, O1) or right (P4, O2) hemisphere do
a better job in discriminating various number/letter information
processing conditions (relevant and irrelevant numbers and letters
at four intratrial positions)?  In the first application of the
technique to be described there are sixteen classes to be discriminated from each other.  To perform this discrimination, there are
available five measures from each of four electrodes (twenty
variates).  The stepwise discriminant analysis (BMDP7M, Dixon, 1975)

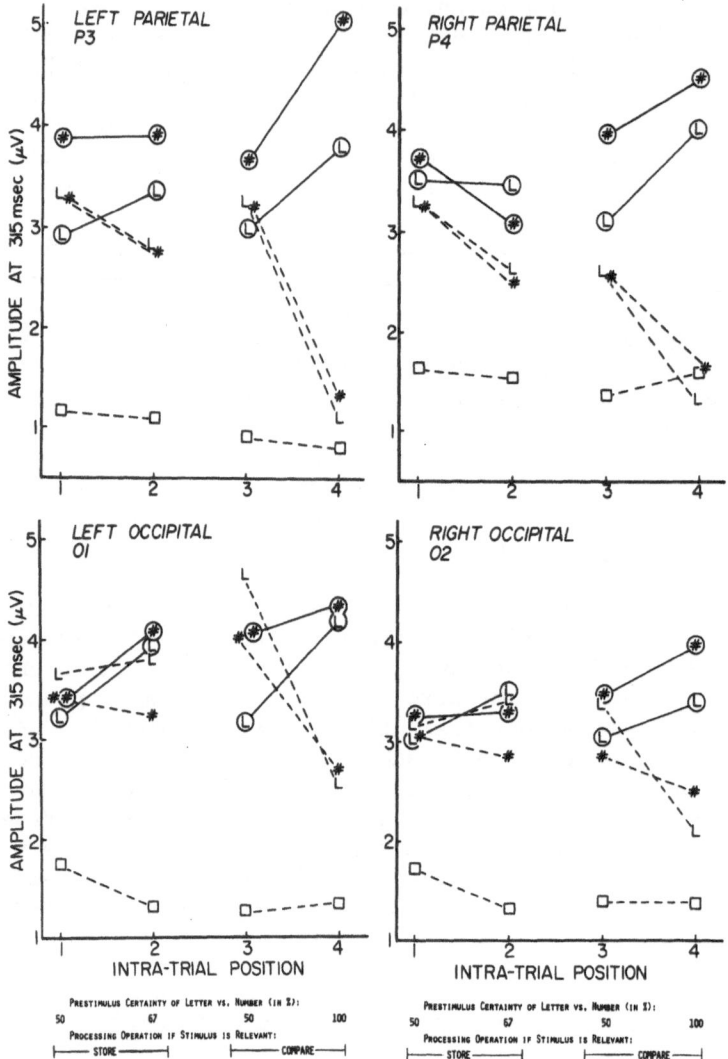

Fig. 4. Amplitude at 315 msec from left and right parietal and occipital electrodes for twenty experimental conditions. Measure is relative to EP level at time of stimulus. Other specifications as for Fig. 2.

selected the measures in the order of their effectiveness in classifying each of the 128 responses into the sixteen experimental conditions. The intercorrelations among the measures are taken into account. For the next measure to be added to the prediction equation the stepwise procedure selected the measure which is most

effective after the influence of the previously selected measures
is taken into account.  When the discriminant analysis is allowed
access to all twenty measures, the single best measure in discriminating the sixteen information processing conditions was the mean
amplitude over 480 msec from P3 (left parietal area).  Of the first
seven measures, six were from the left hemisphere (P3 mean over
480 msec, P3 at 0 msec, P3 at 315 msec, O1 at 315 msec, P4 mean
over 480 msec, O1 at 105 msec, P3 at 105 msec, in order of their
selection).  Since there were 16 conditions to be discriminated,
chance was 1/16 or 6.25%.  The development classification success
using the first seven measures was 47.7%.  A better index of the
generality of the success rate is the jackknifed classification
success which was 28.1% (Table I).  The jackknifed procedure is a
cross-validation technique which assesses the classification success
when each case is left out of the development set and then classified.  This success rate is significantly better than chance (Chi
square = 100.8; df = 1; p << .001).

Another assessment of hemispheric differences involves com-
puting separate discriminant analyses with measures from each side
alone and comparing the classification success rates.  The results
of this procedure also are given in Table I.  When discriminating
the sixteen information processing conditions, the measures from
the left side alone (P3,O1) achieved the same classification
success as when measures from both left and right sides were
available (28.1%).  A lower classification success rate (20.3%) was
obtained when measures from the right side alone (P4, O2) were
used.  These results indicate that measures from both left and right
sides carry information about the information processing conditions,
but that the left-side measures carry more such information than
those from the right side.  The fact that the left side alone does
as well, or nearly as well, as when both sides could contribute to
the classification equations indicates that the measures from the
right side are largely redundant with those from the left side.
The single most important variate of the ten available from each side
was the mean amplitude over 480 msec from the parietal site (P3 for
left side alone, P4 for right side alone).

Essentially the same pattern of results was obtained for
additional groupings of the experimental conditions (Table I).  In
order to provide comparisons which included the blank control flashes,
the information processing design was simplified by ignoring whether
the stimuli were letters or numbers.  When discriminating the blanks
and the resulting eight information processing conditions (relevant
or irrelevant stimuli X 4 intratrial positions) the single best
measure was again found to be the mean amplitude over 480 msec
from P3.  The first four measures selected for inclusion in the
discrimination were from the left hemisphere.  The final set of
variables selected included five from the left and three from the
right and accurately classified (jackknifed) 53.1% of the cases.

TABLE I

Discrimination of Experimental Conditions Using EP Measures
from Both Sides, Left Side, and Right Side

| Groups | Chance | Both Sides | Left Side | Right Side |
|---|---|---|---|---|
| Information Processing 16: number or letter X relevant or irrelevant X 4 intratrial positions | 6.25% | 28.1% (6L,1R) | 28.1% (5P,30) | 20.3% (3P,30) |
| Information Processing 9: relevant or irrelevant X 4 intratrial positions and blanks | 12.0% | 53.1% (5L,3R) | 51.9% (3P,20) | 46.9% (5P,20) |
| Relevance 3: relevant, irrelevant, and blanks | 36.0% | 85.0% (5L,3R) | 81.9% (2P,20) | 76.9% (5P,20) |
| Stimuli, physical 3: numbers, letters, and blanks | 36.0% | 70.6% (6L,2R) | 71.2% (4P,40) | 63.1% (3P,30) |
| Individual Subjects 8: subject | 12.5% | 96.9% (2L,8R) | 92.5% (5P,50) | 94.4% (5P,50) |

Entries are jackknifed classification success rates (maximum for ten or less variates) from stepwise discriminant analyses (BMDP7M). All were significantly better than chance. The values of Chi square (1 df), corrected for discontinuity, ranged from 40.7 to 1033.7 (p << .0001). Below each percentage the number of left and right variates (L and R) or number of parietal and occipital variates (P and O) used in the classification functions are given in parentheses. The response measures were standardized separately for each of the subjects before performing the discriminant analyses except for the individual subject's analyses. Each subject's data for each measure were transformed to z scores with mean equal to 0 and stan. dev. equal to 1. This procedure has been found useful in reducing the effect of individual differences upon subsequent analyses which focus on the effect of experimental conditions (Chapman et al., 1978). The general conclusions reached with the subject-standardized measures are the same as those obtained with the raw measures; the main differences are improved rates of classification success when irrelevant subject differences have been removed.

Restricting selection of variates to the left side reduced the classification accuracy only slightly. Selecting variates only from the right produced a somewhat large reduction (Table I).

Various kinds of functions may be assessed in a similar manner by using appropriate classification groups. For example, the side more related to stimulus relevance, regardless of stimulus or intratrial position, was assessed by discriminant analyses using three groups: relevant, irrelevant and blanks (Table I). The results suggest that the left-side EPs carry more information concerning stimulus relevance (81.9%), but that right-side EPs also do a good job in discriminating relevance (76.9%).

Which side was more related to the different physical stimuli was assessed by discriminating three groups: number, letters and blanks (regardless of relevance or intratrial position). The results indicate that the variates from the left side are more related to differences among the visual stimuli (Table I). The single most important variate was the amplitude at 315 msec from the left occipital area (O1).

It is possible to use this discriminant analysis technique to assess which is more related to individual differences. For this purpose the groups were the eight individual subjects. For these analyses the raw measures, before subject standardization, were used. Classification functions were computed which classified each EP case to one of the subjects, regardless of the experimental conditions (relevant and irrelevant number and letter, and blanks, in four intratrial positions). When measures from both sides were available, 96.9% of the EP cases were correctly classified to the individual subject by discriminant functions using two left variates and eight right variates. Measures from the left side alone did not do as well as measures from the right side alone (92.5% and 94.4%, respectively). This evidence suggests that the right side is more closely related to individual differences.

In general, the results indicate that measures over both hemispheres do a reasonably good job of discriminating various experimental conditions and individuals. The classification accuracy is well above chance in every instance. When discriminating information processing characteristics, variates from the left hemisphere are consistently selected first and and often for inclusion in the discriminant equations. Although the differences are not statistically reliable, accuracy is consistently reduced when only variates from the right hemisphere are used in the discrimination. This consistency suggests that measures from the left side are more related to various information processing distinctions than measures from the right side. Measures from the right side appear to be more related to individual differences.

SUMMARY

In a number-letter information processing experiment, comparing laterally recorded EPs with each other and comparing the lateral
EPs with previously reported midline EPs, the similarities are more
striking than the differences.  However, rather subtle hemispheric
differences which are reasonably consistent have been found.  The
assessment of these lateral effects was facilitated by the use of
control stimuli (blank flashes) and by particular kinds of multiple
discriminant analyses.  These have provided evidence that some kinds
of processes are more strongly related to the left side while other
processes are not.  Information processing, including stimulus
differences, was more discriminated by EP measures from the left
side.  Individual differences were more related to the right side.

ACKNOWLEDGEMENTS

This research was supported in part by USPHS Grants EY01593
and EY01319 and Office of Naval Research Contracts N00014-77-C-0037
and CNA SUB N00014-76-C-0001.  We gratefully acknowledge the aid
and comments of Henry R Bragdon, John A. Chapman, Samuel A. Shelburne, Jr., Don Montabana and Janice K. Martin.

REFERENCES

Chapman, R.M.  Evoked responses to relevant and irrelevant visual
    stimuli while problem solving.  Proc. Amer. Psychol. Assoc.,
    1975, 177-178.

Chapman, R.M.  Human evoked responses to meaningful stimuli.  XVII
    Int. Congr. Psychol., Moscow, 1966, 6, 53-59.

Chapman, R.M.  Discussion on eye movements, CNV and AEP.  In E.
    Donchin and D.B. Lindsley (Eds), Averaged Evoked Potentials:
    Methods. Results and Evaluations, Washington, D.C., NASA
    SP-191, 1969a, 177-180.

Chapman, R.M.  Definition and measurement of "psychological"
    independent variables in an average evoked potential experiment.
    In E. Donchin and D.B. Lindsley (Eds), Averaged Evoked
    Potentials: Methods, Results and Evaluations, Washington, D.C.,
    NASA SP-191, 1969b, 262-275.

Chapman, R.M.  Evoked potentials of the brain related to thinking.
    In F.J. McGuigan and R. Schoonover (Eds.), Psychophysiology
    of Thinking, New York: Academic Press, 1973.

Chapman, R.M.  Latent components of average evoked brain responses
    functionally related to information processing.  In Int.
    Symposium on Cerebral Evoked Potentials in Man, precirculated
    abstracts.  Brussels: Presses Universitaires de Bruxelles,
    1974a.

Chapman, R.M.  Semantic meaning of words and average evoked poten-
    tials.  In Int. Symposium on Cerebral Evoked Potentials in
    Man, precirculated abstracts.  Brussels: Presses Universitaires
    de Bruxelles, 1974b.

Chapman, R.M.  Hemispheric differences in average evoked potentials
    to relevant and irrelevant visual stimuli.  In Int. Symposium
    on Cerebral Evoked Potentials in Man, precirculated abstracts.
    Brussels: Presses Universitaires de Bruxelles, 1974c.

Chapman, R.M. (Chair)  ERPs and language.  Transcript of panel at
    Fourth International Congress of Event Related Slow Potentials
    of the Brain (EPIC IV), David A. Otto, Program Chairman, 4-10
    April 1976, Hendersonville, N.C.

Chapman, R.M.  Light intensity and the "storage" component in
    visual evoked potentials.  Electroenceph. Clin. Neurophysiol.,
    1977, 43, 778.

Chapman, R.M.  Connotative meaning and average evoked potentials.
    In H. Begleiter (Ed.), Evoked Brain Potentials and Behavior,
    New York: Plenum Press, in press.

Chapman. R.M.  On the road to specific information in evoked
    potentials.  In J.C. Armington, J. Krauskopf and B. Wooten
    (Eds.)  Visual Psychophysics: Its Physiological Basis, New
    York: Academic Press, in press.

Chapman, R.M. and Bragdon, H.R.  Evoked responses to numerical and
    non-numerical visual stimuli while problem solving.  Nature,
    1964, 203, 1155-1157.

Chapman, R.M. and Chapman, J.A.  The General Automation 18/30 as
    a system for the general analysis and acquisition of data in
    physiological psychology.  Behav. Res. Methods Instrum., 1972,
    4, 77-81.

Chapman, R.M., McCrary, J.W., Bragdon, H.R. and Chapman, J.A.
    Latent components of event related potentials functionally
    related to information processing.  In J.E. Desmedt (Ed.),
    Progress in Clinical Neurophysiology, Vol. 6, Cognitive
    Components in Cerebral Event Related Potentials and Selective
    Attention, Basel: Karger, in press(a).

Chapman, R.M., McCrary, J.W.  Chapman, J.A. and Bragdon, H.R.  Brain
    responses related to semantic meaning.  Brain and Language,
    1978, 5, 195-205.

Chapman, R.M., McCrary, J.W. and Chapman, J.A.  Short term memory:
    The "storage" component of human brain responses predicts
    recall.  Science, in press(b).

Dixon, W.J. (Ed.)  BMDP Biomedical Computer Programs, Berkeley:
    Univ. of California Press, 1975.

Donchin, E., McCarthy, G. and Kutas, M.  Electroencephalographic
    investigations of hemispheric specialization.  In J.E.
    Desmedt (Ed.), Progress in Clinical Neurophysiology, Vol. 3:
    Language and Hemispheric Specialization in Man:  Cerebral
    Event Related Potentials, Basel: Karger, 1977.

Halliday, A.M., Barrett, G., Halliday, E. and Michael, W.F.  The
    topography of the pattern evoked potential.  In J.E. Desmedt
    (Ed.). Visual Evoked Potentials in Man:  New Developments,
    Oxford: Oxford Univ. Press, 1977.

Jewett, D.L., Romano, M.N. and Williston, J.S.  Human auditory
    evoked potentials:  Possible brain stem components detected on
    the scalp.  Science, 1970, 167, 1517-1518.

# A SYSTEM TRANSFER FUNCTION FOR VISUAL EVOKED POTENTIALS

Richard Coppola

National Institute of Mental Health

Bethesda, Maryland

## INTRODUCTION

The electroencephalogram (EEG) and evoked potentials (EP) have long held the promise of being a way of studying the sensory processing of the brain. If we take the view that the EEG is a continuous output signal, some features of which represent the response to input signals consisting of sensory stimuli, we have an input/output system that seems suitable for application of engineering analysis techniques. Using this approach, Clynes et al. (1964) studied the brain wave responses to step, ramp and sine wave light stimuli. The step stimuli allowed them to obtain the transient response of the "system", and the sine wave stimuli allowed them to obtain the steady state response. These results, as well as the work of other investigators (Donker, 1975; Montagu, 1967; van der Tweel and Verduyn-Lunel, 1965), have demonstrated the nonlinear nature of steady state evoked potentials (SSEP). For stimulation by sine wave modulated light (SML) in the frequency range 5-9 Hz, a persistent second harmonic response is seen even at very low modulation depths. Further evidence of nonlinearity is seen in the poor results in attempting to predict the response to high flash rates based on superposition of responses from low flash rates.

In engineering analysis the transient response is usually characterized in the time domain by the impulse response, whereas the frequency domain is normally used to illustrate the steady state response via a transfer function. For a linear system the steady state frequency response can be obtained by the Laplace transform of the impulse response; thus either the transient or the steady state response is sufficient to characterize the system under investigation. However, in dealing with a nonlinear system the transient

69

response will usually not be sufficient to reveal the steady state response.

Recently several investigators have utilized Wiener's theory of nonlinear systems to develop identification technique for biological systems (French and Butz, 1973; Marmarelis and McCann, 1973; Marmarelis and Naka, 1974; McCann, 1974). This theory gives a description of a nonlinear system that is very general in nature. To call the description a transfer function is usually thought of as referring to frequency characteristics. However, the method does give a closed form function that relates the output to the input in the time domain.

Nonlinear analysis can also be employed when the input to a system is a point process and the output is a continuous signal. Krausz (1975) derived functional representations similar to Wiener for the case of a Poisson process input. This method has been applied to investigation of human somatosensory EEG responses (SER) to electric pulse stimulation (Scalabassi et al., 1977). The method has been termed "functional power series analysis" and involves the assumption that the nervous system operates as a stochastic transformation represented in a manner where the continuous output is an integral expansion of continuous kernels and a discrete input function. The kernels are analogous to Wiener's and have the same properties. This method applied to SERs has revealed that the nonlinear interactions noted may produce a facilatory or an occlusive effect. These results have been useful in the study of multiple sclerosis.

The rest of this paper will give a brief introduction to nonlinear analysis methods and will show how they may be applied to human visual evoked responses to give a transfer function which relates the time waveform of a visual input stimulus to the evoked EEG output signal. Once this function is obtained it can be used to predict the transient and steady state responses to visual stimuli of similar form.

Along with these predictions we can also determine the nonlinear interaction present in the system as is usually obtained by recovery cycles from double pulse stimulation.

NONLINEAR SYSTEMS THEORY

Volterra series have been used to express the output of a nonlinear system with memory by an expansion of integrals of powers of the input (Bedrosian and Rice, 1971). Wiener recognized their usefulness in describing nonlinear circuits and developed an expansion that allows a system characterization similar to linear systems theory (Wiener, 1958).

Here the output is related to the input by a series of functionals:

$$y(t) = \sum_{n=0}^{\infty} G_n[h_n,x(t)]$$

We can view this sytem relationship as in the block diagram shown
in Fig. 1.

The $G_n$ are a complete set of orthogonal functions.  The first
three are:

$$G_0[h_1,x(t)] = h_0$$

$$G_1[h_1,x(t)] = \int_0^{\infty} h_1(\tau)x(t-\tau)d\tau$$

$$G_2[h_2,x(t)] = \int\int_{00} h_2(\tau_1,\tau_2)x(t-\tau_1)x(t-\tau_2)d\tau_1 d\tau_2 - P\int_0^{\infty} h_2(\tau,\tau)d\tau$$

P is the spectral density of a white Gaussian noise input.

The $\{h_n\}$ are the set of a Wiener kernels characterizing the
system.  They are essentially generalized impulse responses; $G_1$ is
equivalent to the linear convolution integral and $h_1$, the linear
impulse response.  The higher order kernels essentially describe
the amount of nonlinear cross-talk in the system.

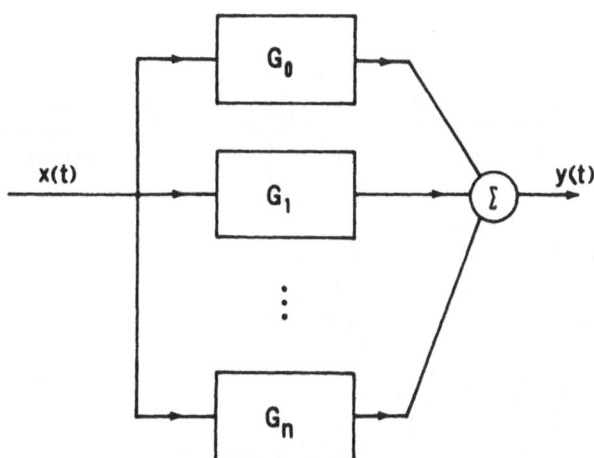

Fig. 1.   System relationship of G functionals.

The system identification problem is now one of finding these kernels. Lee and Schetzen (1975) developed a cross-correlation technique where the general result is:

$$h_n(\sigma_1,\ldots,\sigma_n) = \frac{1}{n!P^n} \cdot [y(t) - \sum_{m=0}^{n-1} G_m[h_m,x(t)]]x(t-\sigma_1)\ldots x(t-\sigma_n)$$

This technique is based on a scheme of delays as shown in Fig. 2 for the second order case.

The actual digital solution is obtained by replacing the time averages by expected values which are estimated by discrete time correlograms. The continuous signals are replaced by their discrete time samples, and the kernels are represented by their values at discrete lag times.

Wiener showed that two nonlinear systems are equivalent if and only if their responses to the same white noise input is the same. This gives a method of testing how successful the system indentification was by comparing the model response to the actual response. This comparison can be made by a mean square error measurement (MSE). Because the functionals of the system model are orthogonal, we know that if the series is truncated after the nth term (order) the result is still the best MSE approximation up to that term.

The theory is, in general, applicable to a wide range of physical systems. There are, however, several preliminary considerations

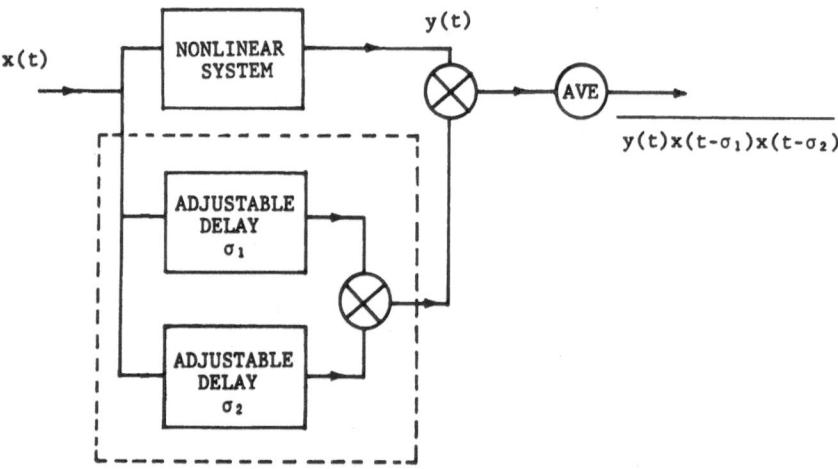

Fig. 2.   Two dimensional delay used for system identification.

before attempting NLTFA (Marmarelis and Naka, 1974). Two main requirements of a system are that it be time invariant and that it
have a finite memory. If ergodicity cannot be assumed, solutions can
still be worked by noting that for random processes the time average
of the ensemble average is equal to the ensemble average of the time
average (French and Butz, 1973). Since the system kernels are deter-
ministic, the cross-correlations can be averaged across replications
to give satisfactory results.

The finite memory consideration means that the system output
must not depend on the infinite past in any significant way. For
all physically realizable systems, this is obviously true. The
problem is one of figuring how much of the past is necessary in
order to determine the output to a desired degree of accuracy. Since
the kernels can be computed only for a finite number of lags, this
length should be chosen according to the system memory.

There are several parameters that must be determined in order
to perform the identifying experiment: (1) bandwidth and dynamic
range of stimulus; (2) length of experiment; (3) averaging or smooth-
ing of input and output signals; (4) sampling rates. The order of
the model depends on the nonlinearities present, and a second order
model can, at most, account for second harmonic responses.

For a complete review of this type of nonlinear analysis see
Hung and Stark (1977). Palm and Poggio (1977, 1978) give a rigorous
discussion of some of the mathematical problems associated with the
Wiener methods. They point out that since discrete time signals are
used in actual practice, many of these difficulties are overcome.


METHODS

The length of the evoked EEG response to a light flash is on
the order of 500 msec as found in standard average evoked potential
studies. A reasonable starting point seems to be a model that would
include the ability to predict such a response. With this in mind,
a 20 sec stimulation period was chosen. This appears to be a good
compromise between having enough length to compute a stable cross-
correlogram and being short enough to have some assumption of
stationarity of the subject's EEG.

It is clear that response averaging would be necessary to bring
the signal-to-noise levels into the region where the analysis might
be able to work. Starting with the assumption that at least as many
trials as are necessary for normal AEP work would be required meant
collecting about sixty trials. An actual trial consisted of 25 sec
of white noise stimulation followed by a few seconds pause. The
light level was left at the average level of the stimulus during
the rest time in order to reduce problems with adaptation and ini-

tial eye blink transients.  The last 20 sec of the EEG response was
recorded for each trial.

Stimulus generation and control of data collection were provided by a PDP-11 computer based system for stimulus-response experiments.  Gaussian noise was generated by averaging twelve values
from a uniformly distributed random process and multiplying by a
desired standard deviation.  This procedure gives noise clipped at
plus and minus 6 standard deviations.  The Gaussian random numbers
were then output at a fixed time rate to a digital-to-analog converter followed by a low pass filter to remove switching transients.
Bandwidth was thus controlled by the rate of output, and dynamic
range was controlled by the choice of standard deviation.  A frequency range of 0-15 Hz was chosen with a mean stimulus intensity
of 60 footlamberts.  The standard deviation was set at a half log
step of the mean value.  The analog signal thus derived was used to
drive an Iconix photostimulator which utilizes hot cathode fluorescent tubes.  These tubes were set behind a rear projection screen of
43 X 55 cm placed at 50 cm from the subject's eyes.

Vertex and midline occipital leads referenced to right ear were
recorded using gold disk electrodes.  The EEG amplifiers used had a
low frequency 3 dB point of 0.5 Hz.  This was followed by an active
low pass filter that was flat to 42 Hz and down 45 dB at 60 Hz.
The filtered output was then converted to 10-bit digital values at
a rate of 100 samples per second per channel.   Each of the trials,
as described above, consisted of the same white noise sequence.
The responses were recorded on disk for later analysis.


RESULTS

Artifact-free trials were averaged together to give a 2000
point data record for both the vertex and occipital responses.
Split half averages revealed very good agreement, indicating the
validity of the response to this type of stimulus.  The stimulus
signal in log foot lamberts was sampled at the same rate to provide
a 2000 point data record of the input signal.  An example of the
stimulus signal and response averages obtained is shown in Fig. 3.

An analysis program was written which performs the cross-
correlogram computations.  The program is set up to calculate the
first and second order kernels and the model responses for each of
them.  It currently is running on a PDP-11/40 and has a limitation
of 90 lags and 1000 data points.  For an analysis with a model of
90 lags, using the first 1000 points of the vertex response, the
resulting first order model response (G1), second order (G2) and the
total model are shown in Fig. 3.  The percent variance accounted
for by the first order model is 16.5, and for the first and second

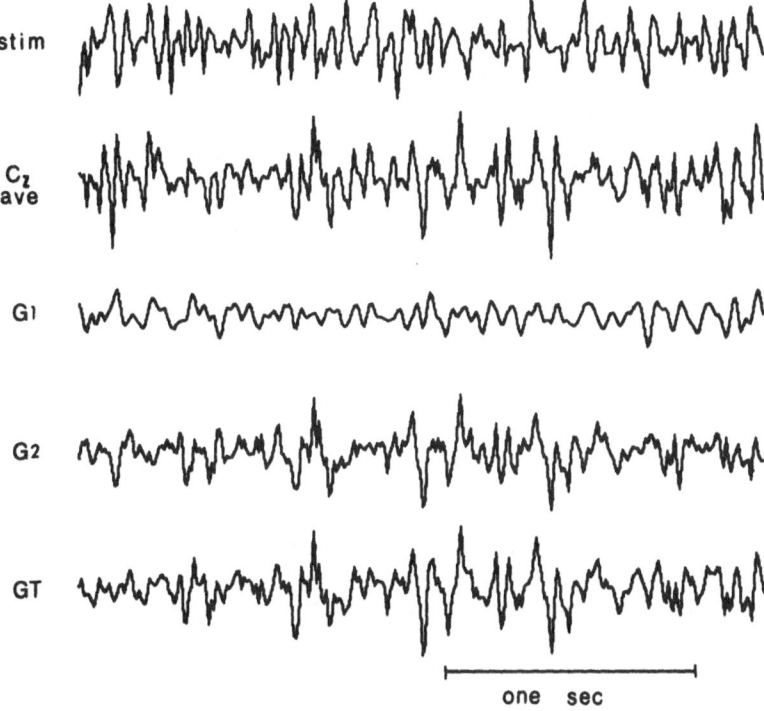

stim

C$_z$
ave

G$_1$

G$_2$

G$_T$

one   sec

Fig. 3.   Stimulus and response records with first and second order
model responses.

order together it is 70.   The visual agreement between the model's
response and the actual response is seen to be quite good.   Considerable nonlinearity is indicated since the percent variance accounted for statistics indicates that the major contribution to the model
is from the second order (i.e., nonlinear) model.

The linear kernel (h1) can be presented as a series of values
at the discrete lag times they correspond to.   The nonlinear second
order kernel (h2), however, is two-dimensional, and so a simple
visual presentation is more difficult.   The kernel may be thought of
as consisting of two parts.   The first is the diagonal values corresponding to equal lag times in each dimension.   These represent
the memory-less features of the nonlinearity.   The off diagonal
elements represent the nonlinear impulse interactions in time.   These
are the memory features of the nonlinearity.   Fig. 4 shows the first
order kernel and the main diagonal of the second order kernel.

The question arises as to whether the distribution of values in

IMPULSE RESPONSE

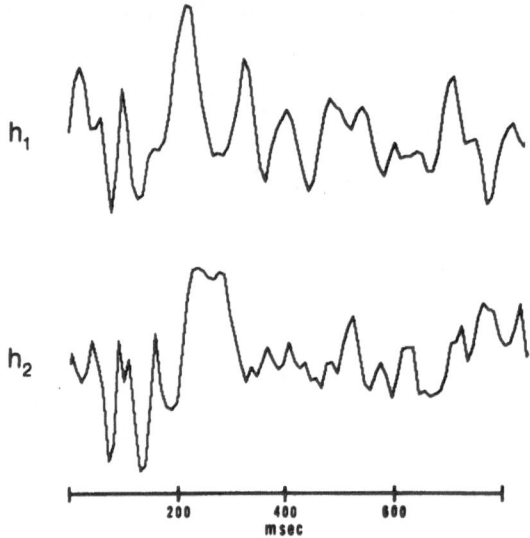

Fig. 4.   First and second order kernel impulse responses.

the second order kernel reveals anything about essential features of
the system under study.   The form of h2 for a memory-less nonlinearity followed or preceded by a linear system is easily computed
(French and Wong, 1977).   For a memory-less nonlinearity, such as a
rectifier followed by a linear filter, the second order kernel has
values only along the diagonal and exhibits no nonlinear interaction
in time.   This also indicates that such a system will still obey
linear superposition.

For a linear system preceding a rectifier, the nonlinear kernel
does have off-diagonal values.   This form clearly gives an increase
in nonlinear interaction times.   Similar results are found if a
general nonlinear kernel is considered to be preceded or followed
by a linear filter.   For a linear system following h2, the effect
is to smear h2 out along lines parallel to the diagonal.   For the
case of a preceding linear system, h2 is spread out both parallel
and perpendicular to the diagonal (Stark, 1968).

For the results here the major values of h2 are seen to be
along the diagonal with the most nonlinear interaction being contained within a relatively short period of time (i.e., close to the
diagonal).   A lot of smearing parallel to the diagonal is also noted.
These indications would suggest that a short response system precedes
the nonlinearity while a longer response time system follows it.

Facilitation Effects of Nonlinear Interaction

The amount of off-diagonal activity in the second order kernel indicates the amount of nonlinear interaction present in the system. In order to more clearly quantify this interaction, a comparison of model responses, with and without nonlinear interaction, was undertaken.  In EP work, recovery cycles are usually studied by looking at the effect of a preceding pulse spaced some variable length of time before another pulse.  If nonlinear interaction is not present, the response to the second pulse will be a linear superposition of the responses to each pulse spaced appropriately in time.  To simulate that situation, the diagonal only of the h2 response was used to

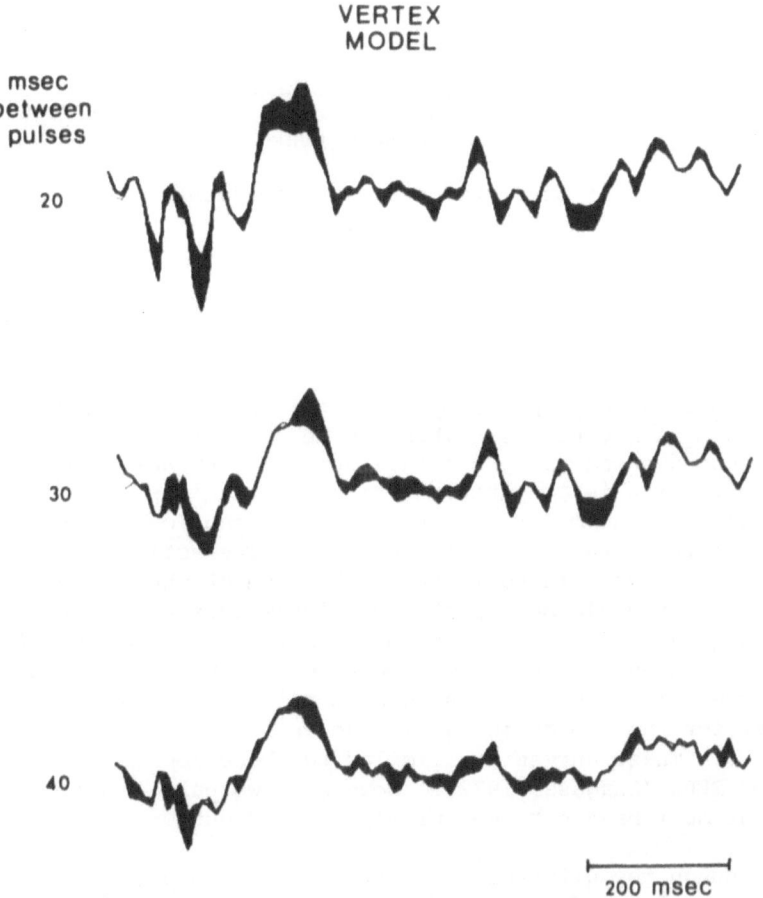

Fig. 5.  Shaded area is the difference between responses to double pulses computed with and without nonlinear interaction.

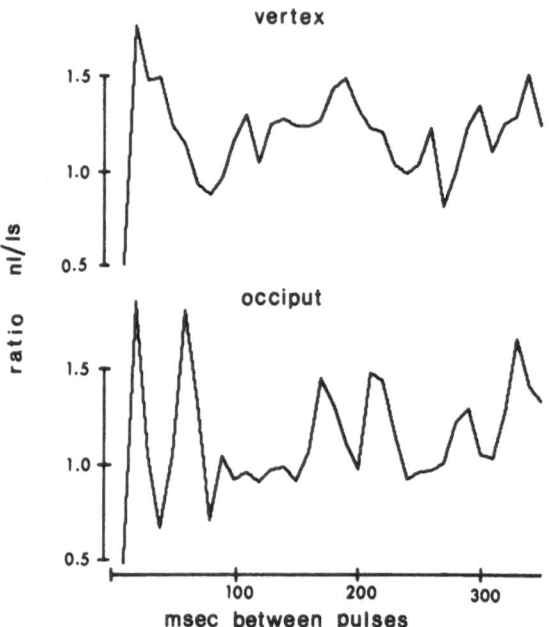

Fig. 6.  Ratio of predicted responses to double pulses computed
with and without nonlinear interaction.

compute an impulse response by superposition with the response to an
impulse some delay before.  This may be contrasted to the response
to the second pulse using the full nonlinear kernel.  Fig. 5 shows
the results of this computation for several values of delay time between pulses.  The major result of the interaction is seen to be
an initial facilitation of the response.  The action of a pulse 20
msec before another is to increase the size of the response considerably over what would be expected by linear superposition alone.
These results may be quantified by comparing some measure of interest
for each response.  The maximum peak-to-peak value of the response
within the first 350 msec was used in this case.  The ratio of these
measures for the two cases is plotted versus the time between pulses
in Fig. 6.  These curves are similar to those reported in the literature for SERs (Shagass, 1972).  However, two pulse experiments using
visual stimuli have not been widely carried out.

Although the difference in the form of the pulse response between the vertex and the occiput is clear, the form of the facilitation curve is similar.  Both show an early peak and then a refrac-
tory period followed by an even response.  As pointed out earlier,
the spreading of the nonlinear kernel perpendicular to the diagonal

may be due to a linear filter preceding the nonlinear element.  In
this case that would suggest that an element common to both the vertex and occipital systems and early in the processing stage might be
responsible for the nonlinear interaction.  The usual source of the
nonlinearity is considered to be rectification at the retinal
ganglion level.  If this is the case, the preceding linear element
would indicate filtering at the retinal level.  Thus caution is urged
in attributing any recovery cycle effects to more central phenomena.

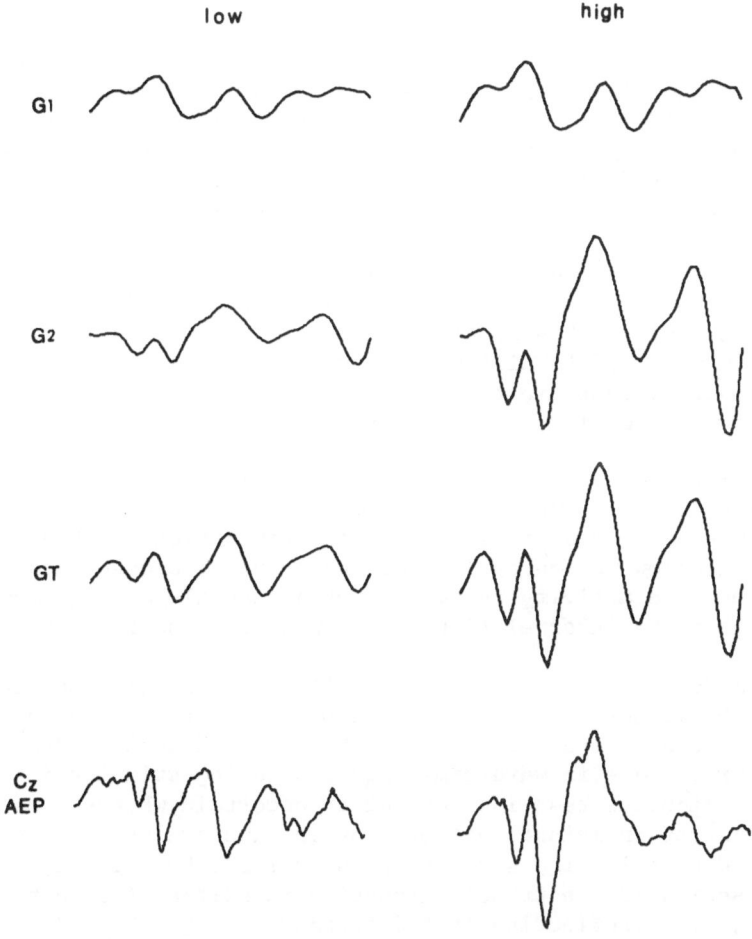

Fig. 7.  Actual vertex AEP and the nonlinear model predicted
response for a high and low intensity stimulus.

Pediction of the Transient Response

Vertex and occipital standard average evoked potentials were
also collected using the same equipment.  The EP experiment was one
designed to study the relation of response measures to stimulus intensity (Buchsbaum, 1978).  Four intensities of light (3, 25, 80 and
220 footlamberts) were presented randomly intermixed but counterbalanced for preceding intensity.  The individual stimulus was a
half second light flash using the Iconix photostimulator.  The EEG
response for 512 msec after stimulus onset was averaged for sixty-
four presentations of each intensity.  Sampling rate was 250 Hz,
giving 128 samples per average.  A computer program was written to
generate the transfer function model's response to similar transient
stimuli.  A half-second step function was used as the input signal,
and the kernel outputs were computed.

When using different size step functions as input to the transfer function, it is seen that the relative contributions to the total
response of the linear (G1) and nonlinear (G2) components are also
different.  This is shown in Fig. 7 for the vertex response.  It
can be seen that while the latencies of the peaks of the predicted
response are quite similar to the actual AEP, the relative sizes of
the peaks depend on the differential contributions from G1 and G2.

In looking at a sequence of AEPs to various intensity stimuli,
similar shifts of peak size are noted (Buchsbaum, 1978).  The suggestion provided by this model is that some of this empirically noted
variation may be due to differential stimulation of separate linear
and nonlinear elements in the system.  This result is quite similar
to that for the model's predicted SSEPs.

More late activity is noted in the model's response than is
usually seen in EPs.  This may reflect the fact that the transfer
function was arrived at by steady state stimulation which does not
adequately follow the decay time of the actual response mechanisms.
Some of the late activity is seen to be at the alpha frequency, suggesting again the interrelation of EPs with ongoing activity.

The model should be adjusted to allow for changing the relative
sizes of the linear and the nonlinear portions of the response. This
would allow closer study of whether the parallel system idea can
account for changes in waveforms with increasing stimulus intensity.
Further, a rigorous test is required to ascertain whether the model
really reflects individual differences in waveform shape.  This could
be achieved by selecting subjects with reliable but clearly different
AEPs and seeing if the transfer function identified for each subject
is successful in reflecting this difference.

SUMMARY

   This study develops a method of nonlinear transfer function
analysis that is applicable to human EEG research.  A white noise
stimulation experiment that allows indentification of the Wiener
kernels of a nonlinear system is shown to be successful in modeling
the human visual EEG system.  Results, which are presented for both
vertex and occipital EEG, show that over 70% of the response variance
is accounted for.  The resulting nonlinear transfer function is
shown to be useful in studying several aspects of EEG.  Nonlinear
interaction in the model accounts for facilitation effects as seen
in recovery cycle studies.  Frequency response characteristics are
also developed which suggest the existence of separate linear and
nonlinear pathways in the visual system.  Prediction of the transient response by the model is found to agree with actual AEPs to
different intensities of stimulation.  The resulting waveform
appears to be a summation of differential contributions of linear
and nonlinear components.


REFERENCES

Bedrosian, E. and Rice, S.O.  The output properties of Volterra
      systems (nonlinear systems with memory) driven by harmonic and
      Gaussian inputs.  Proc. IEEE, 1971, 59, 1688-1707.

Buchsbaum, M.S.  Neurophysiological studies of augmenting/reducing.
      In A. Petries (Ed.), Individuality in Pain and Suffering, in
      press.

Clynes, M., Kohn, M. and Lifshitz, K.  Dynamics and spatial behavior
      of light evoked potentials.  Ann. N.Y. Acad. Sci., 1964, 112,
      468-509.

Donker, D.N.J.  Harmonic composition and topographic distribution
      of responses to sine wave modulated light (SML), their repro-
      ducibility and their interhemispheric relation.  Electroenceph.
      Clin. Neurophysiol., 1975, 39, 561-574.

French, A.S. and Butz, E.G.  Measuring the Wiener kernels of a non-
      linear system using the fast Fourier transform algorithm.  Int.
      J. Control., 1973, 17. 529-539.

French, A.S. and Wong, R.K.S.  Nonlinear analysis of sensory trans-
      duction in an insect mechanoreceptor.  Biol. Cybernetics, 1977,
      26, 231-240.

Hung, G. and Stark, L.  The kernel identification method - review of
      theory, calculation, application and interpretation.  Math.
      Biosci., 1977, 37, 135-190.

Krauaz, H.I.   Identification of nonlinear systems using random im-
    pulse train inputs.   Biol. Cybernetics, 1975, 19, 217-230.

Lee, Y.W. and Schetzen, M.   Measurement of the Wiener kernels of
    a nonlinear system by cross-correlation.   Int. J. Control,
    1965, 2, 237-254.

Marmarelis, P.Z. and McCann, G.D.  Development and application of
    white noise modeling techniques for studies of insect visual
    nervous system.   Kybernetik, 1973, 12, 74-89.

Marmarelis, P.Z. and Naka, K.-I.   Identification of multi-input
    biological systems.   IEEE Trans. Biomed. Eng., 1974, 21, 88-101.

McCann, G.D.   Nonlinear identification theory models for successive
    stages of visual nervous system of flies.   J. Neurophysiol.,
    1974, 37, 869-895.

Montagu, J.D.   The relationship between the intensity or repetitive
    photic stimulation and the cerebral response.   Electroenceph.
    Clin. Neurophysiol., 1967, 23, 152-161.

Palm, G. and Poggio, T.   Wiener-like system identification in
    physiology.   J. Math. Biol., 1977, 4, 375-381.

Palm, G. and Poggio, T.   Stochastic identification methods for non-
    linear systems:  An extension of the Wiener theory.   SIAM J.
    Appl. Math., 1978, 34, 524-534.

Sclabassi, R.J., Risch, H.A., Hinman, C.L.. Kroin J.S., Enns, N.F.
    and Namerow, N.S.  Complex pattern evoked somatosensory responses
    in the study of multiple sclerosis.   Proc. IEEE, 1977, 65,
    626-633.

Shagass, C.   Evoked Brain Potentials in Psychiatry, Plenum Press:
    New York, 1972.

Stark, L. Neurological Control Systems, Plenum Press: New York, 1968.

van der Tweel, L.H. and Verduyn-Lunel, H.F.E.   Human visual responses
    to sinusoidally modulated light.   Electroenceph. Clin. Neuro-
    physiol., 1965, 18, 587-598.

Wiener, N.   Nonlinear Problems in Random Theory, M.I.T. Press;
    Cambridge, 1958.

SOMATOSENSORY EVOKED POTENTIALS IN MAN:   MATURATION, COGNITIVE

PARAMETERS AND CLINICAL USES IN NEUROLOGICAL DISORDERS

John E. Desmedt

Brain Research Unit, University of Brussels

115 Boulevard de Waterloo, Brussels, Belgium

The cerebral somatosensory projection was the first to be mapped in primates and studied in intact man.  While many publications have been dealing with the visual or auditory modalities (cf. Desmedt, 1977a,c) the somatosensory evoked potentials (SEP) have only recently become a topic for the many studies which elaborate on the earlier work (cf. Giblin, 1964; Debecker and Desmedt, 1964; Halliday, 1967).  EPs are smaller and more localized on the scalp than the auditory or visual EPs.  Furthermore the fast early components of the SEP have been distorted or missed in many studies that were done with inadequate amplifier bandpass or computer sampling rate (Desmedt et al., 1974).  When these and other methodology problems are duly considered (Desmedt, 1977d), SEPs offer outstanding opportunities, namely because far field and primary cortical components, as well as later components, can be studied.  Another feature is the remarkable length of the somatosensory pathway extending from peripheral nerves to spinal cord, brain stem and cortex which makes the SEP susceptible to a variety of pathological assaults that can be diagnostically explored by appropriate procedures.  Finally SEPs recorded during perceptual decision tasks can differentiate cognition related changes involving either the early, middle range or later components in somatosensory perception (Desmedt et al., 1965; Desmedt and Robertson, 1977a,b; Desmedt, 1977e).

Normalization of SEP studies is only beginning.  The SEPs recorded at the contralateral scalp over the postcentral gyrus comprise many subcomponents with diverse consistencies across subjects and with different significance.  Many current ambiguities or contradictions appearing in the literature can be related to differences in control of various parameters.  For example, the stimulus used to elicit SEPs is generally an electric shock to a mixed nerve

trunk.  This technique is rather painful for the subject, and it has
more limitations than currently believed because so many nerve
fibers of different significance are simultaneously fired.  It is
wiser to restrict the input to the afferent fibers from a skin area
by delivering the stimulus to fingers, toes or branches of sensory
nerve (Desmedt, 1971).  The SEP latency is affected by stimulus
intensities in a range close to threshold (Desmedt et al., 1976).
Intervals between stimuli in a series should preferably be random,
and the mean frequency should not exceed 1/sec.  When studying slow
component waveforms the intervals should certainly exceed 4 sec to
minimize sequential distortions and interactions (Desmedt and
Debecker, 1972).

     The EP components are conveniently identified by their polarity
and peak latency (Donchin et al., 1977).  Several factors affect
the latency of the early SEP components.  Any lowering of tissue
temperature around the peripheral nerve increases the SEP latency
since the afferent conduction velocity drops with a Q10 of 1.5 to
2.0 with temperature; it is, therefore, important to exclude this
source of variation by checking local temperatures with a thermistor
and by maintaining them at physiological range (Desmedt, 1971).

     Another factor is the body size which influences the distance
actually traveled from the stimulation point to the brain.  For
example, in normal adults the onset latencies of the first cortical
event N22 of the SEP to finger stimulation varies from 15.5 to 22 ms

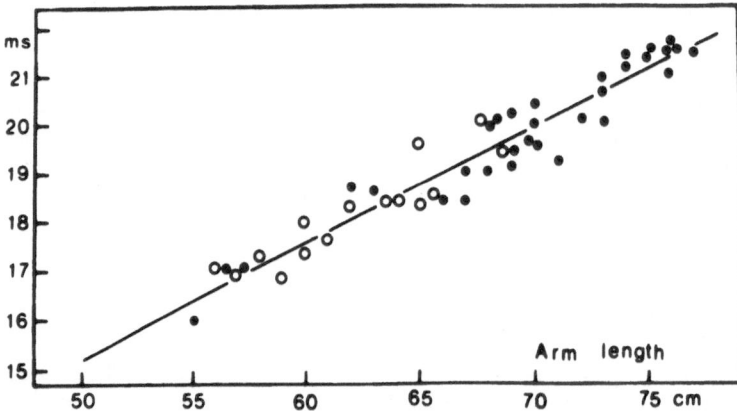

Fig. 1.   Onset latencies (msec, ordinate) of N22 of the SEP to
electric stimulation of fingers of the contralateral hand in normal
dults, fifteen females (circles) and thirty-two males (dots).  The
abscissa represents the arm length in cm, as measured from the stimulating cathode to the shoulder (acromion bone) with the arm stretched.
From J.E. Desmedt and E. Brunko, 1978.

in persons of body size from 1.5 to 2.0 m (Fig. 1). The peak latency of N22 can range from about 19 to 24 msec. For purposes of no-
menclature, one can label the component from its actual peak latency
in the subject (e.g., N21 or N23), or else use N22 throughout with
the understanding that a variation of ± 3 msec can occur for different body builds (cf. Donchin et al., 1977; Desmedt and Brunko, 1978).
The true significance of latency differences for early SEP components
should be carefully considered when comparing subjects of different
ages (Desmedt and Cheron, 1978) or clinical patients with nervous
lesions.

It has not been appreciated that the electric stimulation of
different skin areas elicits SEPs with genuinely different waveforms
either in the normal adult (Desmedt and Brunko, 1978) or in the newborn (Desmedt, 1971). Fig. 2B shows the prominent early N24 cortical SEP component elicited by stimulation of the median nerve in a
normal neonate during slow wave sleep. The N24 component presents
similar features, but slightly longer duration, in the neonate during rapid eye movement sleep (Desmedt and Manil, 1970). This N24
is recorded over the postcentral cortex about 45 mm from the midline,
but it is barely seen at the midline in A.

By contrast, stimulation of the posterior tibial nerve in the
same session elicits an SEP with an early cortical positive component

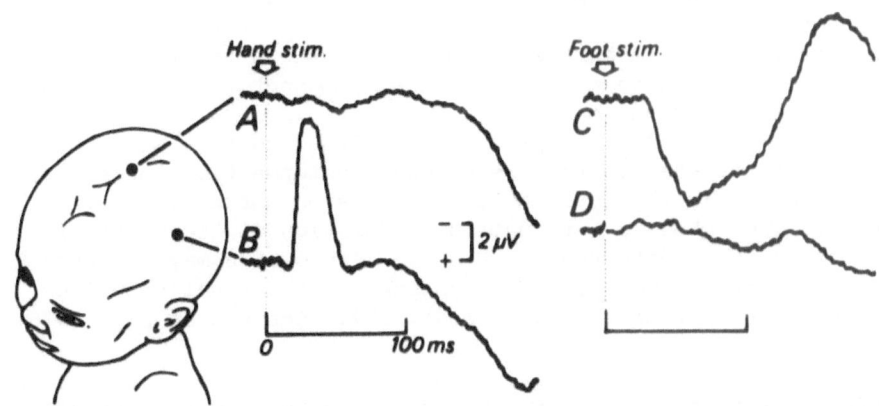

Fig. 2. Normal newborn of three days, slow wave sleep. Comparison
of the early components of the SEP to stimulation of the right median
nerve at the wrist (A,B) or of the right posterior tibial nerve at
the ankle (C,D). The averaged SEPs are simultaneously recorded from
two scalp locations shown on the left side. The reference is a midfrontal electrode. Negativity of the active electrode registers
upwards in all records. From J.E. Desmedt, 1971.

that is not preceded by a large negative component; this early
SEP component to foot stimulation occurs close to the midline (C)
but not at the more lateral scalp location (D). These and other
recent results are in line with Penfield's cortical somatotopy in
man. Extensive data on the profiles and scalp topography of cortical SEPs to stimulation of different skin areas can be found elsewhere (Desmedt and Brunko, 1978).

## MATURATION

The SEP of newborns presents characteristic features related
to the immaturity at birth of both the human brain and the afferent
fibers of the somatosensory pathway. For example, the neonate SEP
to finger stimulation presents a prominent cortical N30 which has
a much slower time course than the corresponding N22 component in
the adult. The mean onset latency of N30 in the newborn is 22 msec,
and its mean duration is 15 msec during rapid eye movements sleeping
or waking and 20 msec during slow wave sleep (Desmedt and Manil,
1970). The mean duration of the homologous N22 in the adult is 4
msec (Desmedt et al., 1976).

During maturation after birth, a gradual change of the N30
component occurs whereby the adult pattern is slowly acquired over
a period of several years. Fig. 3A-C shows typical SEPs to finger
stimulation at eight months. At this age, the large early negative
component presents a rather short latency of 15 msec. For comparison the SEPs of two adults (Fig. 3D,E) present a latency close to
the mean of 19 msec and an N22 of about 4 msec duration. Another
major feature of SEP maturation depicted in these records is the
increase of the subsequent positive P28 component. As discussed
elsewhere, in relation to morphological data in immature mammals
(Purpura et al., 1964), the prominence of the negative N30 at birth
in man can be related to the precocious development of the superfi-
cial axo-dendritic thalamocortical synapses on cortical pyramidal
neurones. The subsequent reduction in duration of the negative
component together with the increase in size of P28 may, in part,
reflect the later development of synapses on the basal dendrites
of the cortical pyramids (cf. Desmedt, 1971; Desmedt et al., 1976).

Shortage of space does not allow a review of data about scalp
topography of these and other SEP components, but it is already
obvious that studies along these lines are uncovering unsuspected
features of maturation of the human brain. For example, the question of the changes of onset latency of the early cortical negative
SEP component with age raises several issues. The mean onset latency is 22.5 msec in newborns and 18.8 msec in adults, a highly significant difference (p < 0.001): however, the onset latency is much
shorter, between 12.5 and 16.0 msec in children from about six

months to nine years (Desmedt et al., 1976). This somewhat surprising finding can be resolved if one takes into account the increase in length of the somatosensory pathway as the child grows. The body size of the twenty-nine subjects we studied is plotted in the lower part of Fig. 4. For roughly assessing the factor of pathway length, we divided the onset latency of N22 by the body size and found a highly consistent profile (Fig. 4, lower part, dots) which is fitted

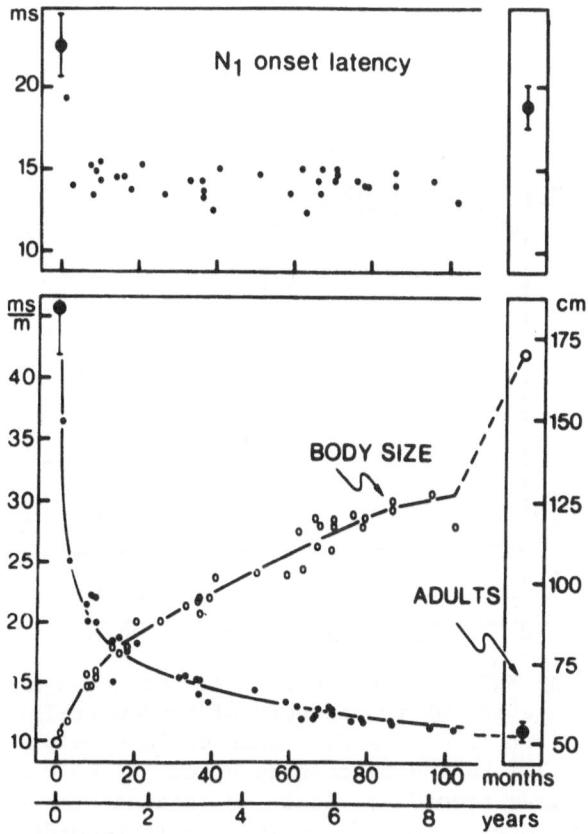

Fig. 4. The changes in onset latency of the early cortical negative component of the SEP with age (abscissa, months or years). Upper graph, onset latency in msec. Only the mean value with the standard deviation is indicated for the newborns and for the adults rectangle of the right. Lower graph, the body size of the same subjects in cm (ordinate on the right side; circles) and the onset latency of SEP divided by the body size (ordinate on the left side; dots). From Desmedt et al. (1976).

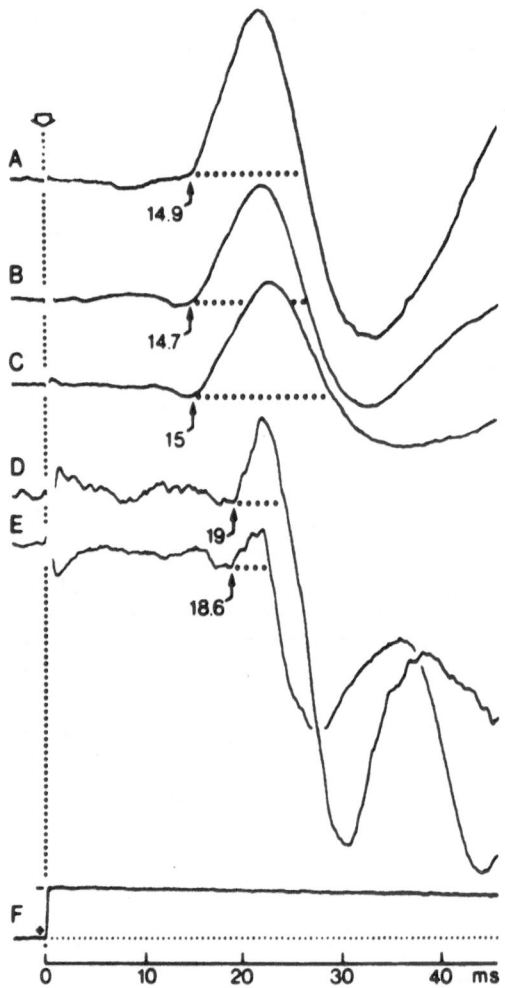

Fig. 3. Different SEP profiles in infants and in adults. SEPs
elicited by stimulation of two fingers of the contralateral hand
with brief pulses of 10 mA. A-C, female child of eight months and
twenty-one days, 7.1 kg and 67 cm body size. A and C are different
runs but same active recording electrode located over the postcentral gyrus 60 mm lateral to the midline. B is recorded with an electrode 50 mm from the midline. The three SEPs consistently show
onset latencies and N22 duration characteristic for that age. D,
SEP recorded in a normal male adult of twenty-seven years. E, SEP
recorded in another male adult of thirty-six years. Finger stimuli
delivered at random intervals with a minimum of 1 sec. Bandpass of
the recording system 0.3 to 3000 Hz. All subjects awake with eyes
open. F, calibrating step function of 0.5 μV for A-C and of 1.25
μV for D and E.

by a negative power function calculated as:

$$y = 32.44 \ X^{-0.221} \ (r^2 = 0.962)$$

This procedure largely eliminates body size as a factor and depicts what is expected in an ideal population that would not grow and would remain at a constant body size of one meter (Desmedt et al., 1976). Then the onset latency of N22 would be 46 msec at birth (for a newborn of one meter body size) and 11 msec in the standard adult (also of one meter body size). The graph is helpful for focusing on true maturational features of the somatosensory pathway, once the effect of distance traveled by the afferent impulses is excluded. Thus it takes about eight years for a child to acquire adult conduction velocities (CV) along the entire somatosensory pathway. These data emphasize the remarkably slow maturation of somatosensory afferent conduction in man (Desmedt et al., 1976).

The above data dissociate pathway length and axonal maturation as factors determining the onset latency of SEP from birth to adulthood. A further study can provide more detail by recording the sensory nerve action potentials (cf. Dawson, 1956; Gilliatt, 1973). The maximum sensory CV estimated from the nerve potentials elicited by finger stimulation is much slower in newborns than in adults (Gamstorp and Shelburne, 1965; Desmedt et al., 1973) in agreement with the differences found for sensory axon diameters (Guthrecht and Dyck, 1970). In normal full-term newborns the sensory CV varies between 21 and 34 m/s and it rapidly increases to the adult range of 60 to 75 m/s in the 12-18 months after birth (Desmedt et al., 1973). This rather fast maturation rate of the peripheral sensory axons cannot account for the much slower changes in corticipetal conduction depicted in the lower graph of Fig. 4.

The problem can be clarified by plotting the progress of the peripheral sensory nerve volley and by extrapolating the calculated peripheral sensory CV to the segment between Erb's point and the dorsal column nuclei at the first cervical level (Fig. 5). The sensory nerve and Erb's point recordings provide consistent CV values of 67, 52 and 21 m/s in the subjects illustrated. The latency extrapolated for the DC nuclei, namely 15, 8 and 9 msec, is a little longer than the onset latency of the neck potential to finger stimulation. As previously suggested (Desmedt, 1971), it is then possible to divide the time interval to the onset of cortical SEP (corrected for three synaptic delays) by the measured distance from the base of the skull to the postcentral area in order to obtain an estimate of the "central" somatosensory CV; this gives 56, 21 and 7.5 m/s, respectively, for the adult, infant and newborn subjects in Fig. 5. Detailed results not reported here indicate that the maturation rate of the central somatosensory axons is, indeed, the major factor for the slow changes of onset latency of SEP as a function of age after

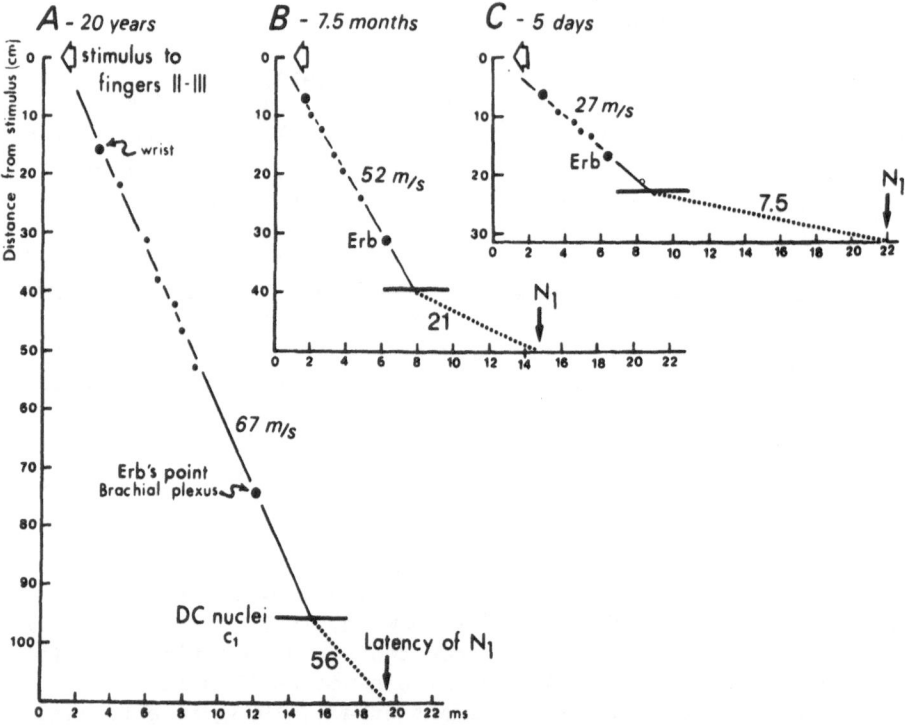

Fig. 5. Peripheral and central afferent conduction of a sensory
volley elicited by stimulation of fingers II and III in an adult of
twenty years (A), an infant of 7.5 months (B) and a newborn of five
days (C). Abscissa, latency in msec of the earliest component recorded at peripheral nerve potential of cortical SEP. Ordinate,
distance in cm traveled by the afferent volley from the fingers.
The same scale is used for each subject to emphasize the different
body sizes. The thicker dots correspond to the latency at the wrist
or at Erb's point (supraclavicular fossa : brachial plexus). The
peripheral afferent CV is extrapolated to the level of dorsal column
nuclei. The dotted line corresponds to conduction from the DC nuclei
to the postcentral cortex. The values proposed for the "central"
conduction, namely 56, 21 and 7.5 m/s have been corrected for three
delays. (From Desmedt et al., 1973.)

birth. This factor had not been disclosed until these evoked potential studies which raise important issues about the kinetics of
maturation of the various pathways of the human brain (Desmedt et
al., 1976). The method is relevant for clinical studies to identify
peripheral versus central disorders.

## COGNITION RELATED SEP COMPONENTS

It is known that the subject's attention to task stimuli influences the waveform of the corresponding evoked potentials.  This
parameter should never be ignored even when no specific task is
given to the subject (as in standard clinical tests) because un-
controlled attention shifts introduce inconsistencies (cf. Donchin
et al., 1977).  The best known cognition related component is the
P300, a positive wave of 250-500 msec peak latency elicited by task
relevant signals which resolve the subject's uncertainty (Sutton
et al., 1965; Desmedt et al., 1965; Vaughan and Ritter, 1970; Hillyard and Picton, 1978).  The P300 can be elicited in purely somatosensory (thus intramodality) paradigms.  For example, random sequences of near-threshold electrical stimuli are delivered to two
fingers of each hand, and the subject is asked to pay attention and
count the stimuli to one designated finger (target signals) in each
run (Desmedt et al., 1977; Desmedt and Robertson, 1977a,b).

Fig. 6 shows positive components of about 400 msec peak latency
in this case (this named P400) elicited by the target signals, no
matter which of the four fingers is designated in any run (A1).  The
P400 does not appear in the SEPs to identical stimuli when these are
not targets in the task and, therefore, remain largely ignored by
the subject (B1).

When the random sequence of four finger stimuli is carried out
at a faster pace (150/min instead of 40/min mean random rate), the
identification by the subject of the target signals becomes quite
difficult, and a new component occurs in the SEP.  A negative wave
with peak latency of 150 msec appears to target signals and also
in the SEP to nontarget signals delivered to the adjacent finger of
the same (attended) hand (Fig. 7).  This N150 reflects a special
cerebral processing that is required to distinguish the target and
nontarget signals arriving from two very close skin areas.  That the
differentiation is efficient is, indeed, indicated by the score of
the subject after each run; it is also interesting that a P400 component only appears in the SEP to target signals which suggests that
the P400 may index completion of somatosensory target identification (Desmedt and Robertson, 1977a,b).

The next problem, whether primary EP components are influenced
by the cognitive tasks, can be submitted to a critical test with
the SEP in which the early cortical components of the postcentral
projection are detected (this is not so readily achieved in auditory
or visual modalities).  Even when large enhancements of N150 or P400
occurred, the earlier N22 and P45 SEP components were not changed
in the somatosensory paradigms at various rates and cognition-related changes started only after 55 msec (Desmedt and Robertson,
1977a,b).  Thus, centrifugal gating at afferent relays (cf. Towe,

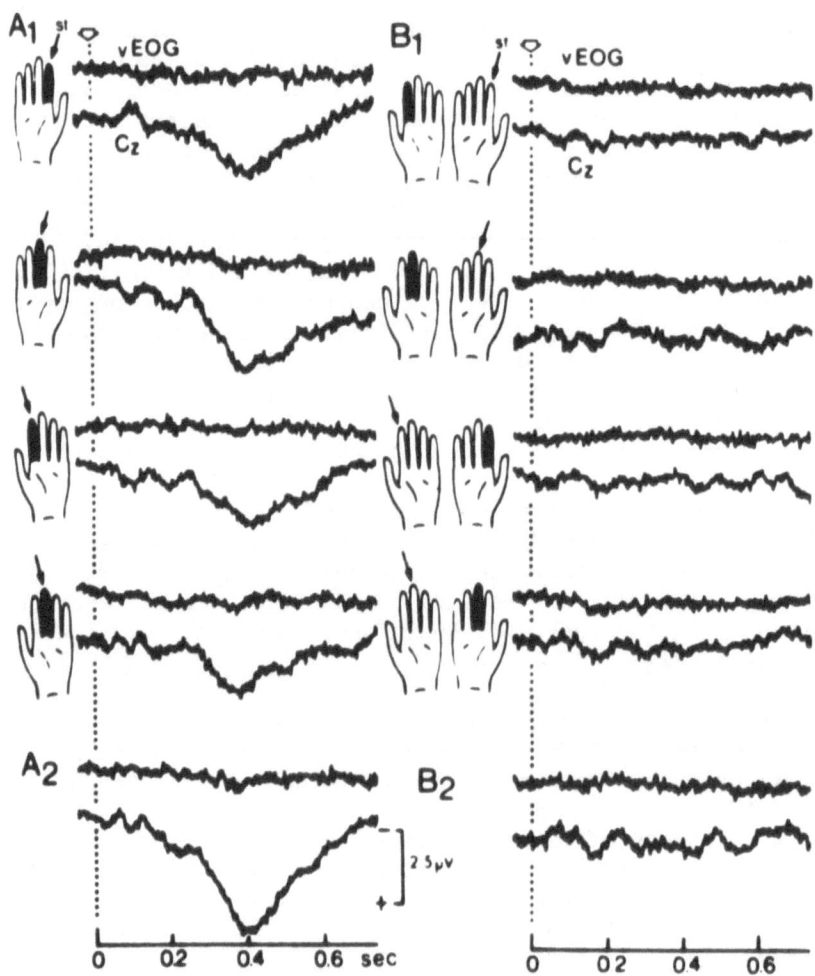

Fig. 6. The P400 component in intramodality selective attention.
Random sequence of electrical stimuli 1 mA above subjective threshold delivered to four fingers. The hand figurines at the left of
each pair of traces indicates in black the finger to which the subject is requested to pay attention in the corresponding run. The
small arrows point to the finger stimulus that elicits the illustrated SEP. Active electrode at the vertex (Cz) with earlobe reference (lower trace of each pair). The upper trace is the vertical
electro-oculogram (EOG) serving as check for lack of eye movement
artifacts. A1, SEPs to target shocks shown for each of the four
fingers (averages of seventy-five samples). A2, sum of these four
averages (N=300). B1, SEPs to nontarget shocks delivered to the
finger symmetrical to that attended in the opposite hand (N=75).
B2, sum of the four averages for nontarget SEPs. The P400 appears
only for the target signals. (From Desmedt et al., 1977).

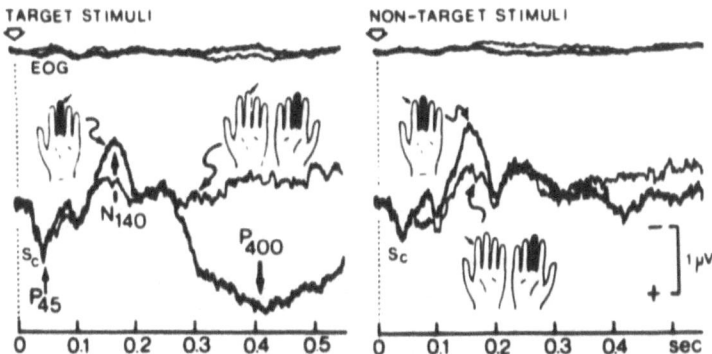

Fig. 7. The N150 and P400 components in intramodality selective attention task carried out at forced pace. Random sequence of electrical stimuli to four fingers. Two average SEP traces are superimposed for comparison, and they both are elicited by identical stimuli to the third (left side) or to the second (right side) finger of the left hand (small arrows). On the left, the third finger is designated as target for the task (thicker trace and black finger in figurines) and large N150 and P400 occur while the earlier P45 is not affected; the control thinner trace corresponds to runs in which the third finger of the opposite hand is the target. Notice that P45 is identical in both traces although N150 and P400 fail to appear in the thinner trace. Right side, nontarget stimuli to the second adjacent finger of the left hand in the same runs; there is virtually no P400, but a large N150 when the third finger of the left hand is a target in the task. The upper traces are EOG controls which exclude eye movement or muscle artifacts. (From Desmedt and Robertson, 1977.)

1973; Desmedt, 1975) is not a mechanism for these effects. However, the data leave it open whether delayed involvement of the powerful thalamocortical gating circuit of Skinner and Yingling (1977) might not participate in the switching on and off of the cognition-related SEP components. The above data must be taken into account when assessing SEP changes in neurological patients.

## SEP USES IN PERIPHERAL NEUROLOGICAL DISORDERS

The conventional recording of sensory nerve potentials (Gilliatt, 1973) is quite sensitive to nerve pathology, but it fails when the nerve potentials are markedly desynchronized. The cerebral SEP then provides a useful alternative because the cortex can achieve a time integration of the decimated and desynchronized afferent impulses (Desmedt et al., 1977; Desmedt, 1971).

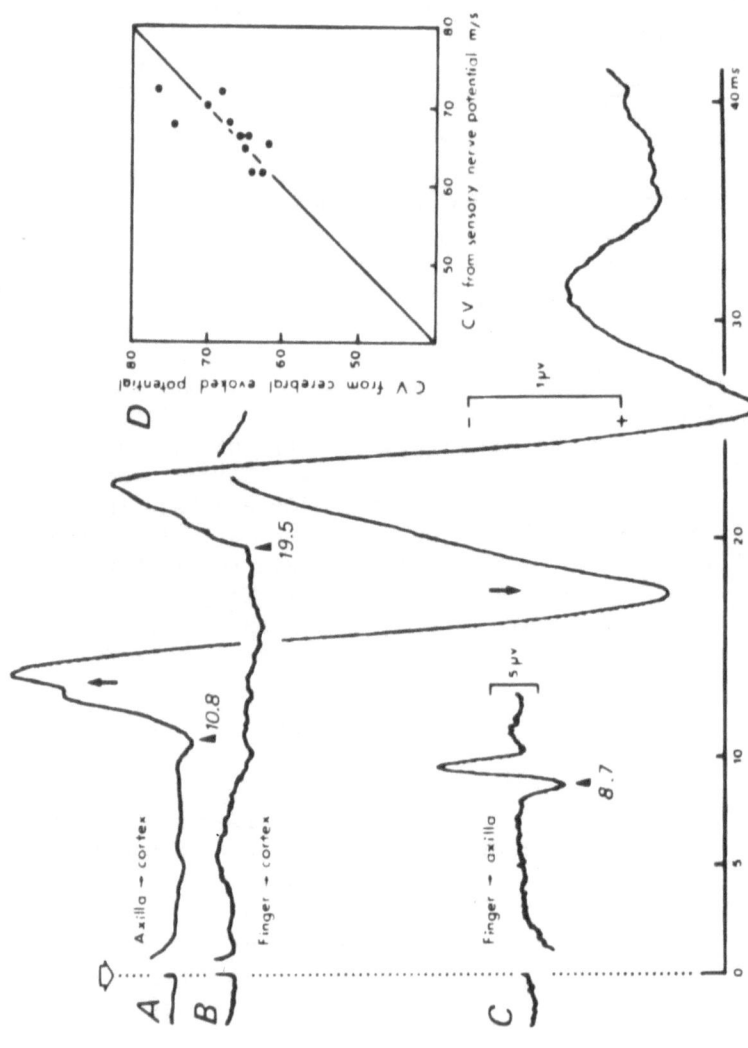

Fig. 8. Evaluation of the maximum afferent CV from the latency difference of SEP (ordinate in D) compared to the method based on recording sensory nerve potentials (abscissa in D) for eleven young normal adults. SEPs elicited by stimulation of the median nerve at the axilla (A) or of fingers II and III (B). Large N22 and P28 components are seen. The nerve potential (C) recorded from the median nerve at the axilla is elicited by the same finger stimulation. (From Desmedt and Noel, 1973).

Because the onset latency of the early cortical SEP component can be accurately estimated, latency differences are provided by SEPs to stimulation of fingers or nerves at different levels (Fig. 8). In normals the sensory CV calculated from SEP agrees well with that provided by direct sensory nerve potentials (Desmedt, 1971; Desmedt and Noel, 1973). The method used in lower limbs opens up useful diagnostic procedures since most common neuropathies involve predominantly the sensory fibers of the legs, and sensory nerve potentials are more difficult to record from these nerves (cf. Gilliatt, 1973; Shiozawa and Mavor, 1969; Desmedt and Noel, 1975). Fig. 9 shows the delays of the early cortical (positive) SEP to stimulation of the sural nerve at three levels which allows a sensory CV of about 50 m/s to be calculated. The diagram (Fig. 9D) depicts the effect of body size in twelve normal young adults for stimulation of the sural nerve at the lateral malleolus (Desmedt and Noel, 1975).

Clinical SEP data are documented elsewhere (Desmedt et al., 1966; Desmedt, 1971; Desmedt and Noel, 1973, 1975) and only one example is shown to illustrate the sensory CV evaluation from SEP in a patient with a section and suture of the median nerve at the wrist (Fig. 10). Five months after suture the SEP to distal finger III stimulation was very small, 0.3 µV, and much delayed, 57 msec (Fig. 10B). The CV of the regenerating fibers was calculated as 5.4 m/s which agrees with animal data for newly regenerating axons. No nerve potentials could be recorded in this case.

SEPs provide unique diagnostic evidence in lesions involving the plexus or spinal roots, such as traction injuries or root compressions. For example, in a twenty-six year old patient with Stage III Hodgkin's disease, the delayed SEPs to femoral stimulation documented a bilateral invasion of the spinal roots by pathological tissue at the lumbar level (Desmedt and Noel, 1975).


SEP USES IN CENTRAL NEUROLOGICAL DISORDERS

There is current interest in searching for subclinical lesions of multiple sclerosis by averaging visual or auditory EPs (cf. Desmedt, 1977a,c) as well as SEPs (Desmedt and Noel, 1973; Matthews et al., 1974). These tests, in fact, can complement each other by exploring different brain areas, thereby increasing the potential yield of diagnostic findings at early stages of the disease. Peripheral CV is normal in multiple sclerosis (Desmedt and Noel, 1973), but the onset latency of SEP is frequently increased, especially for stimulation of limbs with a clinical sensory deficit (Fig. 11D). However, "silent lesions" with normal sensation and position sense in the stimulated area can be accompanied by significant increase of SEP latency (Fig. 11A,C).

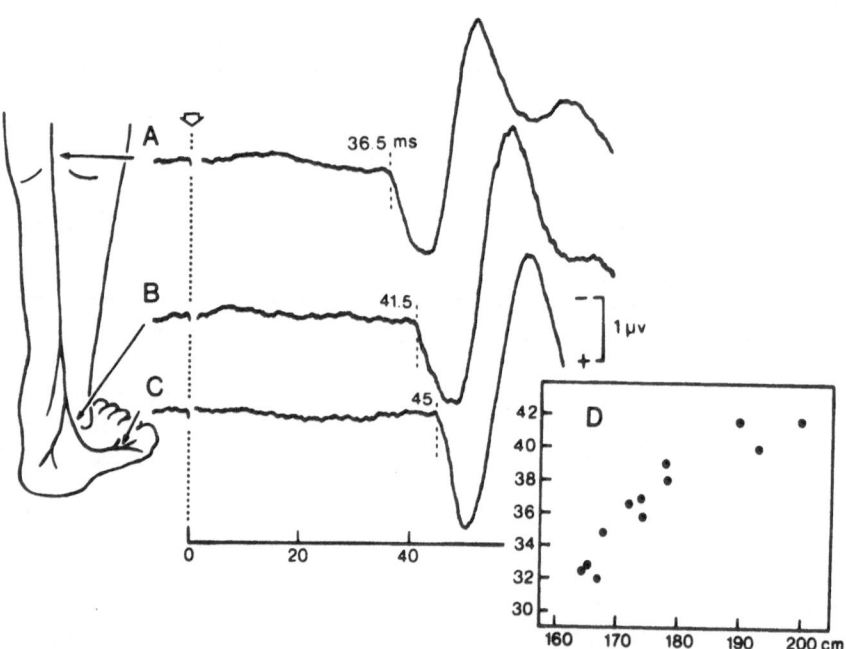

Fig. 9.  Evaluation of maximum sensory CV in the sural nerve of
normal young adults.  SEPs recorded from the midline, 2 cm below Cz.
Midfrontal reference.  The SEPs start with a positive component (see
above).  The effect of body size is shown in D.  (From Desmedt and
Noel, 1975).

        Another major SEP application is in vascular or tumor lesions
of the brain stem.  The afferent volley eliciting the cortical SEP
travels in the dorsal column and median lemniscus pathway (Halliday,
1967; Desmedt, 1971).  No changes of SEP are recorded in the Wallen-
berg syndrome in which the lateral vascular lesion spares the median
lemniscus but involves the spinothalamic pathway (Halliday, 1967;
Noel and Desment, 1975).  In patients with a thalamic syndrome of
Dejerine, the SEP has a reduced voltage and increased latency on the
affected side (Tsumoto et al., 1973; Noel and Desmedt, 1975).  In
patients with a locked-in syndrome who present brain stem quadri-
plegia (infarction of basis ponti) and alert wakefulness, but who
cannot communicate except to a limited extent by eye movements, the
SEP is invaluable in documenting the extent of the lesion and the
actual sensory loss.  The median lemniscus in the ventral pontine
tegmentum is in a critical position above the pontine infarct, and
the SEP anomalies can document the dorsalward extension of the lesion

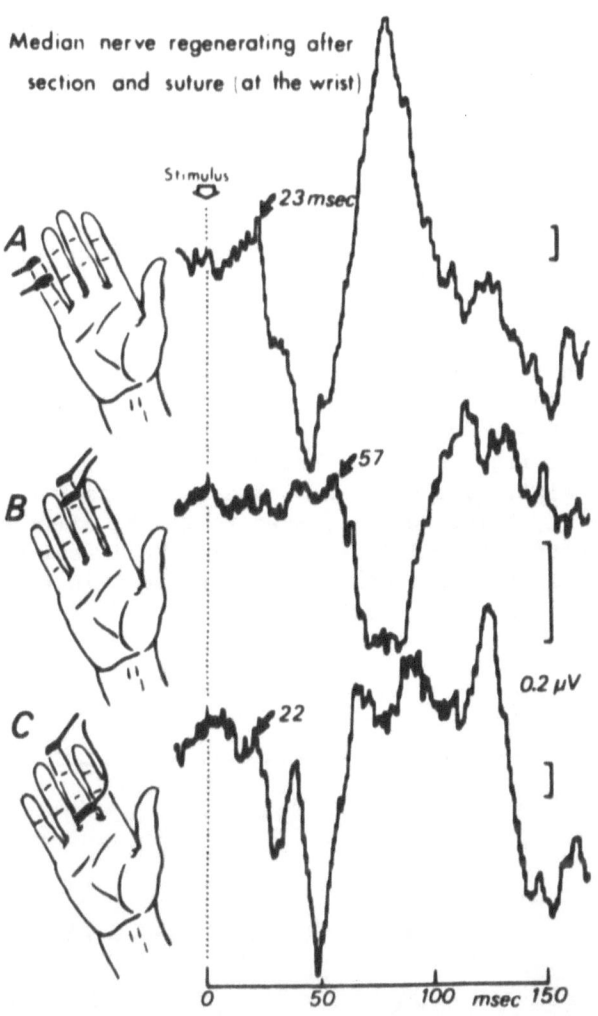

Median nerve regenerating after
section and suture (at the wrist)

Stimulus

23 msec

57

22

0.2 µV

0        50        100  msec 150

Fig. 10.  Patient of thirty-seven years with a complete suture of
the right median nerve at the wrist.  Five months later no sensory
nerve potentials could be recorded above the lesions site from the
median nerve upon stimulation of the tip of the third finger.  The
patient described a faint subjective sensation when the third finger
was tapped (Tinel sign).  SEP recording from contralateral parietal
scalp showed a much delayed and reduced potential (B).  Notice the
increased amplification for this trace.  Controls are provided for
the normal fifth finger (A) and for proximal third finger in the
radial territory (C).  (From Desmedt, 1971.)

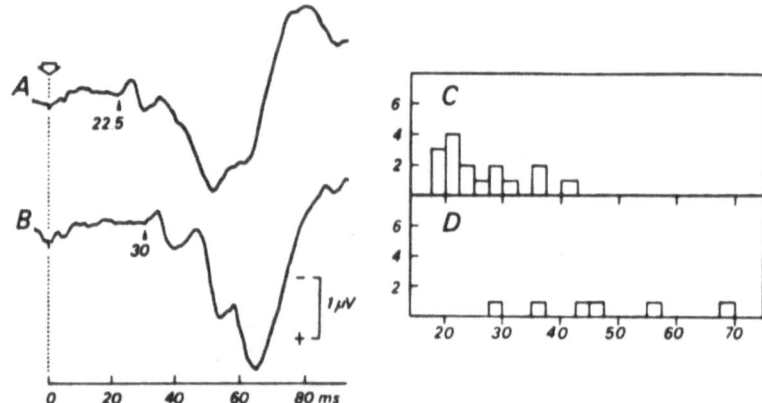

Fig. 11.  SEP in multiple sclerosis.  A, B female patient of thirty-
four years with unilateral sensory deficit for finger position on
the left side.  SEP to stimulation of fingers II and III on the
clinically silent right side (A) has a significantly increased latency for body size.  The delay is larger for stimulation on the
left side (B).  C, D latencies of SEPs to finger stimulation in
seventeen patients with multiple sclerosis.  Clinical sensory deficits are absent in the patients in C and present in the patients in
D.  (From Desmedt and Noel, 1973.)

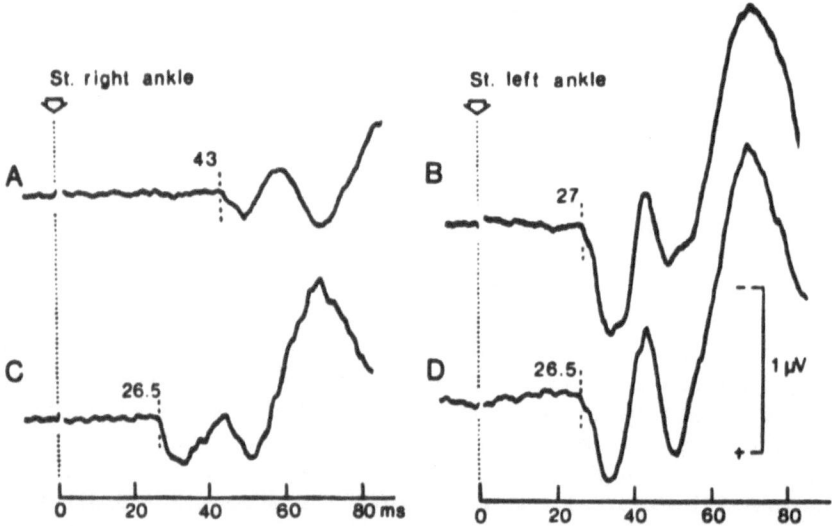

Fig. 12.  SEPs to stimulation of the right (A,C) or left (B,D) posterior tibial nerve at the ankle in a female patient of twenty-five
years with a locked-in syndrome studied either fourteen days (A,B)
or twenty-two months (C,D) after the pontine infarct.  The onset
latencies of the early positive component are indicated.  (From Noel
and Desmedt, 1975.)

(Noel and Desmedt, 1975). For example, Fig. 12 shows the marked
delay of the early positive SEP component to stimulation of the right
(A), but not the left (B), posterior tibial nerve in such a patient.
Twenty-two months later the SEP was still reduced but had acquired a
fairly normal latency (Fig. 12C) while the control SEP for left
stimulation (D) had not changed. These and other data about SEPs to
upper or lower limb stimulation on both sides allow a fairly consistent mapping of the brain stem lesion.

## SUMMARY

Somatosensory evoked potentials (SEPs) recorded from the intact
scalp offer unusual possibilities for probing brain processes since
both the early (primary) and late components can be identified in
average records. The early cortical SEP component presents a latency
that reflects primarily the conduction time from the peripheral
stimulation site up to the parietal projection cortex. For example,
the area of skin innervation which is stimulated influences both
the waveform and scalp topography of the SEP. Between birth and
adulthood the SEP feature presents dramatic changes, and the onset
latency varies systematically in relation to both body growth and
to maturation of the peripheral and central nerve fibers of the
somatosensory pathway. SEPs elicited by stimulation of several
fingers in random order at different mean rates have recently disclosed clear-cut changes during selective attention involving different designated fingers in different runs of the experiment. In
such intramodality cognitive tasks, large P400 components appear
only in the SEPs elicited by target signals. Earlier N150 SEP components are elicited at fast mean rates of the same task, and they
can be seen both in the SEP to target and nontarget (adjacent finger)
signals. Clinical uses of SEPs elicited by stimulation of appropriate areas in upper or lower limbs are documented for both peripheral nerve disorders and for the diagnosis of spinal, brain stem
or cerebral lesions that involve the somatosensory pathway.

## ACKNOWLEDGEMENTS

The work reported in this chapter was supported by the Fonds
de la Recherche Scientifique Medicale and the Fonds National de la
Recherche Scientifique.

## REFERENCES

Dawson, G.D. The relative excitability and conduction velocity of
    sensory and motor nerve fibres in man. J. Physiol., 1956, 131,
    436-451.

Debecker, J. and Desmedt, J.E.  Les potentiels evoques cerebraux et
    les potentiels de nerf sensible chez l'homme.  Acta Neurol.
    Belg., 1964, 64, 1212-1248.

Desmedt, J.E.  Somatosensory cerebral evoked potentials in man.  In
    A. Remond (Ed.), Handbook of Electroencephalography and Clini-
    cal Neurophysiology, Vol. 9, Amsterdam: Elsevier, 1971.

Desmedt, J.E.  Physiological studies of the efferent recurrent audi-
    tory system.  In W.D. Keidel and W.D. Neff (Eds.), Handbook of
    Sensory Physiology, Vol. 5, Berlin: Springer, 1975.

Desmedt, J.E. (Ed.)  Visual Evoked Potentials in Man:  New Develop-
    ments.  Oxford: Oxford University Press, 1977a.

Desmedt, J.E. (Ed.)  Attention, Voluntary Contraction and Event
    Related Cerebral Potentials, Prog. Clin. Neurophysiol., Vol 1,
    Basel: Karger, 1977b.

Desmedt, J.E.(Ed.)  Auditory Evoked Potentials in Man.  Psychophar-
    macology Correlates of Evoked Potentials.  Progr. Clin. Neuro-
    physiol., Vol 2, Basel: Karger, 1977c.

Desmedt, J.E.  Some observations on the methodology of cerebral
    evoked potentials in man.  In J.E. Desmedt (Ed.), Attention,
    Voluntary Contraction and Event Related Cerebral Potentials,
    Progr. Clin. Neurophysiol., Vol 1, Basel: Karger, 1977d.

Desmedt, J.E.  Active touch exploration of extrapersonal space eli-
    cits specific electrogenesis in the right cerebral hemisphere
    of intact right-handed man.  Proc. Nation. Acad. Sci., Washing-
    ton D.C., 74, 1977e.

Desmedt, J.E. and Brunko, E.  Different hemispheric topography of
    somatosensory evoked potential (SEP) to stimulation of fingers
    or of skin of the arm in man.  In J.E. Desmedt (Ed.), Clinical
    Uses of Cerebral, Brain Stem and Spinal Somatosensory Evoked
    Potentials, Progr. Clin. Neurophysiol., Vol. 7, Basel: Karger,
    1978.

Desmedt, J.E., Brunko, E. and Debecker, J.  Maturation of the somato-
    sensory evoked potentials in normal infants and children, with
    particular reference to the early N1 component.  Electroenceph.
    Clin. Neurophysiol., 1976, 40, 43-58.

Desmedt, J.E., Brunko, J., Debecker, J. and Carmeliet, J.  The sys-
    tem bandpass required to avoid distortion of early components
    when averaging somatosensory evoked potentials.  Electroenceph.
    Clin. Neurophysiol., 1974, 37, 407-410.

Desmedt, J.E. and Cheron, G.  Aging, cerebral evoked potentials and the somatosensory pathway.  Neurol., 1978, 28, 347.

Desmedt, J.E. and Debecker, J.  The somatosensory cerebral evoked potentials of the sleeping newborn.  In C.D. Clemente, D.P. Purpura and F.E. Mayer (Eds.), Sleep and the Maturing Nervous System, New York: Academic Press, 1972.

Desmedt, J.E., Debecker, J. and Manil, J.  Mise en evidence d'un signe electrique cerebral associe a la detection par le sujet, d'un stimulus sensoriel tactile.  Bull. Acad. Roy. Med. Belg., 1965, 5, 887-936.

Desmedt, J.E., Franken, L., Borenstein, S., Debecker, J., Lambert, C. and Manil, J.  Le diagnostic des ralentissements de la conduction afferente dans les affections des nerfs peripheriques. Interet de l'extraction du potentiel evoque cerebral.  Rev. Neurol., 1966, 115, 255-262.

Desmedt, J.E. and Manil, J.  Somatosensory evoked potentials of the normal human neonate in REM sleep, in slow wave sleep and in waking., Electroenceph. Clin. Neurophysiol., 1970, 29, 113-126.

Desmedt, J.E. and Noel, P.  Average cerebral evoked potentials in the evaluation of lesions of the sensory nerves and of the central somatosensory pathway.  In J.E. Desmedt (Ed.), New Developments in EMG and Clinical Neurophysiology, Basel: Karger, 1973.

Desmedt, J.E. and Noel, P.  Cerebral evoked potentials.  In P.J. Dyck, P.K. Thomas and E.H. Lambert (Eds.), Peripheral Neuropathy, Vol. 1, Philadelphia: Saunders, 1975.

Desmedt, J.E., Noel, P., Debecker, J. and Nameche, J.  Maturation of afferent conduction velocity as studied by sensory nerve potentials and by cerebral evoked potentials.  In J.E. Desmedt (Ed.), New Develoments in EMG and Clinical Neurophysiology, Basel: Karger,  1973.

Desmedt, J.E. and Robertson, D.  Differential enhancement of early and late components of the cerebral somatosensory evoked potentials during fast sequential cognitive tasks in man.  J. Physiol. Lond., 1977a, 271, 761-782.

Desmedt, J.E. and Robertson, D.  Search for right hemisphere asymmetries in event related potentials to somatosensory cueing signals.  In J.E. Desmedt (Ed.), Language and Hemispheric Specialization in Man: Cerebral Event Related Potentials, Progr. Clin. Neurophysiol., Vol. 3, Basel: Karger, 1977b.

Desmedt, J.E., Robertson, D., Brunko, E. and Debecker, J.   Somato-
    sensory decision tasks in man:  Early and late components of
    the cerebral potentials evoked by stimulation of different
    fingers in random sequences.  Electroenceph. Clin. Neuro-
    physiol., 1977, 43, 404-415.

Donchin, E., Callaway, E., Cooper, R., Desmedt, J.E., Goff, W.R.,
    Hillyard, S.A. and Sutton, S.   Publications criteria for
    studies of evoked potentials (EP) in man.   Report of a commit-
    tee.   In J.E. Desmedt (Ed.), Attention, Voluntary Contraction
    and Event Related Cerebral Potentials., Progr. Clin. Neuro-
    physiol., Vol. 1, Basel: Karger, 1977.

Gamstorp, I. and Shelburne, S.A.   Peripheral sensory conduction in
    ulnar and median nerves of normal infants, children and adoles-
    cents.   Acta. Paediat. Scand., 1965, 54, 309-313.

Giblin, D.R.   Somatosensory evoked potentials in healthy subjects
    and in patients with lesions of the nervous system.   Ann. N.Y.
    Acad. Sci., 1964, 112, 93-142.

Gilliatt, R.W.   Recent advances in the pathophysiology of nerve
    conduction.   In J.E. Desmedt (Ed.), New Developments in EMG
    and Clinical Neurophysiology, Basel: Karger, 1973.

Gutrecht, J.A. and Dyck, P.J.   Quantitative teased fiber and his-
    tologic studies of human sural nerve during postnatal develop-
    ment.   J. Comp. Neurol., 1970, 138, 117-130.

Halliday, A.M.   Changes in the form of cerebral evoked responses in
    man associated with various lesions of the nervous system.
    Electroenceph. Clin. Neurophysiol., 1967, Suppl. 25, 178-192.

Hillyard, S.A. and Picton, T.W.   Event related brain potentials and
    selective information processing in man.   In J.E. Desmedt (Ed.)
    Cognitive Components in Cerebral Event Related Potentials and
    Selective Attention, Progr. Clin. Neurophysiol., Vol. 6, Basel:
    Karger, 1978.

Matthews, W.B., Beauchamp, M. and Small, D.G.   Cervical somatosen-
    sory evoked responses in man.   Nature, 1974, 230-232.

Noel, P. and Desmedt, J.E.   Somatosensory cerebral evoked potentials
    after vascular lesions of the brain stem and diencephalon.
    Brain, 1975, 98, 113-128.

Purpura, D.P., Shofer, R.J., Housepian, E.M. and Noback, C.R.
    Comparative ontogenesis of structure-function relations in
    cerebral and cerebellar cortex.   In D.P. Purpura and J.P.

Schade (Eds.), Growth and Maturation of the Brain, Progr.
Brain Res., Amsterdam: Elsevier, 1964.

Schiozawa, R. and Mavor, H.  In vivo human sural nerve action
potentials.  J Appl. Physiol., 1969, 26, 623-629.

Skinner, J.E. and Yingling, C.D.  Central gating mechanisms that
regulate event related potentials and behavior.  A neural
model for attention.  In J.E. Desmedt (Ed.), Attention, Voluntary Contraction and Event Related Cerebral Potentials,
Progr. Clin. Neurophysiol., Vol. 1, Basel: Karger, 1977.

Sutton, S., Braren, M., Zubin, J. and John, E.R.  Evoked potential
correlates of stimulus uncertainty.  Science, 1965, 150, 1187-
1188.

Towe, A.L.  Somatosensory cortex:  Descending influences on ascending systems.  In A. Iggo (Ed.), Somatosensory Stem.  Handbook
of Sensory Physiology, Vol. 2, Berlin: Springer, 1973.

Tsumoto, T., Hirose, N., Nonaka, S. and Takahashi, M.  Cerebrovas-
cular disease:  Changes in somatosensory evoked potentials
associated with unilateral lesions.  Electroenceph. Clin.
Neurophysiol., 1973, 35, 463-473.

Vaughan, H.G. and Ritter, W.  The sources of auditory evoked responses recorded from the human scalp.  Electroenceph. Clin.
Neurophysiol., 1970, 28, 360-367.

EVENT RELATED POTENTIAL INVESTIGATIONS IN CHILDREN AT HIGH RISK

FOR SCHIZOPHRENIA

David Friedman, Herbert G. Vaughan, Jr. and

L. Erlenmeyer-Kimling

New York State Psychiatric Institute, New York City

## INTRODUCTION

The search for the antecedents of schizophrenia has recently been advanced by the introduction of research in which individuals who are known to be at high statistical risk for schizophrenia are studied prospectively before the onset of disturbances in functioning (Pearson and Kley, 1957; Mednick and McNeill, 1968; Garmezy and Streitman, 1974; Erlenmeyer-Kimling, 1975). Children of schizophrenic parents are chosen as the high risk subjects; if one parent is schizophrenic, some ten to fifteen percent of the children are expected to develop the psychosis in adolescence or adulthood, and if both parents are schizophrenic, the risk increases 36-40 percent (Zerbin-Rüdin, 1967; Erlenmeyer-Kimling, 1968; 1978). The high risk children are compared with children of normal parents for whom the risk estimate is only about one percent, on variables of interest to the investigating team, and, because the comparison is longitudinal, the development of the disorder can be followed. Thus, this research approach eliminates many of the biases prevalent when information is obtained from retrospective reports, although other types of problems may be inherent in the high risk design.

These relatively low risk estimates make it unlikely that large mean differences in any one variable will distinguish the groups. Thus, while group differences, if they occur, are important to examine, the investigator must search for deviant subjects whose scores could be heavily contributing to the differentiation of the groups. Even in the absence of group differences, this strategy should be followed if meaningful interpretation is desired.

105

The majority of hypotheses of how high risk children might perform and the tasks on which they are measured have come, naturally, from research with adult schizophrenics. However, because of the fact that adult schizophrenics are studied after the onset of the illness, it is often not clear whether what one finds is a premorbid characteristic or a consequence of the psychosis. The child at risk offers the researcher a way out of this dilemma, since it is possible to distinguish psychobiologic characteristics that are present before the onset of overt disturbances in functioning from those that appear later.


Event Related Potential (ERP) Studies in High Risk Samples

While autonomic indices have been used with high risk children for the past several years (Fein et al., 1975; Mednick and Schulsinger, 1973; Salzman and Klein, 1978; Venables, 1977), ERP techniques have only recently been utilized. If predisposition to schizophrenia is manifest in disorders of brain function, as many investigators believe, then scalp recorded ERP might be a useful tool in discriminating potential schizophrenics from both their normal control and nonvulnerable high risk counterparts.

Saletu et al. (1975) reported finding no amplitude differences, but did find shorter latency peaks to repetitive auditory stimuli in their high risk group. They concluded that their data supported the hypothesis, consistent with the GSR findings of Mednick and Schulsinger (1973), that the potential schizophrenic, like his adult counterpart, is characterized by a state of hyperarousal. However, their statistical methodology and ERP measurement techniques detract from the forcefulness of this conclusion. We (Friedman et al., 1978b) studied the auditory evoked potentials (AEP) elicited by repetitive tones in twenty high risk and twenty normal control children. Analyses of between groups differences yielded no significant findings. We were, however, able to identify subgroups of both the high risk and normal control samples that differed significantly from each other. In contrast to the findings of Saletu et al. (1975), the high risk subgroup had longer latency P190 and P400 components than the normal control subgroup. No significant amplitude differences were found, although there was a trend for the high risk outliers to have larger amplitude ERP.

In the above studies, there was no task imposed upon the subject, and thus latency shifts could be due to disturbances in either sensory or cognitive information processing. Herman et al. (1977) reported finding no group performance differences but longer latency and larger amplitude N100-P200 responses in their high risk

sample in response to signal and nonsignal stimuli in a version
of the continuous performance test.  They concluded that this reflected a maturational lag in visual information processing.
Herman et al. (1977) recorded between Cz and Oz which could have
reduced their chances of seeing large amplitude late positive
components, as well as obscured any between group topographic
differences.

Potentials recorded from children in a well defined psychological task requiring sustained attention, in which components
can be related to stages of information processing and topographic
data are available to aid in the interpretation of component behavior, should prove more fruitful in the study of high risk children, especially in view of the frequently reported cognitive
dysfunctions in adult schizophrenics.  The data to be reported here
are from a preliminary analysis of the ERP of high risk (HR) and
normal control (NC) children who are part of a longitudinal high
risk study (Erlenmeyer-Kimling, 1970).  These children are measured
on a variety of psychological, biological, psychophysiological and
sociological variables.  The psychophysiologic battery consists of
the measurement of autonomic functioning during two threshold procedures, ERP recording during a combination "odd-ball" and missing
stimulus paradigm, and during two versions of the continuous performance test (CPT).  Previous versions of the CPT have been shown
to differentiate adult schizophrenics from other psychiatric samples,
as well as HR from NC children (Kornetsky and Orzack, 1978; Rutchmann et al., 1977; Grunebaum et al., 1974).  It is the data from
the CPT tasks that are the subject of this paper.

METHODS

Subject Selection

The "at risk" children were obtained through their parents in
a screening of consecutive admissions at six psychiatric hospitals
in the greater New York area between June, 1971 and December, 1972.
In order to be included in the study, the patients had to be white,
English speaking, married at the time of admission and still
living with the spouse, and have two or more children between the
ages of seven and twelve.  The hospital records of patients meeting
these criteria were independently evaluated for schizophrenia by
two senior psychiatrists and a resident at New York State Psychiatric Institute without knowledge of the hospital diagnoses or
the medications prescribed.  No family was taken for study without
a unanimous diagnosis of schizophrenia in the patient.

NC children were obtained through the cooperation of the Nassau and Rockland County School systems. Parental criteria for inclusion were the same as those for the HR sample, with the exception that any child who had a parent with a history of psychiatric hospitalization was eliminated from the study.


## Laboratory Procedures

The first time they were seen, the children were given a large battery of psychologic, psychophysiologic, psychiatric and neurologic tests. The visual ERP procedure which is the subject of this report was not given until the third round of testing (1977-1978) some six to seven years later. This is a preliminary analysis performed on the data of roughly one-third of this cohort of subjects, some of whom are still being seen in our laboratory. In all aspects of the testing procedure, the experimenters were blind with respect to whether a child was HR or NC.


## CPT Tasks and EEG Recording Procedures

The tasks used were modifications of the CPT originally described by Orzack and Kornetsky (1966). Our current versions of these tasks have been fully described elsewhere (Friedman et al., 1978c), and only a brief description will be given here. In Task A, the subject had to respond to the number 08, which occurred fifteen times per block, and withhold his response to any other number (45 per block); in Task B, the subject had to respond to the repetition of any immediately preceding number, which occurred sixteen times per block, and withhold his response to numbers that did not repeat (48 per block). The signal to nonsignal ratio was 1:4 in each task. Fifty msec duration stimuli were flashed at moderate intensity with an ISI of 1 sec. Task B imposed greater processing demands than Task A in that subjects had to sequentially store and compare successive non-signals as potential targets, whereas in Task A the target stimulus was pre-determined and each trial required a simple match or mismatch decision. Eight blocks of stimuli were delivered for each task, with tasks alternated two blocks at a time. The subject was instructed to respond as quickly as possible with a fingerlift which activated a reaction time (RT) key. RTs greater than 1200 msec were considered misses.

EEG was recorded from a midline montage at Fz, Cz, Pz and Oz, and vertical EOG was recorded from above the right eye with a reference electrode on the right earlobe. Data were recorded on a Beckman Dynograph Type RM recorder, amplified 20,000 times with a time constant of 1 sec and high frequency cutoff at 30 Hz, and were stored along with RT on digital tape. Data acquisition and stimulus presentation were controlled by a PDP 11/10 computer which digitized the EEG at 4 msec intervals for a period of 1000 msec (100 pre- and 900 post-stimulus). Averages of signal and non-signal stimuli were computed across blocks. There was a total of 120 signals and 360 nonsignals for Task A, and 128 signals and 384 nonsignals for Task B, but removal of extracerebral artifacts attenuated these numbers in most subjects.

The data of the first 60 HR and NC children seen for this round of testing were selected for preliminary analysis. These subjects were divided into age bands of 11-13, 14-15 and 16-18. Table I presents the characteristics of the two groups. As can be seen, age and sex are well balanced between the groups. #SM and #SF refer to the number of children of schizophrenic mothers and fathers respectively. #Both refers to the number of children whose parents were both diagnosed as schizophrenic and #Mixed refers to the number of children in which one parent was schizophrenic and the other was diagnosed as psychotic depressive.

TABLE I: CHARACTERISTICS OF THE HIGH RISK AND NORMAL CONTROL GROUPS

|       | Mean Age | #Males | #Females | #SM | #SF | #Both | #Mixed |
|-------|----------|--------|----------|-----|-----|-------|--------|
| 11-13 |          |        |          |     |     |       |        |
| HR    | 12.6     | 5      | 2        | 4   | 2   | 0     | 1      |
| NC    | 12.5     | 5      | 6        |     |     |       |        |
| 14-15 |          |        |          |     |     |       |        |
| HR    | 14.5     | 6      | 5        | 7   | 2   | 2     | 0      |
| NC    | 14.5     | 7      | 2        |     |     |       |        |
| 16-18 |          |        |          |     |     |       |        |
| HR    | 16.8     | 7      | 5        | 9   | 1   | 0     | 2      |
| NC    | 16.8     | 6      | 4        |     |     |       |        |
| TOTALS |         |        |          |     |     |       |        |
| HR    | 14.6     | 18     | 12       | 20  | 5   | 2     | 3      |
| NC    | 14.6     | 18     | 12       |     |     |       |        |

## ERP Measurements

Because of the complex nature of the waveforms elicited during
these tasks (Friedman et al., 1978c) and the need for objective,
quantitative ERP indices in evaluating abnormalities in ERP morphology and topography, principal components factor analysis (PCA),
factoring the covariance matrix, was employed.  This method allows
us to associate factors with specific ERP components that are affected by the experimental variables and affords objective confirmation of components we have visually identified in the grand
mean and individual data (see also Squires et al., 1977).  Since
the factors are extracted due to their association with experimental
variance (cf., Donchin and Heffley, 1978; Glaser and Ruchkin, 1976),
abnormalities in waveform morphology can be directly related to
the experimental variables.  We use the factor scores as the baseline to peak measures.

To determine if the group factor structures were the same,
this analysis was done separately for the HR and NC groups.  The
data base for each analysis was an 83 time point (at 12 msec per
point) by 480 waveform data matrix (30 subjects by two tasks by two
stimuli by four electrode sites).  Six factors were varimax rotated
using the BMDP4M computer program (Dixon, 1975).

## RESULTS AND DISCUSSION

Figure 1 presents the grand mean data averaged across the 30
subjects in each group by task and stimulus.  The waveforms from
both tasks consisted of a complex of positive waves which appear to
differ for the two tasks, and, to some extent, for the two groups.
The visual evoked potential (VEP), clearly visible at Oz, consisted
of a positive-negative-positive complex, consistent in latency and
amplitude across tasks and stimuli.  N150 appears to be more negative
to the Task B waveforms.  In order of increasing latency, the remaining positive peaks are: (a) P240, maximal at Cz, present to both
stimuli of both tasks.  (b) P350, maximal at Pz, clearly seen in the
nonsignal waveforms of each task.  (c) As RT increases, the signal
waveforms become increasingly differentiated, so that P350 can be
seen in the Task B signal, but is not discernible in the Task A
signal.  This peak appears to be larger to the nonsignals of Task B.
(d) P450, with a parietal focus, is seen in the ERP of both stimuli
in both tasks, with much larger amplitude to signals than nonsignals,
and of larger amplitude to the nonsignals of Task B than those of
Task A.  (e) P550 is seen most clearly in the Task B nonsignals, and
is not visible at all in the Task A nonsignals.

The vertical lines mark mean RT, which was significantly longer
in Task B than in Task A (p<.0001).  In general, the HR group shows

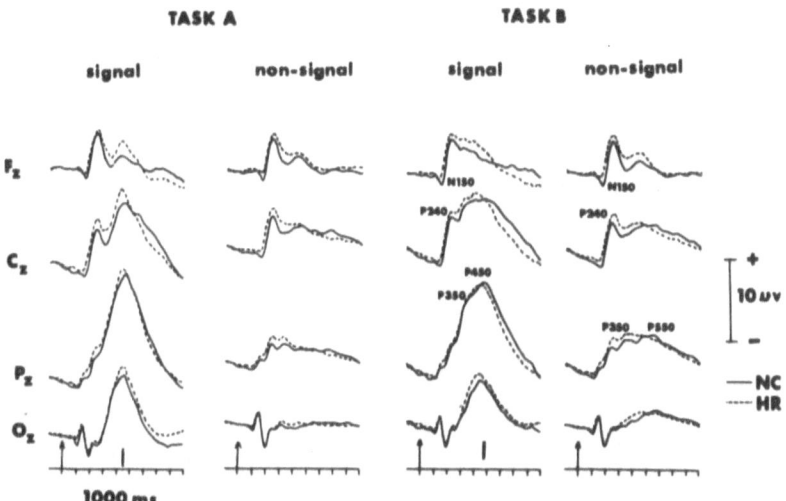

Figure 1.  Grand mean ERP recorded from 30 HR and 30 NC children in response to the stimuli from both tasks at the four electrode sites.

more frontal activity in the P240-P450 region, less initial negativity (N150) and a faster return to baseline following the late positive complex (LPC) than do the NC.  The HR group shows somewhat less very late positive activity, especially in response to the nonsignals of Task B.

## Principal Components Analysis

Figure 2 presents the loading functions after varimax rotation for both groups of subjects.  It is clear that the shapes of these functions are identical, with the main difference occurring in their latencies, which are approximately 50 msec longer to peak for the HR group for factors 3 through 6.  With the exception of Factor 2, each loading function is associated with a component seen in the grand mean: Factor 1 with P450, Factor 3 with P240, Factor 4 with P550, Factor 5 with P350 and Factor 6 with the increasing negativity preceding the stimulus and culminating frontally in N150. Factor 2 has large positive loadings at a point in time when P450 is decrementing, and appears to represent return to baseline following this late positive activity.

At the present time, we are beginning to explore the sources of latency variance which are evident in the factor loading functions.  Our method has been to systematically reduce the data set

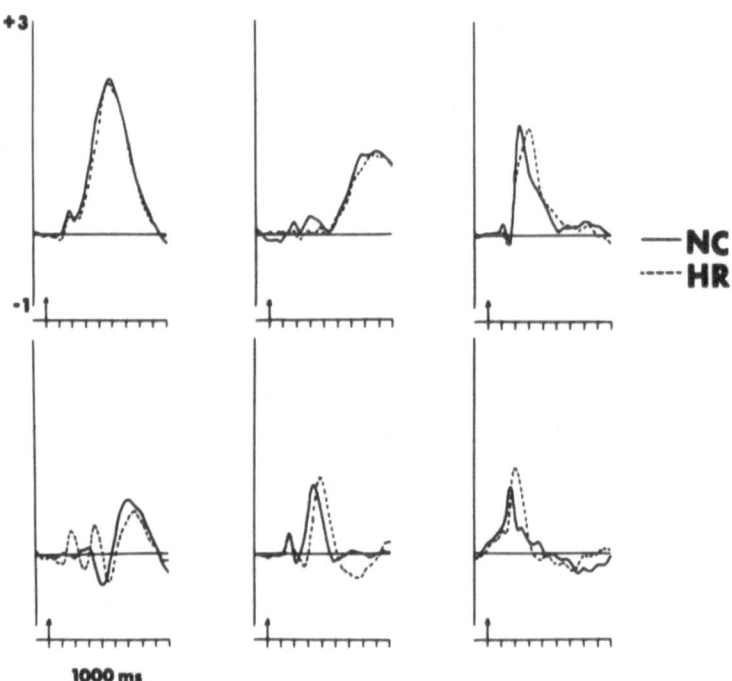

Figure 2.  Rotated factor loading functions resulting from PCAs
performed separately for each group across tasks, stimuli and
electrodes.

of performing PCA for each group separately by task demonstrated
replication of the factor structures seen when the analysis was
done across tasks, and demonstrated that the longer latency N150,
P240 and P350 factors seen for the HR group occurred within the
Task A waveforms only.  We are now attempting to further pinpoint
the source of these latency shifts by performing PCA separately
for type of stimulus within a task.  The results should tell us
whether the source is in the signal, nonsignal or both.

## Factor Score Analyses

Repeated measures ANOVA were used to assess the effect of risk
group, age group, task, stimulus and electrode location on the
factor scores resulting from a PCA pooling the data from both
groups of subjects.  All findings reported below are significant
at the .05 level or better, unless noted.  All factors showed

topographies extremely similar to the ERP components with which
they were associated.  Consistent with the increased processing
demands of Task B, the waveforms of this task were marked by significantly greater P350 and P550 amplitude factors, with a large
effect on P450 amplitude elicited by nonsignals of Task B.  The
P550 component appears independent of the P450 component, which is
larger to signals than nonsignals, since it behaves differently,
being larger to nonsignals and has a more posterior distribution,
especially in the Task B waveforms.  It appears similar in latency
and distribution to the P4 component recently reported by Stuss
and Picton (1978).  P240 appears to be a visual P2, and as such,
its greater amplitude in the Task B waveforms can be attributed to
the greater attentional requirements of this task, since others
have shown that P2 is affected by attentional demands (e.g., Picton
and Hillyard, 1974; Friedman et al., 1973).  This factor showed a
trend towards greater amplitude in the HR group (p<.09).  Consistent with the greater attentional requirements of Task B is the
finding of more initial negativity (N150 factor) in this task than
in Task A.  This factor was less negative in the brain potentials
of the HR group, but this did not attain statistical significance
(p<.07).  Both CNV and N100 have been shown to be greater under
conditions requiring greater attentiveness (Hillyard et al., 1973;
Picton and Hillyard, 1974; Friedman et al., 1973; Tecce, 1972).
The baseline factor, which appears similar in topography and temporal relationship to the LPC to the slow wave factor of Squires
et al. (1977), behaves differently.  Their slow wave was affected
by probability.  Our baseline factor was larger to nonsignals, the
frequent stimulus, than to signals, the infrequent stimulus.  The
HR group produced faster returns to baseline than the NC group, as
did the oldest group of subjects compared to the younger subjects.

    The current data confirm our previous findings (Friedman et
al., 1978c) and those of others (e.g. Squires et al., 1975; Adam
and Collins, 1978; Stuss and Picton, 1978; Thatcher, 1977; Keselica
et al., 1977) in demonstrating multiple positivities within the
latency range of P300, and their greater amplitude elicited by Task
B (Friedman et al., 1978a).


                    Identification of Deviant Subjects

    Because not all children with a schizophrenic parent are ge-
netically at risk, it is necessary to search, within the HR sample,
for a subgroup of individuals whose deviance on selected measures
suggests that they are the vulnerable members of the group.  To
begin with, we assessed the effects of the variables of stimulus,
task and electrode locus on the factor scores obtained from separate PCAs performed for each group, using repeated measures ANOVA.
Despite the differences in the peak latencies of the factors be-

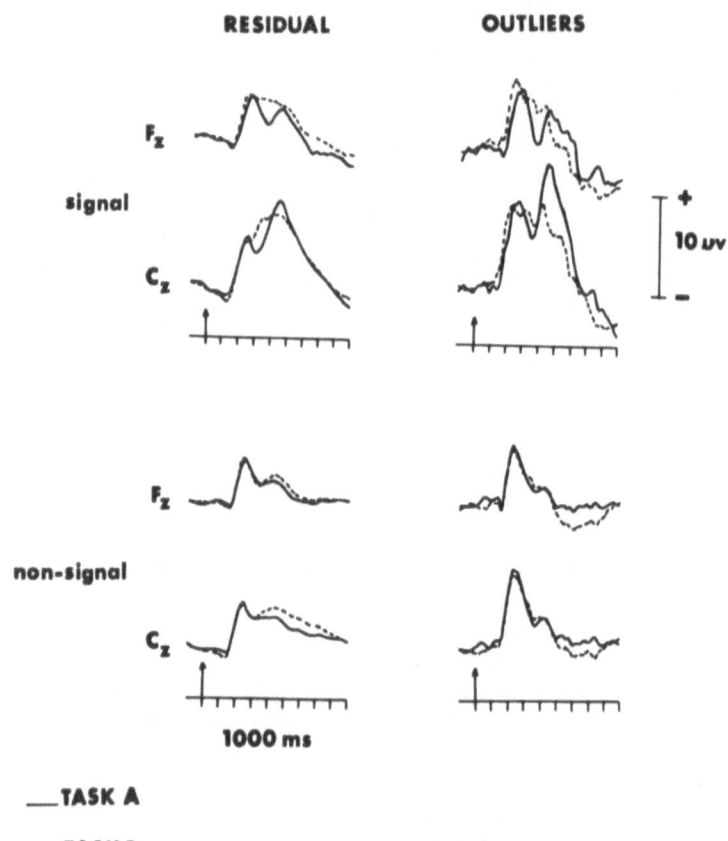

Figure 3.   Grand mean ERP averaged across the four outliers and across the remaining 26 HR subjects (Residual) in response to both stimuli from each task.


tween groups, these factors behaved similarly in each group, supporting the conclusion that these factors were the same.  The fact
that they behaved similarly for both groups allowed us to use the
NC factor score coefficients to compute factor scores for the HR
group.  Theoretically, this method should produce more deviant HR
than NC subjects.  The distribution of factor scores for each factor was inspected, and, using a criterion of a score of $\pm$ 2, subjects were chosen as outliers, and the number of subjects outlying
on one or more factors was tabulated.  There were ten HR and two NC
that were outliers on four or more factors, and this difference was
highly significant ($X^2=6.12$, p<.02).  Within this group, four subjects, all of whom were HR, showed a consistent pattern of factor
scores: large-amplitude frontal P450 to signal stimuli; large-

amplitude P240 activity to both stimuli and tasks; little initial
negativity; the absence of very late positive activity and faster
returns to baseline.  The ERP at Fz and Cz where these effects were
greatest, averaged across the four subjects, are shown in Figure 3.
Also shown is the residual HR grand mean (N=26) after these four
subjects were subtracted.  Note that the outliers' LPC to nonsignals
is not well defined and is of smaller amplitude than the residual
mean.  The outliers do not show a difference in LPC amplitude between the nonsignals of the two tasks, which is clearly seen in the
residual mean, nor do they show a difference in initial negativity
between tasks, a result which is also prominent in the residual
mean.

### Relationship to Adult Schizophrenic Waveforms

In reviewing the adult schizophrenia ERP literature, Buchsbaum
(1977), Roth (1977) and Shagass (1976) concluded that consistent
features of the adult schizophrenic's waveform were: large amplitude
components prior to 100 msec, reduced amplitude LPCs, low amplitude
CNV and a tendency towards reduced N100-P200 amplitude.  The outliers demonstrate large amplitude P240 components, but this peak
is later than those reported to be of large amplitude in adult
schizophrenics.  However, the outliers do show low amplitude LPCs
to nonsignals of both tasks, which might be indicative of deficient information processing or a difference in the way in which
they analyze the relevant information from the two tasks.  The absence of very late positive activity (P550) adds strength to this
hypothesis.  Stuss and Picton (1978) and Thatcher (1977) have reported a late positive wave, which they have labelled P4, which
has a timing and topography similar to our P550, and which Stuss
and Picton (1978) have related to the processing of feedback information in a learning task.  The absence of this component in the
outlier waveforms might be indicative of a failure to use this
information and to make perceptual adjustments while performing the
task.  The reduced negativity seen in these subjects, and the lack
of difference in this factor between tasks, could reflect a failure
to differentially direct attention between tasks, each of which
appears to require a different level of sustained attention.

### CONCLUSIONS

The major similarities between the outliers' waveforms and
the morphology most often reported for the adult schizophrenic
was seen in low amplitude LPC and early negativity to nonsignals
and reduced negativity to signals.  Marked differences were also
noted: these subjects exhibited large amplitude P240 components
to all stimuli and large amplitude LPCs to signals.  Inasmuch as

the various ERP components reflect different aspects of information processing, it is to be anticipated that each component will have differential importance as an index of potential psychopathology. It is also likely that the child at risk who eventually manifests schizophrenia may show a different premorbid ERP response pattern than the adult schizophrenic. It will only be upon follow-up of these individuals that one should be able to detect ERP character- istics that are true premorbid indicators and those that are a consequence of mental dysfunction.

Our strategy is to follow those children whose ERP waveforms are found to be deviant to determine whether they will also be identified as outliers by other components of our psychophysiolog- ic and psychologic test batteries. One of the outliers reported here was also an outlier on an auditory evoked potential measure of deviance during an earlier round of testing (Friedman et al., 1978b), and three of the four current outliers were also deviant on attentional measures given during the first round of testing (Erlenmeyer-Kimling et al., 1978). However, not all of the chil- dren seen during the first two rounds of testing have been seen for the third round, and any conclusions regarding overlap on measures of deviance would be premature at this time. This analysis of our data serves to point up our more cognitively oriented approach to ERP research with HR children and to outline our methods for de- termining which children might be the most vulnerable. Inherent in this methodology is the fact that even if a small number of children are chosen on this basis, it will not be until several years later, at an age when onset is expected, that validation of the selection process will occur.

SUMMARY

Visual ERP were recorded from thirty children at high risk for schizophrenia (HR) and from thirty normal controls (NC) during two versions of a continuous performance test which differed in their task demands. Task A required a simple target identification, while Task B, the more complex of the two, required comparison of successive stimuli. Multiple late positive components were seen in the brain potentials of both groups of subjects in both tasks. Principal components analysis (PCA) confirmed the existence of these components, yielding identical factor structures for both groups of subjects. Late positive components were generally of larger amplitude in the Task B waveforms, while N150 and P240 factor amplitudes appeared to be influenced more by the difference in attentional requirements between the tasks. There was a ten- dency for N150 to be less negative and P240 of larger amplitude in the HR than in the NC group. Four children at high risk for schizo- phrenia were selected on the basis of extremely deviant factor scores. Their brain potentials were characterized by low amplitude N150, small LPCs to nonsignal stimuli, large LPCs to signal stimuli and high amplitude P240 components. While differences between their pattern of response and those of the adult schizophrenic were seen, similarities were also evident. Those components which were deviant in these HR children have also been shown to differ from normal in the adult schizophrenic and are components that have been implicated in mechanisms of selective attention and cognitive processing.

## ACKNOWLEDGMENTS

The authors would like to express their deep appreciation to the following people who participated in various phases of this project: Mr. James Wilson, Jr. for running subjects and preparing the data for analysis; Mr. Tom Chin for preparation of the data for analysis; Mr. Jim Hollenberg, Ms. Henrietta Wolland and Mr. John Nee for computer programming. Drs. Rainer, Stone and Cowan provided the diagnoses of the parents of our high risk children. We are grateful to Dr. Jacques Rutchmann for his help in the design of the tasks. We thank Drs. Barbara Cornblatt, Walter Ritter, Dan Ruchkin, Yvonne Stellingwerf and Samuel Sutton for productive discussions regarding the data. This research was supported by USPHS Grant MH 19560 and the Department of Mental Hygiene of the State of New York.

## REFERENCES

Adam, N. and Collins, G. I. Late components of the visual evoked potential to search in short-term memory. Electroenceph. Clin. Neurophysiol., 1978, 44, 147-156.

Buchsbaum, M. S. The middle evoked response components and schizophrenia. Schiz. Bull., 1977, 3, 93-104.

Dixon, W. J. BMDP Biomedical Computer Programs, Univ. Calif. Press, 1975.

Donchin, E. and Heffley, E. F. Multivariate analysis of ERP data: a tutorial review. In, D. Otto (Ed.), New Perspectives in ERP Research. Washington: U.S. Government Printing Office, in press.

Erlenmeyer-Kimling, L. Studies on the offspring of two schizophrenic parents. In, D. Rosenthal and S. S. Kety (Eds.), The Transmission of Schizophrenia. New York: Pergamon Press, 1968.

Erlenmeyer-Kimling, L.   A prospective study of children of schizo-
     phrenic parents.   USPHS Grant MH-19560, 1970.

Erlenmeyer-Kimling, L.   A prospective study of children at risk
     for schizophrenia: methodological considerations and some
     preliminary findings.   In, R. D. Wirt, G. Winokur and M. Roff
     (Eds.), Life History Research in Psychopathology, Vol. 4.
     Minneapolis: University of Minnesota Press, 1975, 23-46.

Erlenmeyer-Kimling, L.   Issues pertaining to prevention and inter-
     vention in genetic disorders affecting human behavior.   In, G.
     W. Albee and J. M. Joffe (Eds.), Primary Prevention in Psycho-
     pathology.   Hanover: University Press of New England, in
     press.

Erlenmeyer-Kimling, L., Cornblatt, B. and Fleiss, J. L.   Cognitive
     test data on children of schizophrenic parents.   Psychiatric
     Annals, in press.

Fein, G., Tursky, B. and Erlenmeyer-Kimling, L.   Stimulus sensi-
     tivity and reactivity in children at high risk for schizophrenia.
     Psychophysiol., 1975, 12, 226.

Friedman, D., Hakerem, G., Sutton, S. and Fleiss, J. L.   Effect of
     stimulus uncertainty on the pupillary dilation response and the
     vertex evoked potential.   Electroenceph. Clin. Neurophysiol.,
     1973, 34, 473-484.

Friedman, D., Vaughan, H. G., Jr. and Erlenmeyer-Kimling, L.   Task
     related cortical potentials in children in two kinds of vigi-
     lance tasks.   In, D. Otto (Ed.), New Perspectives in Event
     Related Potential Research.   Washington: U.S. Government Print-
     ing Office, in press (a).

Friedman, D., Frosch, A. and Erlenmeyer-Kimling, L.   Auditory
     evoked potentials in children at high risk for schizophrenia.
     In, H. Begleiter (Ed.), Evoked Potentials and Behavior.   New
     York: Plenum Press, in press (b).

Friedman, D., Vaughan, H. G., Jr. and Erlenmeyer-Kimling, L.   Stim-
     ulus and response related components of the late positive com-
     plex in visual discrimination tasks.   Electroenceph. Clin.
     Neurophysiol., in press (c).

Garmezy, N. and Streitman, S.   Children at risk: the search for
     the antecedents of schizophrenia.   Part I: Conceptual models
     and research methods.   Schiz. Bull., 1974, 8, 14-90.

Glaser, E. M. and Ruchkin, D. S.  Principles of Neurobiological
    Signal Analysis.  New York: Academic Press, 1976.

Grunebaum, H., Weiss, J. L., Gallant, D. and Cohler, B. J.  Atten-
    tion in young children of psychotic mothers.  Am. J. Psychiat.,
    1974, 131, 887-891.

Herman, J., Mirsky, A. F., Ricks, N. L. and Gallant, D.  Behavioral
    and electrographic measures of attention in children at risk
    for schizophrenia.  J. Abn. Psychol., 1977, 86, 27-33.

Hillyard, S. A., Hink, R. F., Schwent, V. L. and Picton, T. W.
    Electrical signs of selective attention in the human brain.
    Science, 1973, 182, 177-180.

Keselica, J., Petrasek, J. and Vaughan, H. G., Jr.  Topographic
    analysis of cortical potentials associated with intramodal and
    intermodal discrimination tasks.  Paper presented at the Inter-
    national Neuropsychology Society Conference, Sante Fe, 1977.

Kornetsky, C. and Orzack, M. H.  Physiological and behavioral corre-
    lates of attention dysfunction in schizophrenic patients.  In,
    L. C. Wynne (Ed.), The Nature of Schizophrenia.  New York:
    John Wiley and Sons, 1978, 196-204.

Mednick, S. A. and McNeill, T. F.  Current methodology in research
    on the etiology of schizophrenia: serious difficulties which
    suggest the use of the high risk group method.  Psychol. Bull.,
    1968, 70, 681-693.

Mednick, S. A. and Schulsinger, F.  Studies of children at high
    risk for schizophrenia.  In, S. R. Dean (Ed.), The First Ten
    Dean Award Lectures.  New York: MSS Information Corporation,
    1973, 247-293.

Orzack, M. H. and Kornetsky, C.  Attention dysfunction in chronic
    schizophrenia.  Arch. Gen. Psychiat., 1966, 14, 323-326.

Pearson, S. and Kley, I. B.  On the application of genetic expec-
    tancies with age specific base rates in the study of human be-
    havior disorders.  Psychol. Bull., 1957, 54, 406-420.

Picton, T. W. and Hillyard, S. A.  Human auditory evoked potentials.
    II.  Effects of attention.  Electroenceph. Clin. Neurophysiol.,
    1974, 36, 191-199.

Roth, W. T.  Late event related potentials and psychopathology.
    Schiz. Bull., 1977, 3, 105-120.

Rutchmann, J., Cornblatt, B. and Erlenmeyer-Kimling, L.   Report
    on a continuous performance test of sustained attention in
    children at risk for schizophrenia.  Arch. Gen. Psychiat.,
    1977, 34, 571-575.

Saletu, B., Saletu, M., Marasa, J., Mednick, S. A. and Schulsinger,
    F.  Acoustic evoked potentials in offsprings of schizophrenic
    mothers ("high risk" children for schizophrenia).  Electro-
    enceph. Clin. Neurophysiol., 1975, 6, 92-102.

Salzman, L. F. and Klein, R. H.  Habituation and conditioning of
    electrodermal responses in high risk children.  Schiz. Bull.,
    1978, 4, 210-222.

Shagass, C.  An electrophysiological view of schizophrenia.  Biol.
    Psychiat., 1976, 11, 3-30.

Squires, K. C., Donchin, E., Herning, R. I. and McCarthy, G.   On
    the influence of task relevance and stimulus probability on
    event related potential components.  Electroenceph. Clin.
    Neurophysiol., 1977, 42, 1-14.

Squires, N., Squires, K. C. and Hillyard, S. A.  Two varieties of
    long latency positive waves evoked by unpredictable auditory
    stimuli in man.  Electroenceph. Clin. Neurophysiol., 1975, 38,
    387-401.

Stuss, D. T. and Picton, T. W.  Neurophysiological correlates of
    human concept formation.  Behav. Biol., 1978, 23, 135-162.

Tecce, J. J.  Contingent negative variation (CNV) and psychological
    processes in man.  Psychol. Bull., 1972, 77, 73-108.

Thatcher, R. W.  Evoked potential correlates of hemispheric later-
    alization during semantic information processing.  In, S. Harnad,
    L. Goldstein, R. Doty and J. Jaynes (Eds.), Lateralization in
    the Nervous System.  New York: Academic Press, 1977.

Venables, P. H.  The electrodermal psychophysiology of schizophre-
    nics and children at risk for schizophrenia: controversies and
    developments.  Schiz. Bull., 1977, 3, 28-48.

Zerbin-Rüdin, E.  Endogene psychosen.  In, P. E. Becker (Ed.), Human-
    genetik, (Handbuch, Vol. 2).  Stuttgart: Thieme, 1967.

# LATE POSITIVE COMPONENT (LPC) AND CNV DURING PROCESSING OF LINGUISTIC INFORMATION

H. Goto, T. Adachi, T. Utsunomiya and I.-C. Chen

Department of Internal Medicine, Tokyo Metropolitan

Police Hospital, Tokyo 102, Japan

## INTRODUCTION

The late positive component of the evoked potential (LPC) and the contingent negative variation (CNV) have been investigated with visual and acoustic stimuli by many researchers studying linguistic processing. CNVs were investigated during word category discrimination by Burian et al. (1972). LPCs were studied during information processing in sentences by Friedman et al. (1975) and during semantic information processing of words by Thatcher and April (1976). Different lateralization for noun- and verb-evoked EEG scalp potential fields was reported by Brown and Lehmann (1977). Both Burian and Thatcher tried to apply ERPs evoked by words in testing aphasic patients. We studied CNV and LPC during processing of linguistic information to find out if ERPs can be useful for testing the recognition of Japanese sentences and words.

## METHODS

### I. Examination of Sentence Recognition

The experimental subjects included three healthy right-handed persons, three aphasics and one person with auditory agnosia. Three meaningful sentences and three meaningless sentences (which were composed by exchanging the predicates of the three meaningful sentences with one another) were used as acoustical or visual stimuli. Each sentence comprised five spoken syllables or four visually presented characters (two Kanji and two Kana). The subject

was able to determine whether the sentence had a meaning or not by
understanding the key information (the fourth syllable or the third
character) in the acoustically or visually presented sentence.

The acoustically presented sentences were delivered by a simple,
random aural-stimulator (Goto et al., 1976) which consisted of a
conventional 4-channel tape recorder, an endless tape, a control
signal detector, a memory, an analog switch and a motor drive con-
troller.  With this stimulator, the examiner could choose one of
either three meaningful or three meaningless sentences for repro-
duction through monaural headphones with exact timing (100 msec
monosyllable voice, 900 msec interval).  One second after the last
word of the meaningless sentence a red lamp, placed 130 cm in front
of the subject, was lit as the imperative stimulus for the CNV task.

The 9 X 9 or 11 X 11 red light emitting diode (LED) matrix,
viewed binocularly, was used to present sequentially each character
in the visual sentences (40 msec character, 960 msec interval).
One second after the last word of the meaningful sentence, nine LEDs
in the center of the matrix were lit as the imperative stimulus for
the CNV task.  The LED matrix subtended a visual angle of $2^{\circ}$.

The three meaningful and three meaningless sentences were presented in a random sequence with approximately the same number of
occurrences of each sentence.  The subject, lying comfortably in a
supine position, had been told previously that each meaningful
sentence was followed by a sign, and he was ordered to press a switch
as fast as possible after the task signal.

The recording electrodes were placed at C3 and C4.  The reference electrodes were placed at the ipsilateral mastoid processes.
A ground electrode was placed on the forehead.  EEGs were amplified
using 3.0 second time constant amplifiers, stored on a data recorder
and analyzed using an electronic averager.  EOG artifacts were
checked.

II.  Exmination of Word Recognition

Seven right-handed, healthy subjects and three slightly impaired aphasics served in the experiments.  The 11 X 11 red LED matrix
was used as the visual stimulator similar to the sentence examinations (Fig. 1).  Since the ability of Japanese aphasics to use
Kanji and Kana can be selectively impaired, we examined LPCs during
information processing in semantic match and mismatch between either
two successive Kanji or two successive Kana words presented in
Thatcher's paradigm (Thatcher and April, 1976).

In the Kanji experiments a series of visual displays (20 msec

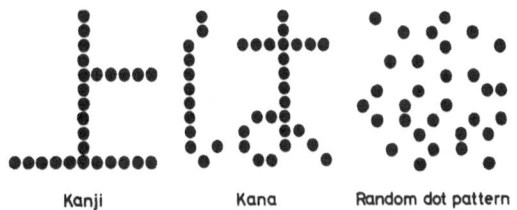

Kanji          Kana          Random dot pattern

Fig. 1.   Kanji, Kana and random dot pattern presented on 11 X 11 LED matrix.


stimulus duration, 1 stimulus/sec) were presented.  A given trial comprised, sequentially, a variable number (two to six) of random dot displays (RDDs), then a first Kanji, then another variable number (two to six) of RDDs, then a second Kanji, then two RDDs (Fig. 2).  Ninety to 120 trials were presented.  The second Kanji was the same, antonymous or semantically unrelated to the first Kanji.  Five pairs each of identical, antonymous and semantically neutral single Kanji words were used as the two successive Kanji words (Table 1).  The subjects were told to press one switch as fast as possible after a trial with semantic match, and another key for mismatch between two successive Kanji.  The recording electrodes were placed at T3, T4, T5, T6, P3 and P4.  The linked ears served as a reference.  A ground electrode was placed on the forehead.  The ERPs were averaged separately for semantic match and mismatch cases. EOG artifacts were checked.

In the experiments of Kana words, each Kanji or one RDD in the above mentioned trial was replaced by three sequential Kanas or RDDs of 30 msec in duration with 80 msec intervals (Fig. 3).  Eight pairs

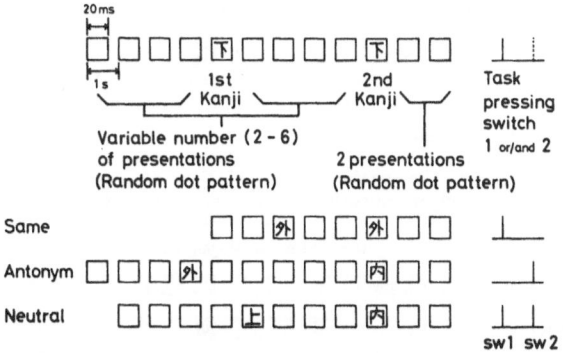

Fig. 2.   Trial sequences in Kanji experiment.

Table 1.  First and second Kanji pairings.  S: same; A: antonymous;
N: semantically neutral.

| 1st Kanji | 2nd Kanji | |
|---|---|---|
| 明 (light) | 上 (up) | (N) |
| 上 (up) | 下 (down) | (A) |
| 暗 (dark) | 上 (up) | (N) |
| 暗 (dark) | 暗 (dark) | (S) |
| 下 (down) | 下 (down) | (S) |
| 外 (out) | 外 (out) | (S) |
| 下 (down) | 上 (up) | (A) |
| 内 (in) | 外 (out) | (A) |
| 下 (down) | 明 (light) | (N) |
| 外 (out) | 内 (in) | (A) |
| 外 (out) | 下 (down) | (N) |
| 内 (in) | 内 (in) | (S) |
| 明 (light) | 明 (light) | (S) |
| 明 (light) | 暗 (dark) | (A) |
| 上 (up) | 内 (in) | (N) |

each of equal, antonymous and semantically neutral Kana words were
used as the two successive Kana words (Table 2).  Tasks for semantic
match and mismatch between two successive words, EEG recording and
data processing were the same as in the Kanji experiments.

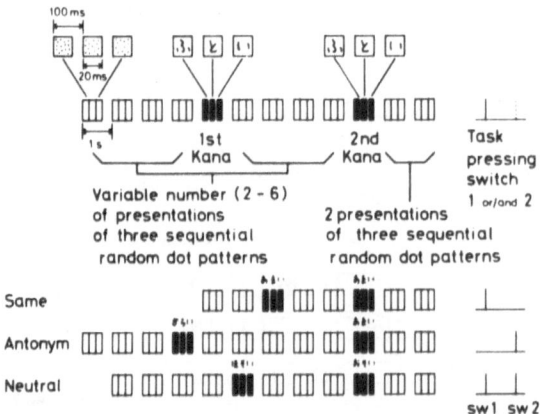

Fig. 3.  Trial sequences in Kana-words experiment.

Table 2.  First and second Kana-word pairings.  S: same; A: antonymous; N: semantically neutral.

| 1st Kana | 2nd Kana | |
|---|---|---|
| おもい (heavy) | あまい (sweet) | N |
| たかい (high) | ひくい (low) | A |
| よわい (weak) | ひろい (wide) | N |
| ふとい (thick) | ふとい (thick) | S |
| ひくい (low) | ひくい (low) | S |
| かるい (light) | おもい (heavy) | A |
| あまい (sweet) | あまい (sweet) | S |
| せまい (narrow) | ひろい (wide) | A |
| ふかい (deep) | あさい (shallow) | A |
| ほそい (thin) | おそい (slow) | N |
| からい (salty) | あまい (sweet) | A |
| たかい (high) | よわい (weak) | N |
| ひろい (wide) | ひろい (wide) | S |
| ほそい (thin) | ふとい (thick) | A |
| かるい (light) | かるい (light) | S |
| あさい (shallow) | はやい (quick) | N |
| おそい (slow) | からい (salty) | N |
| つよい (strong) | よわい (weak) | A |
| ふかい (deep) | ふかい (deep) | S |
| はやい (quick) | はやい (quick) | S |
| はやい (quick) | おそい (slow) | A |
| からい (salty) | あさい (shallow) | N |
| つよい (strong) | つよい (strong) | S |
| せまい (narrow) | たかい (high) | N |

## RESULTS

### I.  Sentence Recognition

Healthy subjects.  In the experiments with acoustic stimulation, evoked potentials were obtained to each spoken syllable.  The amplitude of the N1 component of the evoked potential to the first syllable was the largest.  The amplitudes of P300 to the first and the fourth syllables were larger than those to the others.  In the experiments with visual stimulation, the amplitude of N1 to each character was small.  P200 was observed for every character.  The amplitudes of P300 to the first and the third characters were much larger than those to the second and the fourth characters.  P300 latency to the third character was longer than any of the other P300 latencies.  P650 to the first and the third characters tended to appear, but were not observed in responses to the second and the fourth characters (Fig. 4).  In both acoustic and visual experiments,

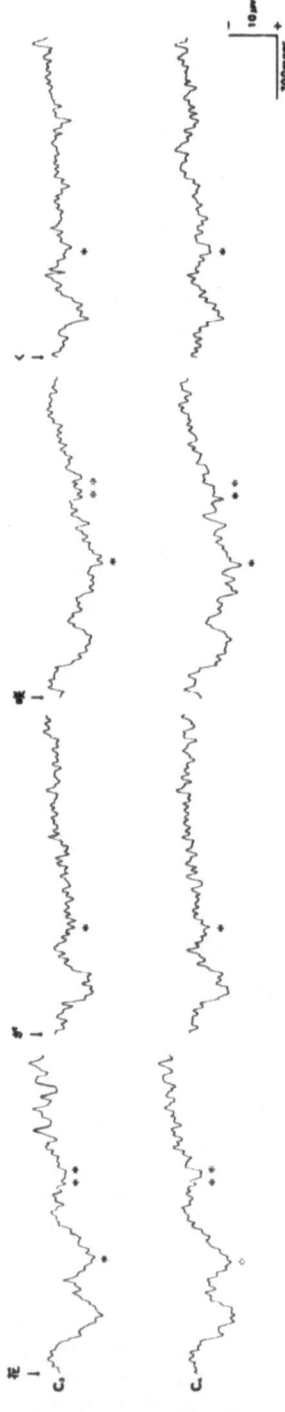

Fig. 4. Visual evoked responses to each character in a sentence. (*)=P300; (**)=P650.

CNV began to develop at the first information (the first syllable
or character) and continued until the subject pressed the switch in
response to the meaningful sentences.  However, when the subject
was stimulated by the meaningless sentences, a CNV began to develop
at the first information, continued until the key information was
given (the fourth voice or the third character) and then disappeared
(Fig. 5, Fig. 6).

In the examination of the aphasic patients, confused responses
were observed in sentence differentiation.  Confused responses to
the acoustically presented sentences were observed in 0-40% of the
aphasic patients in comparison with 0-4% of the healthy subjects.
The confused responses to the visually presented sentences were
observed in 0-68% of the aphasic patients in comparison with 0% of
the healthy subjects.  The evoked potential components N1 and P300
were observed, but the CNV amplitudes were very small or at zero
level in the aphasic patients.  There was no difference between the
CNVs produced by the meaningful and meaningless sentences (Fig. 7).

In the investigation of the auditory agnostic patient, the
evoked potential N1, P300 and CNV were not observed when the patient
was stimulated with the acoustically presented sentences (Fig. 8).
But N1, P300 and CNV were very similar to those in healthy subjects
during visual sentence stimulation (Fig. 9).

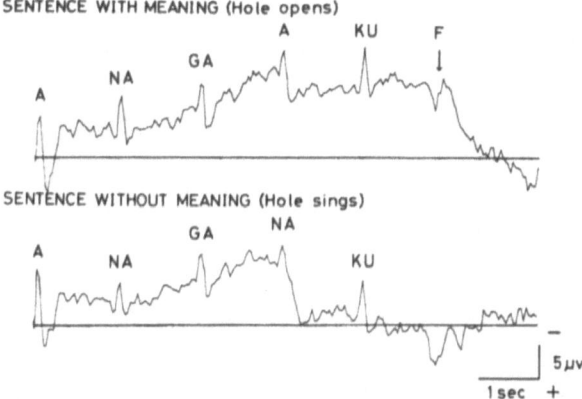

Fig. 5.  Evoked potentials and CNV obtained by aural sentence stimulation.  F: flash; Top record: CNV accompanied by stimulation of
meaningful sentence; Bottom record: CNV accompanied by stimulation
of meaningless sentence.

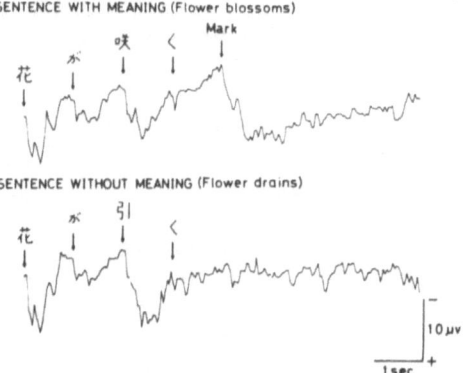

Fig. 6.  Evoked potentials and CNV obtained by visual sentence
stimulation.  Top record: CNV accompanied by stimulation of meaningful sentence; Bottom record: CNV accompanied by stimulation of
meaningless sentence.

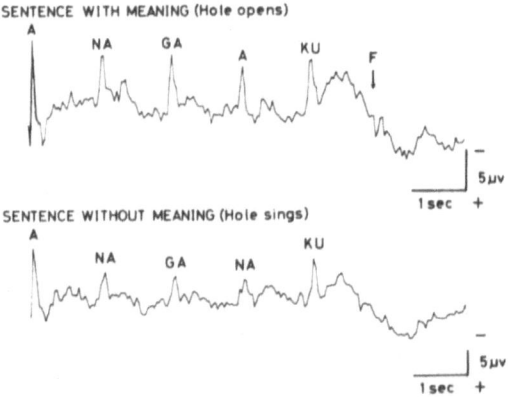

Fig. 7.  Evoked potentials and CNV obtained by auditory sentence
stimulation in an aphasic patient.

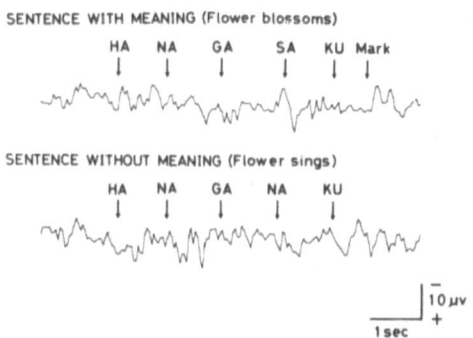

Fig. 8.   Evoked potentials N1, P300 and CNV were not observed in
the auditory sentence stimulation experiment in an auditory agnostic
patient.


## II.   Word Recognition

Healthy subjects.   In the Kanji word experiments, in temporal
leads N1 amplitudes to the second Kanji were not marked, but P200,
P300 and P650 to the second Kanji were observed.   The amplitudes
of P300 and P650 in right side derivations were larger than those
in left side derivations (Fig. 10).   N1, P200 and P300 to the first
Kanji were similar to those to the second Kanji, but P650 to the
first Kanji was not marked.   In the evoked responses to the RDD
just before and after the second Kanji, N1 amplitudes were not
marked.   P200 was observed, but neither P300 nor P650 appeared.

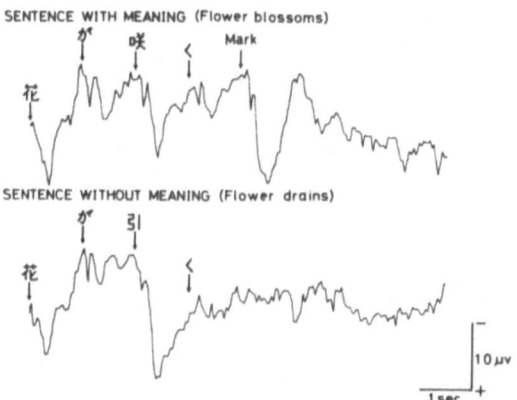

Fig. 9.   Evoked potentials and CNV observed in the visual sentence
stimulation experiment in an auditory agnostic patient.

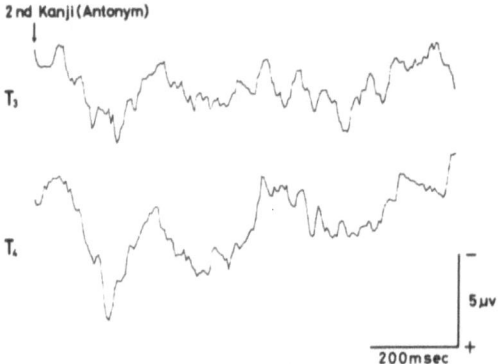

Fig. 10.  Evoked response to the second Kanji (antonymous).

Latencies of P200 to these RDDs were shorter than those of P200 to
the second Kanji (Fig. 11).  In the Kana word experiments, N1
amplitudes to the second Kana words were not marked, but P300 and
P650 were observed.  P300 amplitudes to the second Kana words in
right-sided derivations were larger than those in left-sided
derivations (Fig. 12).  N1, P300 and P650 to the first Kana words
were similar to those to the second Kana words, but not marked.  In
the evoked responses to three sequential RDDs just before and after
the second Kana words, P300 was observed, but P650 was not observed
(Fig. 13).  Evoked responses at P3 and P4 were similar to those at
T3, T4, T5 and T6.

     In the examination of aphasics confused responses were fre-
quently observed in recognition tests of Kanji and Kana.  In

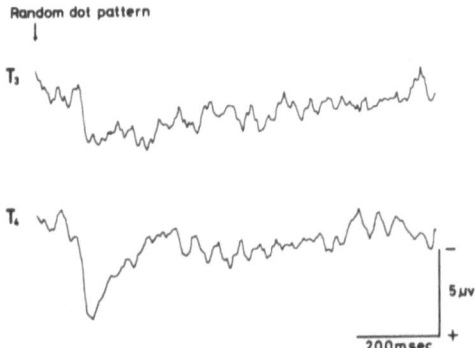

Fig. 11.  Evoked response to random dot pattern (just before the
second Kanji).

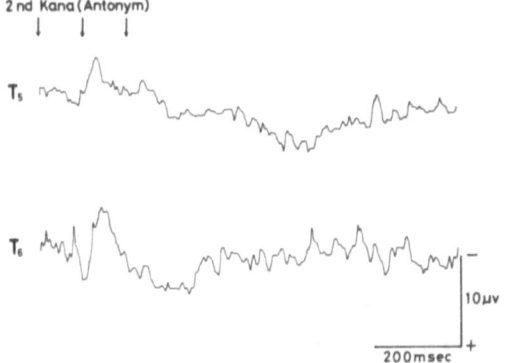

Fig. 12.  Evoked response to the second Kana-word (antonymous).

slightly impaired aphasic patients evoked responses to the second
Kanji tended to be similar to those observed in healthy subjects,
but the amplitudes of P300 and P650 were smaller.  Peak latencies
of P300 and P650 in aphasic patients were much longer than those in
healthy subjects.

## DISCUSSION

Friedman et al. (1975), in a study of averaged visual evoked
potentials to sequentially flashed words comprising sentences of
two conditions, reported that P300 latencies to words which delivered information (last or second word according to condition) were
longer than P300 latencies to any of the other words in the sentence.  In our experiment with visually presented sentences, P300

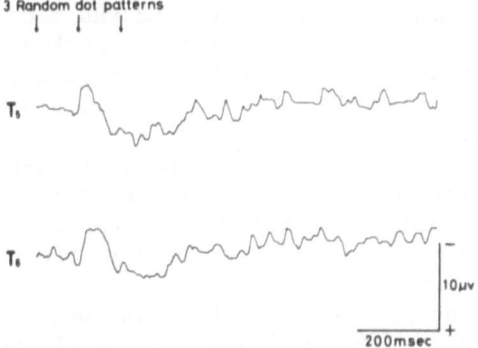

Fig. 13.  Evoked response to three sequential random dot patterns
(just before the second Kana-word).

latency to the key (third) character was longer than that to the other characters. This result is compatible with the result obtained by Friedman's group. They observed the presence of CNVs in some circumstances but not in others. In our experiments a difference between CNVs produced by meaningful and meaningless sentences was observed whenever the subjects discriminated the sentences. When the subjects could not discriminate the sentence, recognition response in the CNV was not observed, and CNV amplitudes were small or zero.

Burian et al. (1972), using two different word groups as warning and non-warning stimuli and following only one group with a flash, argued that the appearance of the CNV following only one group was positive, objective proof that the subjects understood the test words. In our experiments, using not word groups but sentence groups, such a difference between CNVs was observed in the healthy subjects. The recognition response in CNV was not observed in the examination of the aphasic patients who could not discriminate the sentences. In the study of the auditory agnostic patient, it was not observed in the responses to acoustically presented sentences but was observed in responses to visually presented sentences. These facts suggest the usefulness of the CNV as a test for sentence discrimination.

Thatcher and April (1976), using a delayed semantic-matching procedure involving synonym, antonym and semantically neutral English word pairs, demonstrated hemispheric asymmetries (left greater than right) in evoked potentials to the second word at latencies of 300 to 500 msec. In their opinion these major, long latency phenomena indicate that the asymmetries represent processes occurring at the level of memory or semantic representations.

In our experiments of word recognition, using Thatcher's paradigm, evoked response components N1, P300 and P650 to the second word were observed. P650 amplitudes to the second Kanji showed right greater than left asymmetries, but those to the second Kana words showed left greater than right asymmetries. Evoked responses to the first word were similar to those to the second word, but not marked. P650 was not observed in evoked responses to RDDs just before and after the second words of either Kanji or Kana. This suggests that P650 is attributed to semantic match-mismatch task-related brain activities. It is interesting to compare the P650 to the first word, to the second word and to the RDD in the semantic match-mismatch experiments with the P650 observed in the sentence experiments. P650 was observed in evoked responses to the first (subject) and the third (verb stem) characters but not observed in evoked responses to the second (ga-particle) and the fourth (verb ending) characters in the experiments of syntactic match and mismatch between subject and verb.

In the Japanese orthography two types of nonalphabetic symbols, Kana (phonetic symbols for syllables) and Kanji (essentially non-phonetic, logographic symbols representing lexical morphemes) are used in combination.  In studies of Japanese aphasic patients, it has been reported that various types of dissociation between the ability for Kana and Kanji processing may occur (Sasanuma, 1971, 1975).  From the results of studies on Japanese aphasics and tachis-toscopic recognition experiments of Kanji and Kana in left and right visual fields in healthy subjects (Sasanuma et al., 1977; Hatta, 1977), the following hypothesis has been deduced:  Kanji is mainly processed in the left hemisphere.  The discrepant results between asymmetry of P650 amplitudes to the second Kanji and that to the second Kana-word are compatible with the above mentioned hypothesis.

It is very interesting to compare our work with Brown and Lehmann's (1977) which suggests that noun and verb in English are processed in different hemispheres from the observations of noun- and verb-auditory evoked EEG scalp potential fields.

In the examination of aphasics frequent confused responses for recognition of Kanji and Kana-words, smaller amplitudes of P650, and longer peak latencies of P300 and P650 were observed.  It is assumed that information processing of words is more effective and takes a longer time in aphasic patients than in healthy subjects.

SUMMARY

To find out if ERPs can be useful for testing recognition of sentence and word, LPCs and CNV were investigated as follows:  For sentence recognition subjects were required to respond with different key presses when sequentially presented sentences, visual or aural, were recognized as meaningful or meaningless by key information in the presentation.  In healthy subjects P300 ampli-tudes (C3, C4) to the beginning of information and to the key information were larger than those to the other parts of the presented information.  The difference between CNVs produced by meaningful and meaningless sentences was observed after the key information. In aphasia the recognition response in CNV after the key information was not observed.  In auditory agnosia it was observed in responses to visual sentences but not in those to auditory sentences.  For word recognition, subjects were required to press a different switch according to semantic match or mismatch between either two success-ive Kanji or two successive Kana words, presented in Thatcher's (1976) paradigm.  In healthy, right-handed subjects P300 and P650 amplitudes (temporal and parietal leads) to the second Kanji showed a right greater than left asymmetry.  P300 amplitudes to the second Kana words showed the same, but P650 amplitudes to the second Kana words showed a left greater than right asymmetry.  These findings of P650 are compatible with the hypothesis that Kanji (logographic symbols) and Kana (phonetic symbols) are processed differentially in the hemispheres. In aphasics, P650 showed less marked amplitudes and longer peak latencies. These results of two experiments suggest that CNV and LPCs can be useful for testing sentence and word recognition.

## REFERENCES

Brown, W.S. and Lehmann, D. Different lateralization for noun- and verb-evoked EEG scalp potential fields. Abstract. Electroenceph. Clin. Neurophysiol., 1977, 43, 469.

Burian, K., Gestring, G.F., Gloning, K. and Haider, M. Objective examination of verbal discrimination and comprehension in aphasia using the contingent negative variation. A pilot study. Audiology, 1972, 11, 310-316.

Friedman, D., Simson, R., Ritter, W. and Rapin, I. The late positive component (P300) and information processing in sentences. Electroenceph. Clin. Neurophysiol., 1975, 38, 255-262.

Goto, H., Adachi, T., Utsunomiya, T. and Nakano, H. Simple and random aural-stimulator for study of evoked potential, late positive component (P300) and contingent negative variation (CNV). Dig. Eleventh Int. Conf. Med. Biol. Eng., Ottawa, 1976, 444-445.

Hatta, T. Recognition of Japanese Kanji in the left and right visual fields. Neuropsychologia, 1977, 15, 685-688.

Sasanuma, S. and Fujimura, O. Selective impairment of phonetic and non-phonetic transcription of words in Japanese aphasic patients: Kana vs. Kanji in visual recognition and writing. Cortex, 1971, 7, 1-18.

Sasanuma, S. Kana and Kanji processing in Japanese aphasics. Brain and Language, 1975, 2, 369-383.

Sasanuma, S., Itoh, M., Mori, K. and Kobayashi, Y. Tachistoscopic recognition of Kana and Kanji words. Neuropsychologia, 1977, 15, 547-553.

Thatcher, R.W. and April, R.S. Evoked potential correlates of semantic information processing in normals and aphasics. In R.W. Rieber (Ed.), The Neuropsychology of Language, New York: Plenum Press, 1976.

THE MACULAR AND PARAMACULAR SUBCOMPONENTS OF THE PATTERN EVOKED

RESPONSE


A.M. Halliday, G. Barrett, L.D. Blumhardt and A. Kriss

Medical Research Council, Institute of Neurology

National Hospital, Queen Square, London WC1


The studies to be presented have been carried out on healthy subjects, recording the pattern evoked response to a black and white reversing checkerboard stimulus, back-projected onto a circular translucent screen viewed monocularly by the subject at a distance of 1 meter. The full-field stimulus extends out from a central fixation point to an eccentricity of 16 degrees, and the individual checks subtend 50'. The pattern is reversed every 600 msec by moving it rapidly sideways through one square (10 msec transition time), and the response to 200 such reversals has been averaged in each run. For half-field stimulation, one side of the screen is masked off, and smaller areas of the remaining half-field stimulus could be masked off in the same way to test central or peripheral stimulation. The position of the central fixation light remains the same throughout.

The pattern evoked potentials are recorded from a transverse row of five occipital electrodes, the central one placed 5 cm above the inion in the midline and the lateral ones 5 and 10 cm out on each side. All are referred to a common midfrontal reference. Other electrodes have also been used, but the present account will be limited to these five channels.

The response to the full 0 to 16 degree field has a characteristic distribution over the occiput with a maximum amplitude in the midline falling off at the electrodes to either side. Its most prominent feature is the major positive component, designated P100 which is usually preceded and followed by smaller negative peaks, giving the whole response a triphasic negative/positive/ negative (NPN) character (Fig. 1). We have shown in previous studies (Barrett, et al., 1976; Blumhardt, et al., 1977) that the

135

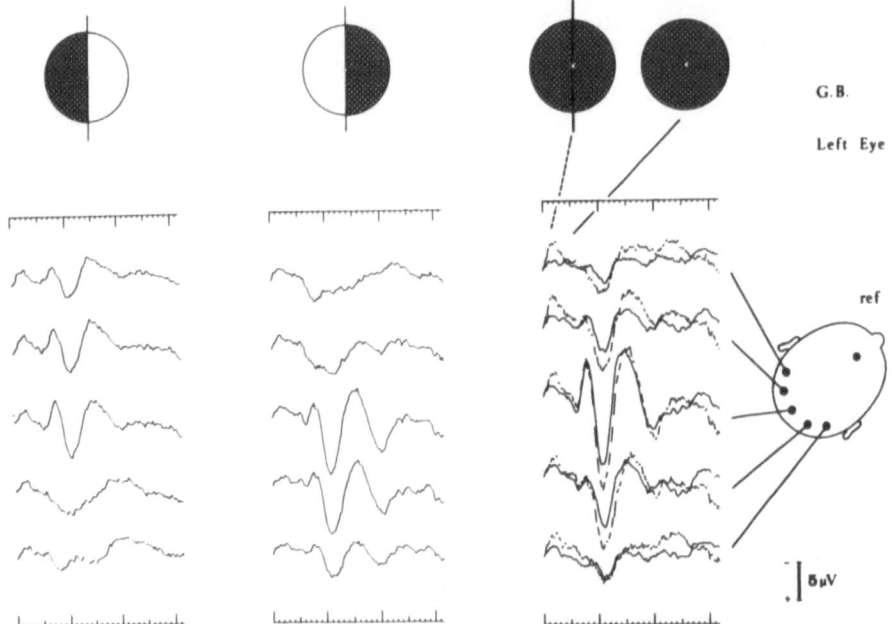

Fig. 1.  Pattern evoked responses to left and right half-field and
whole field reversing checkerboard stimuli presented to the left
eye of a healthy subject.  The subject fixates a small spot of
light situated in the center of the screen, and the stimuli, which
are made up of 50' black and white squares, extend out to an eccentricity of 16 degrees.  Time scale in 10, 50 and 100 msec marks.
In the right-hand record the full-field response is compared with
the sum of the two half-field responses (dotted line).  (From Blumhardt et al., 1977.)

whole-field response is made up of two highly asymmetric half-
field responses.  In each of these, the major positivity with its
accompanying negative peaks is seen at the midline and ipsilateral
electrodes, while the contralateral channels show a relatively flat
record (Fig. 1).  The full-field response approximates closely to
an algebraic summation of the half-field responses recorded in the
same subject, and the midline maximum is due to the addition of the
ipsilateral components from both half-fields at this particular
electrode (Blumhardt et al., 1977; Blumhardt and Halliday, in press).
Although there are quite marked individual variations in the detail
of the waveform, the same asymmetric features are seen in all
healthy subjects, irrespective of which eye is being stimulated.

     There is good evidence that the response recorded from the
electrodes ipsilateral to the half-field stimulated is coming from

the contralateral hemisphere, since hemispherectomized patients
show exactly the same asymmetric distribution for the response
from their preserved half-field (Blumhardt and Halliday, in press).
The reason for this curious lateralization of the major positivity
appears to be the position and orientation of the cortical projection areas generating the response on the medial and postero-medial
surface of the contralateral occipital lobe (Barrett et al., 1976).
However, as we have previously demonstrated (Michael et al., 1971),
the position of the reference in relation to the occipital electrodes is a critical factor in determining what one records.

   In many healthy subjects, a smaller additional triphasic complex of similar latency but reversed polarity (PNP) can be recorded
in the half-field response at the contralateral electrodes.  This
PNP complex shows much more variability in amplitude and waveform
and is often inconspicuous or absent.  When present, it is largest
at the contralateral electrode 10 cm out from the midline.  It can

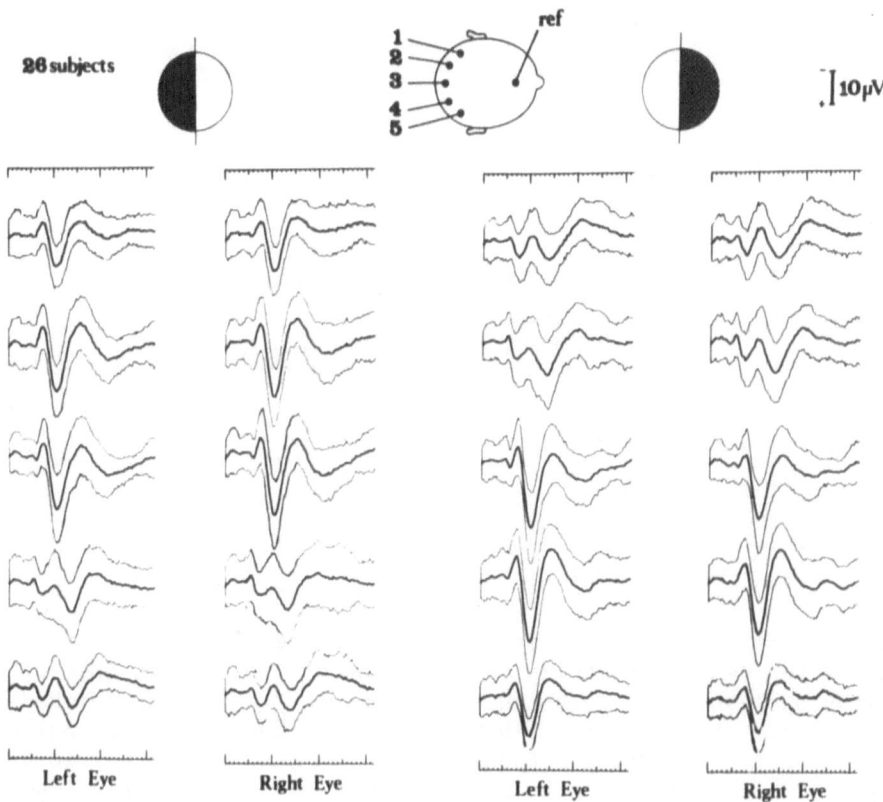

Fig. 2.  Mean waveform and standard deviation for the half-field
responses of twenty-six healthy individuals.  The responses to stimulation of each half-field are shown separately for each eye.  (From
Blumhardt et al., 1978.)

be clearly seen in the mean half-field responses from a large group
of healthy subjects (Fig. 2). The response recorded from the
electrode 5 cm out on the contralateral side appears to be
"transitional" between the large ipsilateral NPN complex and the
smaller, more variable contralateral PNP complex, and it consequently has a larger variance.

At first sight the contralateral PNP complex of the half-
field response looks as if it might be just a phase reversal of the
ipsilateral NPN complex recorded from the other end of the genera-

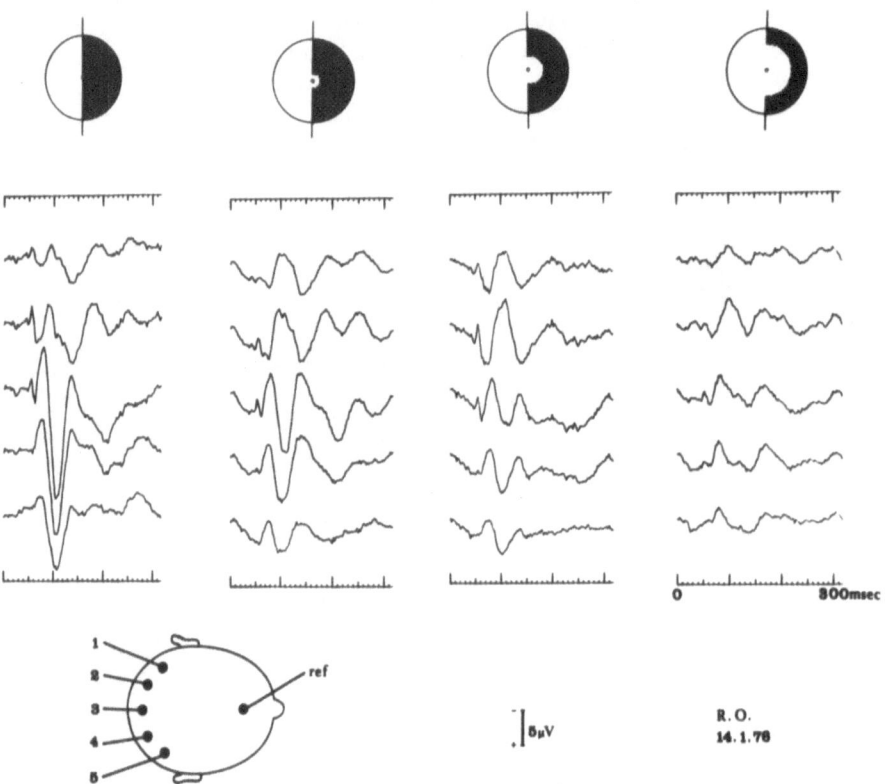

Fig. 3. The effect of removing a progressively increasing propor-
tion of the central stimulus on the right half-field response of a
healthy subject. The left-hand record shows the response evoked
by the full 0 to 16 degree right half-field checkerboard stimulus.
In the other three records the stimulus has been masked off in the
central 2.5 degrees, 5 degrees and 10 degrees, respectively. Note
that the ipsilateral NPN complex is rapidly attenuated when the
central stimulus is removed, whereas the contralateral PNP complex
is actually enhanced for the 2.5 degree and 5 degree "scotoma".
(From Blumhardt et al., 1978.)

tor.  The mean latencies of the subcomponents for a large group of
healthy subjects are, in fact, roughly similar, particularly for the
first two components.  In a group of twenty healthy individuals
Blumhardt et al. (1978) found that the initial ipsilateral negativity (N75) and the corresponding contralateral positive wave (P75)
both had a mean latency of between 76.5 to 78.1 msec.  Corresponding means for the major ipsilateral positivity (P100) and the
contralateral negative wave (N105) similarly fell within the
range 103.7 to 106.3.  There was, however, a greater discrepancy
for the third subcomponent of the two complexes, the ipsilateral
negativity (N145) having a mean peak latency within the range
143.6 to 145.4, while the contralateral positivity (P135) had a
mean latency of 134.6 to 137.5.  Each range consists of four mean
values, one for each half-field of each eye.  These mean latencies
conceal a much higher degree of variability in the individual responses, and an examination of individual records shows that the
ipsilateral and contralateral components can vary independently
in latency.  The peak latency of the contralateral negativity
(N105) may occur a few milliseconds before or after the corresponding ipsilateral positive wave (P100) in the same individual (see
Blumhardt et al., 1978), Fig. 4).

     Further evidence of the independence of the ipsilateral NPN
and the contralateral PNP complexes is provided by a study of the
effect of stimulating separately the central and more peripheral
areas of the 0 to 16 degree half-field.  This demonstrates not
only that the ipsilateral and contralateral components depend to
some extent upon stimulation of different areas of the half-field
but also that the contralateral components can be "masked" by the
ipsilateral ones (Blumhardt et al., 1978).  The response to the
full 0 to 16 degree right half-field shown in the left-hand record
of Fig. 3 has a large ipsilateral NPN complex and a rather small
and insignificant contralateral PNP complex.  When the stimulating
checkerboard is removed from the central 2.5 degrees of the right
half-field, however, the ipsilateral positive components are much
reduced in size, and a much larger contralateral PNP complex
appears (see second record in Fig. 3).  When the central 5 degrees
is masked, leaving the checkerboard stimulus in only the peripheral
portion of the right half-field from 5 to 16 degrees, the ipsilateral NPN complex is even more attenuated while the contralateral
PNP component has shown a slight further increase in amplitude
(third record, Fig. 3).  Only when the checkerboard stimulus is
masked out to 10 degrees is there a significant reduction in the
size of the contralateral PNP response.  It appears, therefore, as
if the ipsilateral NPN complex is evoked particularly by stimulation of the macular parts of the field, while the contralateral PNP
complex, which appears to be hidden in the full-field response in
many individuals, only becomes apparent when the central stimulus
is occluded.

Left Half Field Stimulus

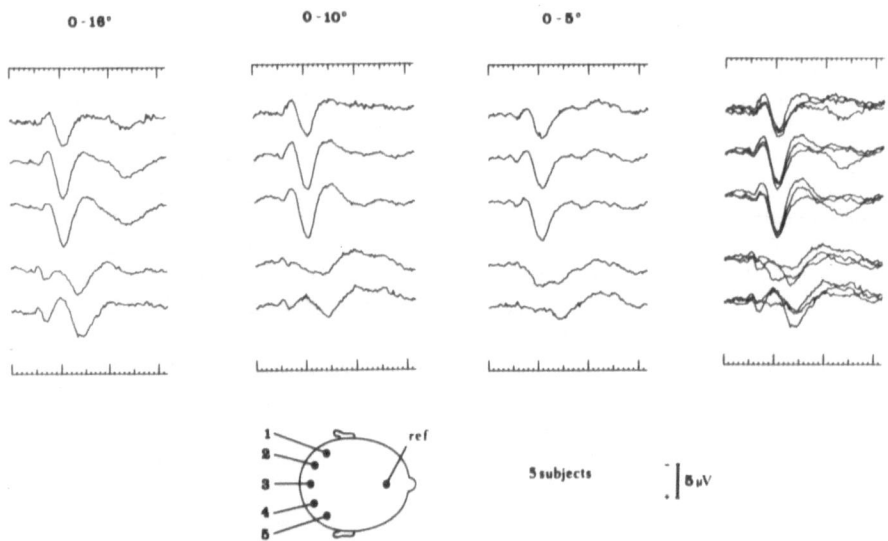

Fig. 4.   The effect of reducing the peripheral area of the left
half-field stimulus on the mean response waveform for five healthy
individuals.  The ipsilateral NPN complex is little affected by
the elimination of the peripheral checkerboard stimulus beyond 10
or 5 degrees (see superimposed responses in the right-hand column).
The contralateral PNP complex is, however, markedly attenuated.
(From Blumhardt et al., 1978.)


The dependence of the contralateral PNP complex on stimulation
of the paramacular areas of the half-field is well seen if the converse experiment is done, progressively occluding the peripheral
extent of the half-field stimulus (Fig. 4).  Since some individuals
show little or no contralateral complex in their normal half-field
response, this effect is best seen in the group mean response.
Reducing the half-field stimulus from 16 degrees to 10 and 5 degrees
has little effect on the ipsilateral NPN complex, since this depends
predominantly on stimulation of the macular area.  The contralateral
complex is, on the other hand, markedly attenuated when the peripheral areas are occluded (Fig. 4).

These results in healthy individuals help to explain the
characteristic changes in the pattern response which are encountered in patients with central scotomata (Halliday et al., 1976).  In
such patients, the normal major positive component of the pattern
reversal response is often completely replaced by a negative component at approximately the same latency.  Significantly, this nega-

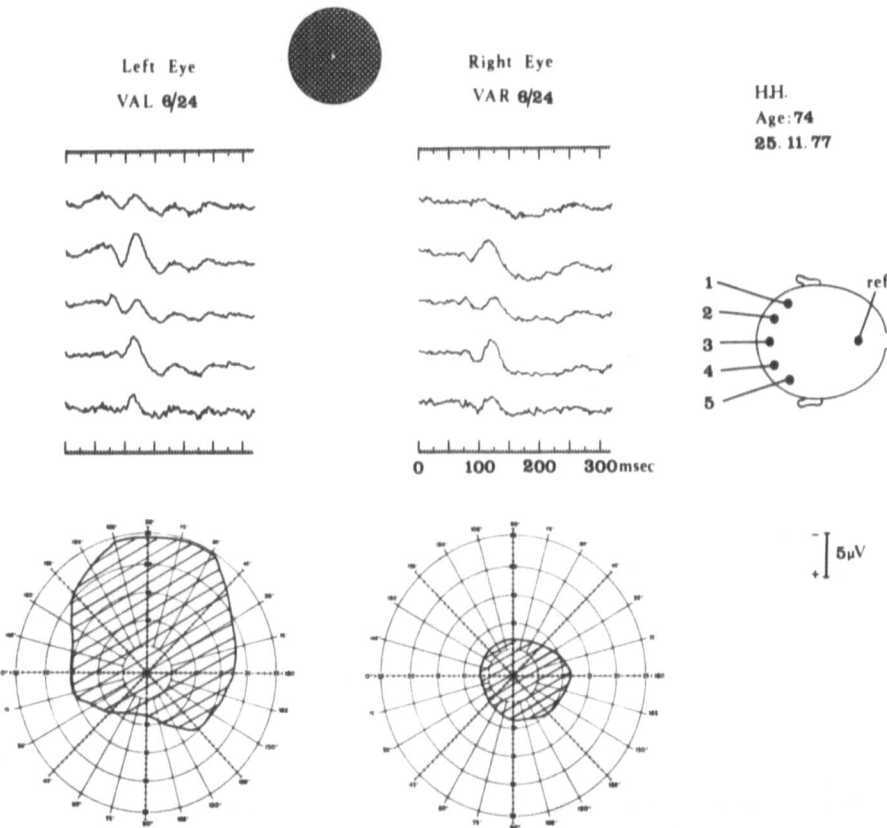

Fig. 5.   Response evoked by the full 0 to 16 degree checkerboard
stimulus from each eye of a 74 year old man with dense binocular
central scotomata due to toxic amblyopia.  Note the replacement
of the normal NPN complex, which has a midline maximum, by the
PNP complex at about the same latency which is of largest amplitude
at the electrodes on either side of the midline.


tivity no longer has a midline maximum but is larger at the lateral
electrodes, usually at the electrode 5 cm out on each side.   It
is, in fact, made up of a combination of the contralateral PNP complexes from the two half-fields (Fig. 5).   This can be clearly
demonstrated by half-field stimulation (Fig. 6).   The PNP complex
of the full-field response is then seen to have a contralateral
distribution for each half-field, while the ipsilateral channels,
where the major positivity normally appears as part of the NPN
complex, are relatively flat.  Lateralization of the responses by
half-field stimulation is, therefore, an important method of analyzing the components of the pattern evoked potential.

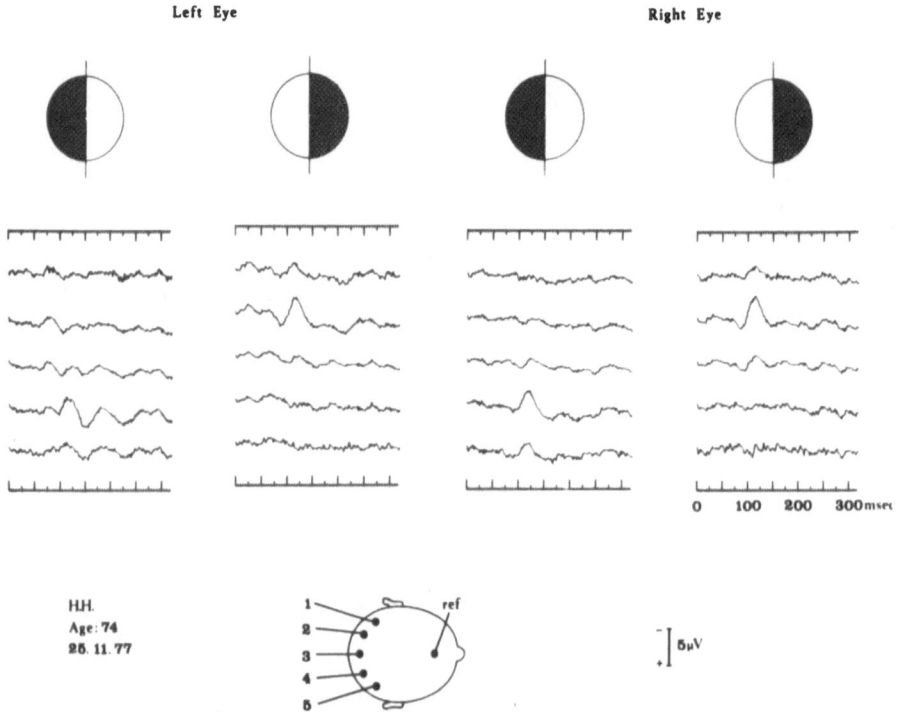

Fig. 6.  Half field responses from the patient whose full-field response was shown in Fig. 5.  Note that the PNP complexes of the full-field response are shown to have a contralateral distribution for each half-field stimulus.


However, a word of caution is necessary.  If correct lateralization is to be achieved, it is essential to adopt a suitable electrode montage.  The half-field response is so widespread over the back of the head that the choice of any reference within this area, such as the ipsilateral ear or mastoid, is liable to distort the record.  If the reference is to be truly indifferent, a location must be chosen which is well outside the area of the scalp from which the response comes.  Fig. 7 shows the same right half-field response recorded in a healthy individual with three different reference electrodes placed respectively on the left ear, midfrontally and on the right ear.  In this instance the standard transverse chain of five occipital electrodes spaced 5 cm apart has been augmented by two extra electrodes 2.5 cm out from the midline.  With the reference on the right ear, the amplitude of the ipsilateral NPN complex is greatly attenuated, because this is also picked up by the reference electrode.  Conversely, when the left ear reference is used, the contralateral PNP complex is slightly attenuated, because this, in turn, is picked up at the left ear.

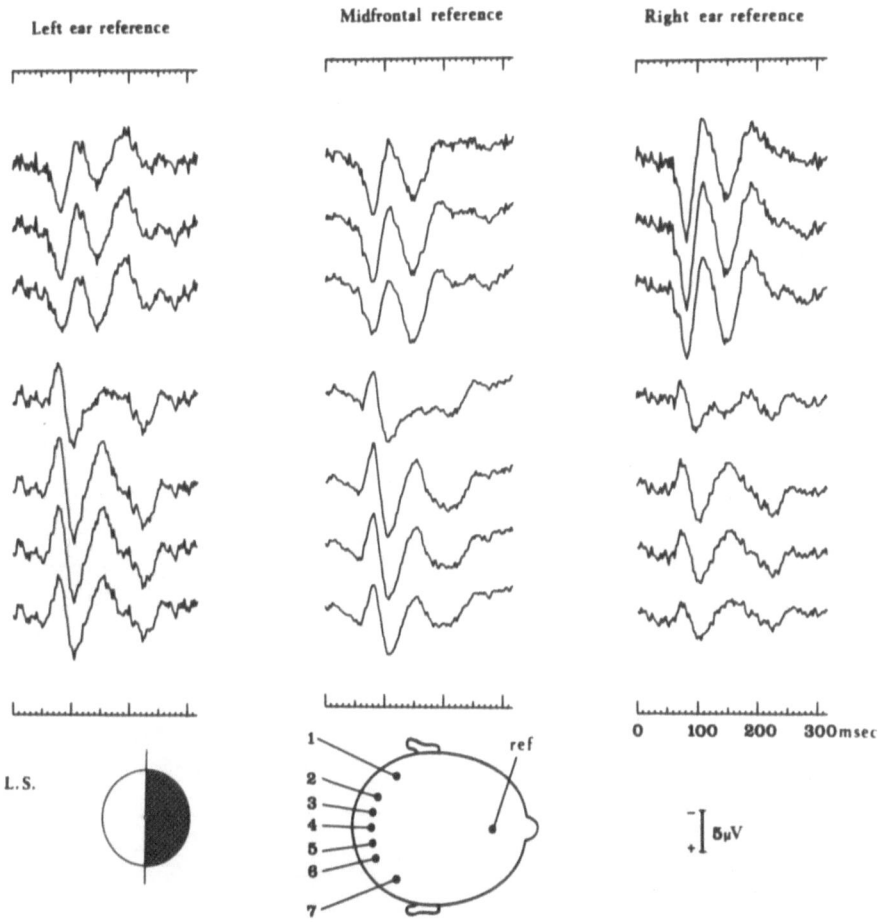

Fig. 7.  Right half-field response recorded from a healthy subject
with three different references.  Two extra electrodes, 2.5 cm out
from the midline, have been used to augment the standard transverse
row of five electrodes spaced 5 cm apart.  Note that the use of a
right ear reference greatly attenuates the ipsilateral NPN complex,
while the contralateral PNP complex is larger when this reference
is used.


     One can actually reverse the apparent lateralization of the
half-field response by the injudicious use of a lateralized reference and a less than optimum electrode montage.  Fig. 8 shows the
left half-field response recorded in a healthy subject in a variety
of ways.  The upper row of five records illustrates the response
recorded with the standard montage used in this study, the transverse row of five occipital electrodes, spaced at 5 cm intervals,

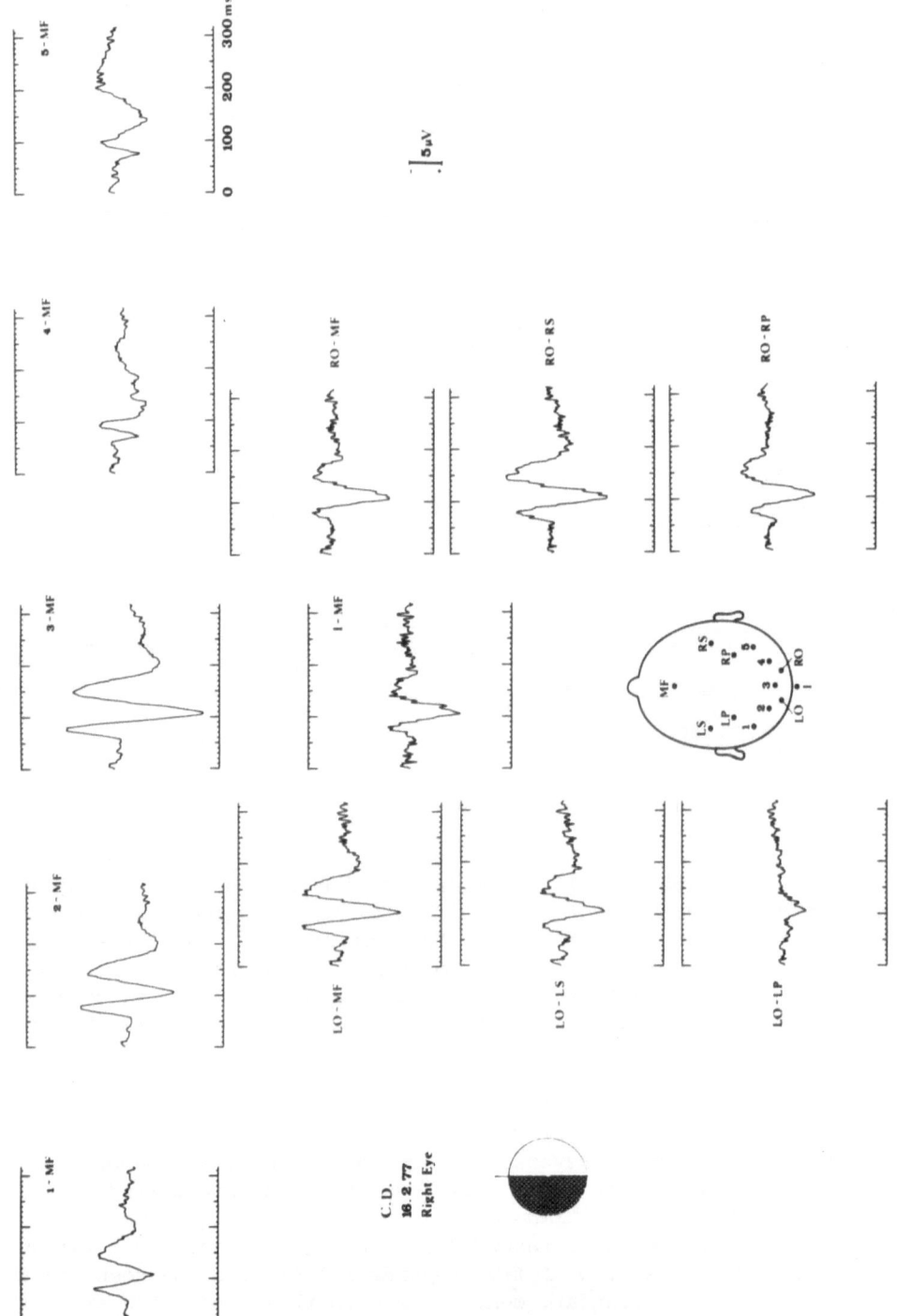

being all referred to a midfrontal reference.  With this montage
the major positive NPN complex is clearly lateralized ipsilaterally
to the half-field stimulated, although the maximum amplitude is
obtained at the midline electrode.  The two contralateral channels
record a typical PNP complex within the same latency range.  When
left and right occipital electrodes much nearer the midline are
used (as in the locations about 2 cms up and out, favored in the
modified Maudsley montage, and the slightly higher and more lateral
locations of the 10-20 system), the lateralization of the major
positivity of the NPN complex is much less clearly seen, because
there is some spread of the positivity over the midline, the transitional zone between ipsilateral and contralateral complexes being
well to the contralateral side of the midline.  This is evident in
the second row of records where the Maudsley left occipital (LO)
and right occipital (RO) electrodes are referred to the midfrontal
reference; the positivity is still larger for the ipsilateral
channel, but the amplitude difference is not very great.  When a
choice of electrodes too near the midline is compounded by the use
of a reference electrode on the same side of the head and within
the wide area from which the occipital response can be picked up,
a false impression of the lateralization of the response may be
obtained (cf. Holder, 1977, 1978).  In the third line of records the
left and right occipital electrode of the Maudsley montage have
been referred to Sylvian reference electrodes on the same side of
the head, and in the fourth line of records the same occipital
electrodes have been referred to left and right parietal references.  In both cases the lateralization of the major positivity
is apparently reversed and appears to be recorded from the side of

---

Fig. 8.  Pattern response from the left half-field of a healthy
subject recorded with different electrode montages.  The upper
five records are for the standard montage used throughout this
study, a transverse row of five occipital electrodes, spaced at
5 cm, referred to a common midfrontal reference.  Note the distribution of the NPN complex in the midline and ipsilateral channels
and the smaller PNP complex seen at the two contralateral electrodes.
The lower records are taken with the left occipital (LO) and right
occipital (RO) electrode of the modified Maudsley montage referred
(from above down) to a common midfrontal reference to a Sylvian
electrode on the same side of the head and to a parietal electrode
on the same side of the head.  Note that the NPN complex is seen
for both channels with the midfrontal reference because the electrodes are only 2 cm from the midline.  With the ipsilateral Sylvian
or parietal reference the NPN complex is mislateralized, appearing
larger in the contralateral channel.  This is because the response
is picked up and partially cancelled by the Sylvian and parietal
references on the left side of the head, but not on the right.

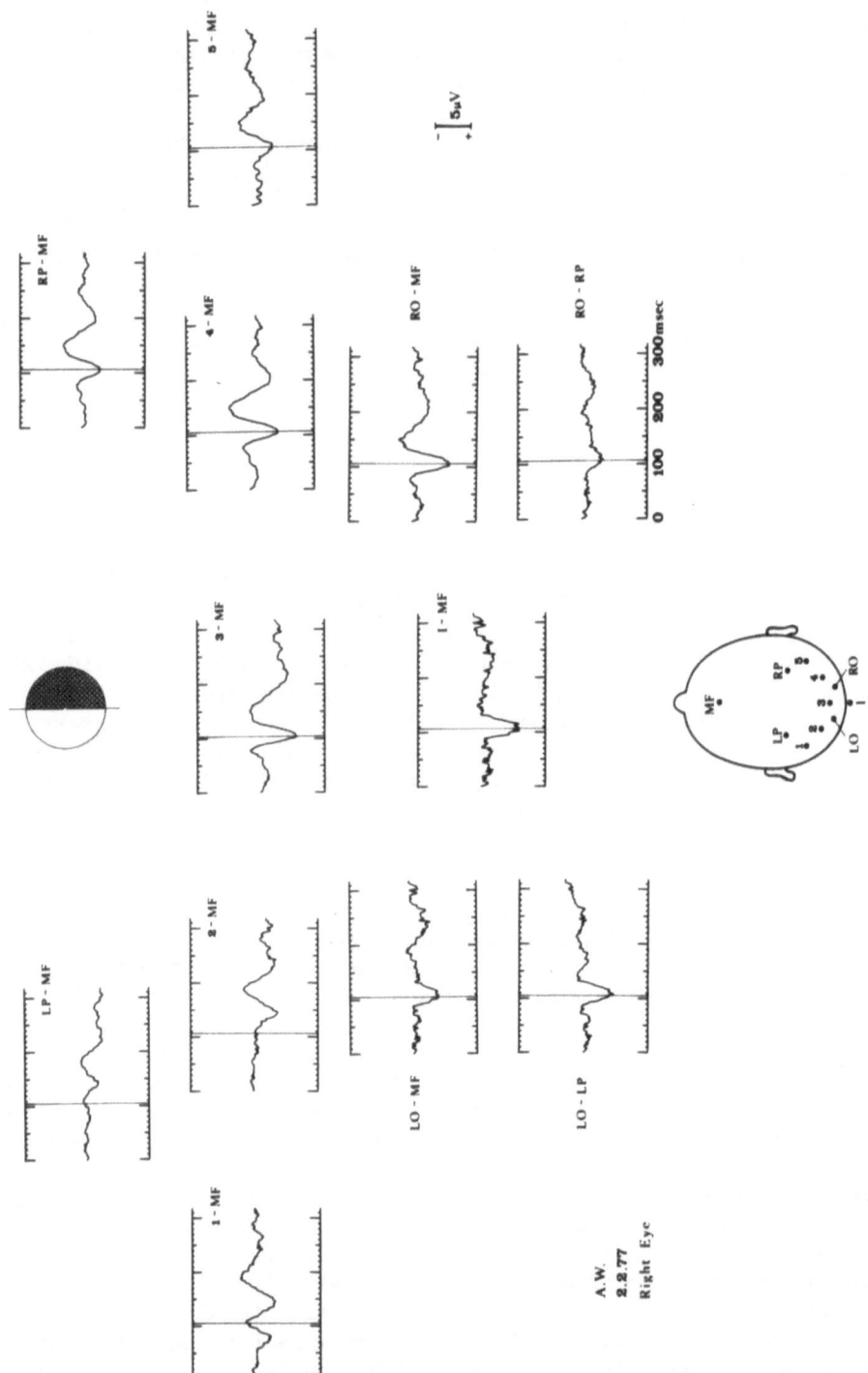

the head contralateral to the half-field stimulated.  This is
because both parietal and Sylvian references on the left side of
the head are picking up something of the ipsilateral response.
The response is, therefore, attenuated in the left occipital channel,
which uses this reference, but is unattenuated in the right occipital channel, because this is referred to the right-sided
reference.  The parietal electrode picks up more of the response
than the Sylvian, owing to its more posterior location, and there
is a correspondingly more marked attenuation of the NPN complex
at the ipsilateral occipital electrode.

Fig. 9 shows a similar example for right half-field stimulation in another healthy subject.  Again the choice of occipital
electrodes too near the midline, referred to a parietal electrode
on the same side, leads to an apparent mislateralization of the
response.  It can be demonstrated by recording the parietal
"references" against the midfrontal electrode that this effect is
due to the ipsilateral parietal electrode picking up the response
(see top right channel) and, thus, attenuating it when it is used
as a reference for the occipital electrode.  The left parietal
electrode produces no such attentuation when used as a reference
for the left occipital channel, because it is on the side of the
head contralateral to the half-field stimulated.  The net result
again is that the major positivity appears to be larger at the
occipital electrode contralateral to the half-field stimulated.
This, however, is misleading, being entirely due to the cancellation occurring between pairs of ipsilateral electrodes because of
the widespread distribution and large amplitude of the response
over the ipsilateral half of the back of the head.

The use of half-field stimulation enables the subcomponents
of the response to be identified as being either ipsilateral or
contralateral.  This can help to resolve many of the ambiguities
which arise in interpreting abnormal pattern response records in
clinical practice.  Fig. 10 shows a typical "crossed" asymmetry
recorded in a 48 year-old man with a suprasellar mass and bitemporal hemianopia.  The P100 component is seen for each eye on the
side ipsilateral to the preserved nasal field, i.e., in the midline

---

Fig. 9.   Pattern response from the right half-field of another
healthy subject to illustrate the effect of electrode montage and
reference.  Note, as in Fig. 8, the apparent mislateralization of
the major positivity for the parietal reference montage (lower
pair of records).  The upper pair of records, from the parietal
references referred to the common midfrontal electrode, demonstrate
that the response is picked up by the parietal reference electrode
on the right side of the head.

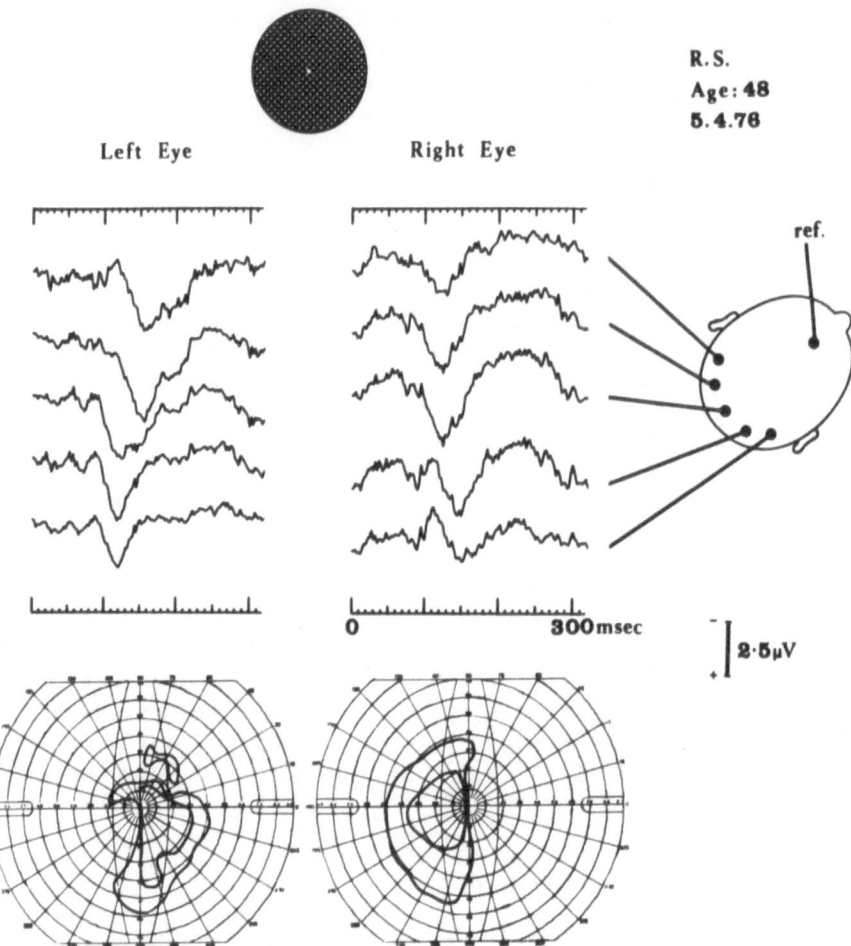

Fig. 10.   Crossed asymmetry in a 48 year old man with a suprasellar
mass and bitemporal hemianopia.   The P100 component is seen ipsilateral to the preserved nasal field from each eye.   Note the large
later positivity recorded from the two channels on the other side
of the head.

and right-sided channels for the left eye response and in the midline and left-sided channels for the right eye response.   There is
also a large, somewhat later positivity on the contralateral side,
particularly prominent in the response from the left eye.   Such
large contralateral positivities have been previously observed and
commented on in the records of patients with compressive lesions
affecting the chiasma (Halliday et al., 1976).   In the absence of
information about the half-field responses, this contralateral

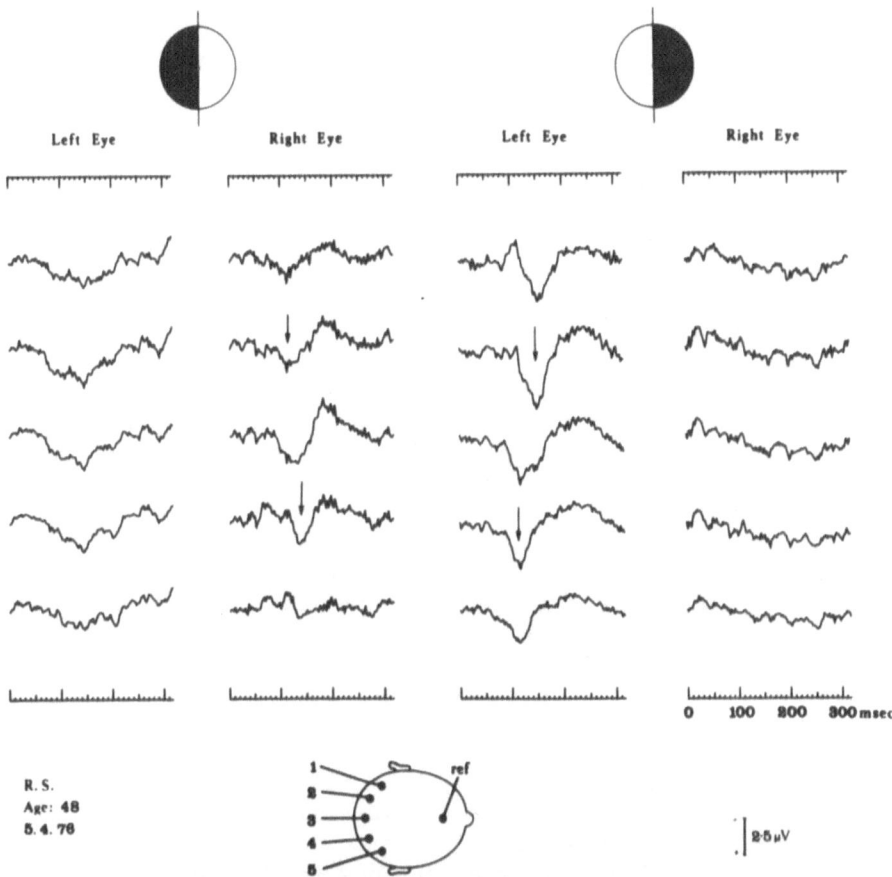

Fig. 11.   Half-field responses from the same patient as in Fig. 10.
Note that all the major features of the full-field response, shown
in Fig. 10, are arising from stimulation of the nasal half-field of
each eye.   In particular, the later contralateral positive wave is
seen to be the P135 component of the contralateral PNP complex of
the half-field response, and not a delayed P100 component arising
from the temporal half-field.

positivity can be interpreted as a delayed P100 from the temporal
half-fields consequent upon the compression of the fibers crossing
in the optic chiasma.   Stimulation of the two half-fields separately (Fig. 11) shows conclusively that this is not the case.   The
"contralateral" positivity, like the ipsilateral P100, is seen in
the responses from the preserved nasal half-fields, and not in the
temporal half-fields.   This component, therefore, represents a large
third component of the contralateral PNP complex (P135).   Since the

evidence from hemispherectomized patients establishes that both
ipsilateral and contralateral components of the half-field response
are produced in the same hemisphere, there is no question of
invoking a delay in the chaismal fibers to explain this response.
This is simply one example of the clarification which can be gained
by the use of half-field stimulation.  We are now using it routinely in clinical practice.


                              SUMMARY


    The occipital potential evoked by a reversing black and white
checkerboard is made up of the addition of the left and right
half-field responses, each originating from the contralateral
hemisphere.  Since the whole field response closely approximates
the algebraic sum of the two half-field responses, there is no
evidence of any significant interaction between the generators in
each hemisphere.

    Within each half-field response, the three components of the
triphasic NPN complex recorded from midline and ipsilateral
electrodes (N175, P100, N145) appear to behave independently from
the components of the PNP complex recorded contralaterally (P75,
N105, P135).  The "ipsilateral" P100 component is evoked particularly by pattern stimulation of the foveal area, while the
"contralateral" N105 component depends on parafoveal stimulation.
The components can be independently enhanced or attenuated by
varying the area stimulated in each half-field.  Occlusion of the
central stimulus attenuates the P100 component, with a consequent
enhancement of the N105.  The same changes in the pattern response
occur pathologically in patients with central scotoma.  A converse
attenuation of the contralateral negativity can occur when the
stimulus is removed from the parafoveal region.

    Many of the ambiguities arising in the clinical use of pattern
EPs can be resolved if the nature of these components is understood.
Correct lateralization of the half-field components depends on the
use of a truly indifferent reference, such as a midfrontal electrode, while misleading appearances may result from reliance on
more posteriorly or laterally placed references, such as an earlobe
or parietal electrode.  Clear identification of the components by
lateralization also enables one to distinguish between the P100 and
the P135 components, which may otherwise be confused and lead to
ambiguity when the problem is one of differentiating delays from
scotomatous changes.

REFERENCES

Barrett, G., Blumhardt, L., Halliday, A.M., Halliday, E. and
    Kriss, A.  A paradox in the lateralisation of the visual
    evoked response.  Nature, 1976, 261, 253-255.

Blumhardt, L.D., Barrett, G. and Halliday, A.M.  The asymmetrical
    visual evoked potential to pattern reversal in one half-field
    and its significance for the analysis of visual field defects.
    Brit. J. Ophthal., 1977, 61, 454-461.

Blumhardt, L.D., Barrett, G., Halliday, A.M. and Kriss, A.  The
    effect of experimental "scotoma" on the ipsilateral and
    contralateral responses to pattern-reversal in one half-field.
    Electroenceph. Clin. Neurophysiol., 1978, 45, 376-392.

Blumhardt, L.D. and Halliday, A.M.  Hemisphere contributions to
    the composition of the pattern evoked potential waveform.
    Exp. Brain Res., in press.

Halliday, A.M.  Visually evoked responses in optic nerve disease.
    Trans. Ophthal. Soc. U.K., 1976, 96, 372-376.

Halliday, A.M. Halliday, E., Kriss, A., McDonald, W.I. and Mushin,
    J.  The pattern evoked potential in compression of the
    anterior visual pathways.  Brain, 1976, 99, 357-374.

Holder, G.E.  The pattern VER in chiasmal compression.  Electro-
    enceph. Clin. Neurophysiol., 1977, 43, 772-773.

Holder, G.E.  The effects of chiasmal compression on the pattern
    visual evoked response.  Electroenceph. Clin. Neurophysiol.,
    1978, 44, 278-280.

Michael, W.F. and Halliday, A.M.  Differences between the occipital
    distribution of upper and lower field pattern evoked responses
    in man.  Brain Res., 1971, 32, 311-324.

# THE EFFECTS OF METHYLPHENIDATE DOSAGE ON THE VISUAL EVENT RELATED POTENTIAL OF HYPERACTIVE CHILDREN

R. Halliday, E. Callaway, J. Rosenthal and H. Naylor

Langley Porter Neuropsychiatric Institute

University of California, San Francisco, California 94143

Hyperkinetic children have a disorder of attention, and that disorder can be reduced by giving stimulant drugs (Barkley, 1977). Unfortunately, the process of attention itself remains something of a mystery. So, naturally both the disorder of attention in hyperkinesis and the beneficial effects of stimulants are also unclear. The sensory ERP reveals something of the sequence of brain operations that follow a stimulus and thus provides a temporal dissection of operations potentially involved in attention. We have been employing ERP to study the interaction of attention and stimulants in hyperkinetic children in the hope of clarifying the nature of attention, its disorder in hyperkinesis and the effect of the stimulant methylphenidate.

## METHOD

### Subjects

The subjects in this experiment were nineteen hyperactive boys referred to us by the Learning Disabilities Clinic, Kaiser Permanente Medical Center, Oakland, California. Diagnostic criteria were similar to those applied to a previous series of children (Halliday et al., 1976). In addition, however, each child in the experiment was rated by his teacher on the Conners Teacher Rating Scale (Conners, 1969) at least two standard deviations above current norms. This scale has been found to differentiate hyperactive children from normals (Cohen et al., 1974) and is sensitive to the effects of methylphenidate even at relatively low doses.

Parents of the children were referred to our project if the pediatrician felt that a clinical trial of methylphenidate was indicated. The project was then explained to the parents and voluntary consent obtained. Treatment was not contingent on participation in the project. Preliminary to actual acceptance, the pediatrician administered 5, 10 and 20 milligrams of methylphenidate to test for possible allergic or other deviant responses.

## Evoked Potential Procedures

Visual evoked potential (VEP) activity, heart rate and reaction time during the attended portions of the experiment were recorded from each child on four different sessions. A placebo capsule was always administered on Session #1. In the remaining sessions the child took three different dosages of methylphenidate 45-60 minutes before the start of a run. The active dosages were 0.16 (low), 0.33 (medium) and 0.66 (high) milligrams methylphenidate/kilograms body weight (mg/kg). For an 80 pound youngster (36 kg), this dosage would be 5, 10 and 20 mg of Ritalin. Order of drug administration was randomly assigned to one of three possible sequences.

The entire experiment was controlled by a small laboratory computer (NOVA 1220). A schematic of this system is shown in Fig. 1. Visual evoked potentials were recorded from a single vertex electrode (Cz) referred to linked ears in the first eight children. In the next eleven children, parietal (Pz) and frontal (Fz) electrodes were added to this montage. Eye movement and cardiac activity were monitored by Beckman electrodes. The EEG was amplified by standard EEG electronics with filters set at 1 and 35 Hz. The trial sequence was initiated by the R-wave of the cardiac cycle which triggered a brief pulse to the computer. A 50 msec flash of light followed 150 msec after this initializing pulse. This delay prevented the R-wave from contaminating the VEP activity. The next trial was randomly initiated after the second, third or fourth R-waves. The interbeat intervals between R-waves on each trial were stored and the means and standard deviations printed out at the termination of the experimental condition, but this data will not be reported here.

The EEG was sampled every 4 msec beginning 50 msec prestimulus and continued over a 1000 msec interval. Individual trials and the averaged VEP were stored on the computer floppy disk system for subsequent analysis. Reaction time and response accuracy in the attending tasks were also stored.

The within-sessions conditions consisted of an active-attending task (ATT) and a passive-observing task (PAS). Whenever possible, one or both tasks were repeated. The number of replications was, however, unequal due to the fact that some children found it diffi-

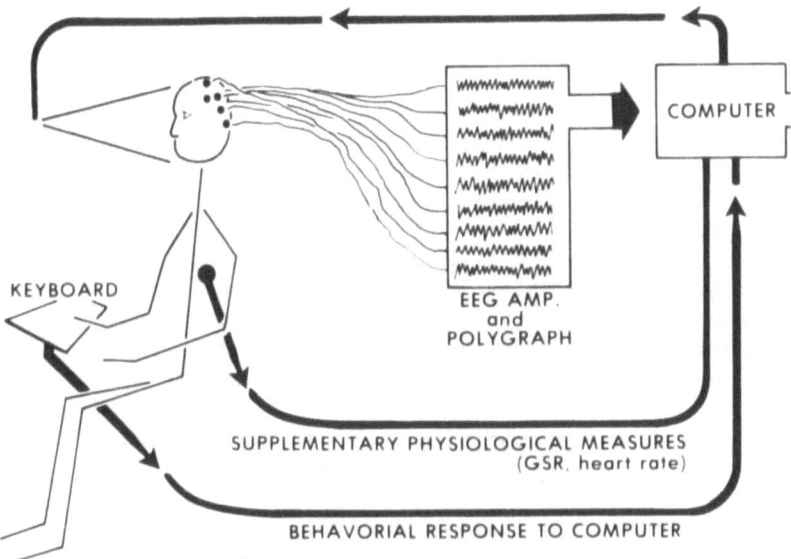

Fig. 1.   Schematic of ERP system

cult to stay attentive during the later portions of the experiment.
For the ATT task, the child was asked to press a microswitch whenever he detected a dim flash (signal) embedded in a series of bright-
er flashes (nonsignals).  Signal events occurred in 10% of the trials,
and each correct detection earned a 10¢ reward.  Heart rate and VEP
data for approximately 100 nonsignals were collected in each attending sequence.  In the PAS task, the child was requested to simply
observe the flashes.  A special eye movement algorithm continuously
computed activity from the eye electrodes and tagged records that
exceeded present levels.  These records were excluded from the computation of the averaged VEP.  Intertrial interval varied between
two and four seconds.  Each attentional run took approximately ten
minutes.  Thus, each session, with appropriate rest periods, required
30-45 minutes to complete.

     The child was seated in a comfortable chair in a sound atten-
uated, electrically shielded room.  Signal and nonsignal stimuli
were delivered by a small box located 153 cm from the child.  Before
the start of each session the child was given sufficient practice to
ensure that he understood the procedures.  He was encouraged to sit
quietly during the run and cautioned against irregular breathing or
looking around the room.

RESULTS

Prior to any analysis, the data for each child was examined
trial by trial, and any records with obvious contaminants were
tagged and excluded from analysis.  In general, very few artifacts
were observed, suggesting that our on-line artifact rejection procedure was adequate.  The ERP data were analyzed in several ways.
Only the data for the Cz electrode will be reported.  We followed
the traditional procedure of having an experienced psychophysiolo-
gist pick the large negative (N1) and positive (P2) peaks visually
while blind to dose and type of attention.  The computer then recorded amplitude from prestimulus baseline and latency from stimulus.
Then, for each measure, an ANOVA was done with AGE (under ten years
and over ten years), DOSE (none, low, medium, high) and ATTENTION
(active or passive) as conditions.  To reduce the amount of missing
data, the data were averaged over replications.

The amplitude of N1 (N159) showed a significant AGE X DOSE X
ATTENTION effect (F = 3.2; df = 3,51) and a near significant (P<.07)
AGE X DOSE effect.  These effects are shown in Figs. 2 and 3.  In the
younger children, increasing doses of methylphenidate increased the
N1 although this effect was more dramatic in the passive-observing
condition.  In the older children, the effects of dosage were quite  ·
different for the two tasks.  N1 in the attending condition showed
a significant increase up to the medium (.33 mg/kg) dose.  Further
increases in dosage precipitated a dramatic decrease in amplitude.
In the passive task, N1 amplitude declined gradually throughout
the dosage range.

Latency of N159 showed a significant linear AGE X DOSE component (F = 7.57; df = 1,17).  This effect is shown in Fig. 4.
Younger children showed an increase in latency up to the medium
dose while older children showed a decrease.

The P228 amplitude showed a significant DOSE X ATTENTION interaction (F = 3.0; df = 3,51) and is shown in Fig. 5.  Amplitude
dropped with increasing dosage with the major effects occurring in
the attending condition.  P228 latency showed no significant effects.

The ERP data from the first eight subjects had been previously
studied by factor analytic technique, and this was repeated on this
larger group.  Each subject supplied up to sixteen ERPs (four doses,
two replications, two attention conditions).  The set of ERPs from
each subject was normalized to remove individual characteristics.
To do this, a mean ERP was computed over all of the subject's ERPs,
as well as the standard deviations.  Thus, there was a mean and a
standard deviation at each time point.  Then for each individual
ERP at each time point, that appropriate mean was subtracted, and
the results were divided by the appropriate standard deviation.

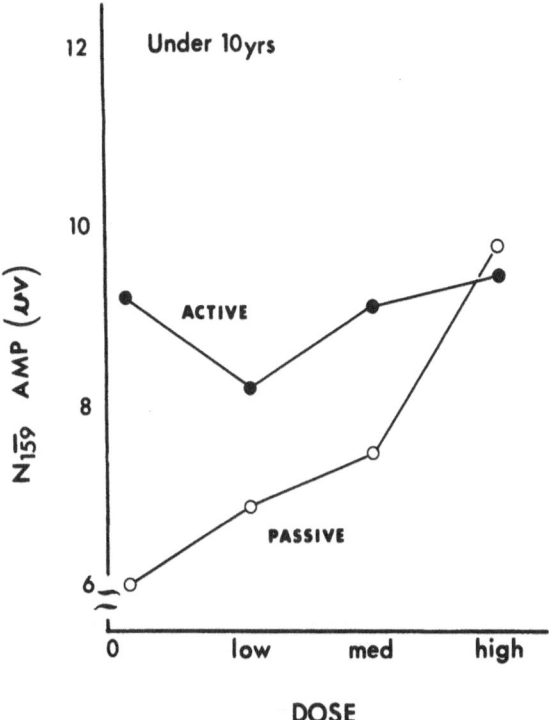

Fig. 2.   Methylphenidate dose/response curves for N159 amplitude
in hyperactive children under ten years.


The result was an ERP measured in standard scores rather than in
voltage.   The correlation matrix of these normalized ERPs was then
factored by principal components analysis.   Nine factors were extracted to account for 81% of the variance, and these were treated
by Varimax rotation.   Factor scores were then derived to characterize each component of the experimental paradigm, and these scores
were submitted to ANOVA.   Of the nine factors, six yielded F ratios
in their respective ANOVAs at the .05 level or better.   These factors
are illustrated in Fig. 6.

     Before discussing these factors, one thing should be noted.
Factor #9, which is not shown, seems to represent the N159 msec component which in our previous factor analysis performed much as the
N1 peak amplitude performed in this analysis.   While in the present
factor analysis this particular factor showed an effect of attention
which was significant at the .06 level, it showed no significant
interaction with dose or age.

     Returning to the figure, Factor #1 behaves much as the P2 com-
ponent in the conventional analysis.   There is a significant DRUG X

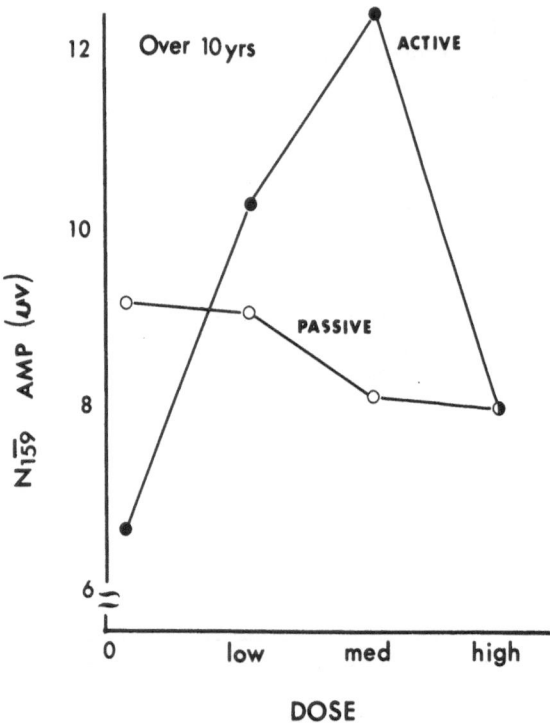

Fig. 3.  Methylphenidate dose/response curves for N̄159 amplitude in
hyperactive children over ten years.

ATTENTION effect (F = 2.9; df = 3,51) that decreases linearly with
dose.  This effect is best seen in the older subjects in the attending condition.  Factor #4 (approximately 400 msec) is principally an
age effect which is consistent with the increase in amplitude of
later components in older children that has been noted by many other
observers.  Factor #5 (approximately 50 msec) is something of a surprise.  This very early component shows a strong DOSE effect (F = 3.8;
df = 3,51) and an AGE X DOSE X ATTENTION effect (F = 3.6; df = 3,51).
This is a complex factor and will require replication before too much
is made of it.  Factor #6 (approximately 300 msec) is a pure
ATTENTION effect (F = 4.9; df = 1,17).  It appears to be the usual
P300.  Factor #7 (approximately 750 msec) is a very late component
which shows a significant quadratic DOSE effect (F = 7.1; df = 1,17)
and an AGE X DOSE effect (F = 2.8; df  3,17).  These effects are
highly significant and unexpected.  They are illustrated in Fig. 7.
Finally, Factor #8 yields both a linear DOSE (F = 7.5; df = 1,17)
and an AGE X DOSE X ATTENTION (F = 3.2; df = 3,51) effect.  This 450
msec component appears principally as a linear dose increase that
is most marked in the younger subjects during the active attention
task.

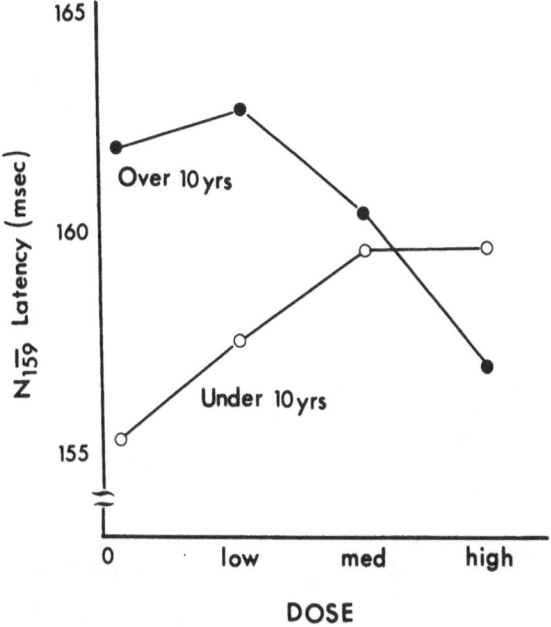

Fig. 4.   Methylphenidate dose effects on N̄159 latency in two age
groups of hyperactive children.

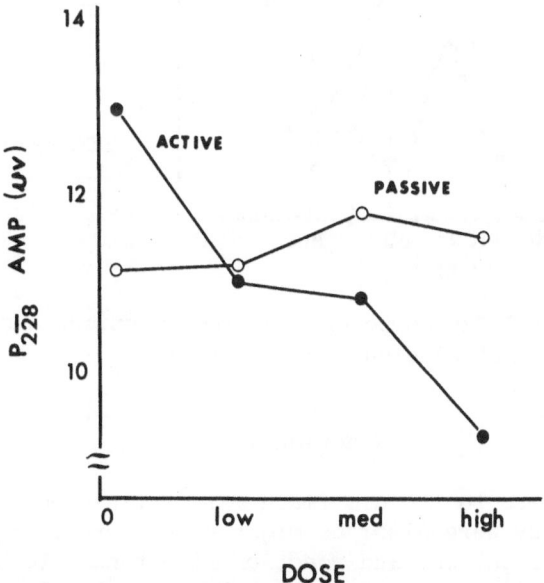

Fig. 5.   Methylphenidate dose/response curves for P̄228 amplitude
in active and passive observing conditions.

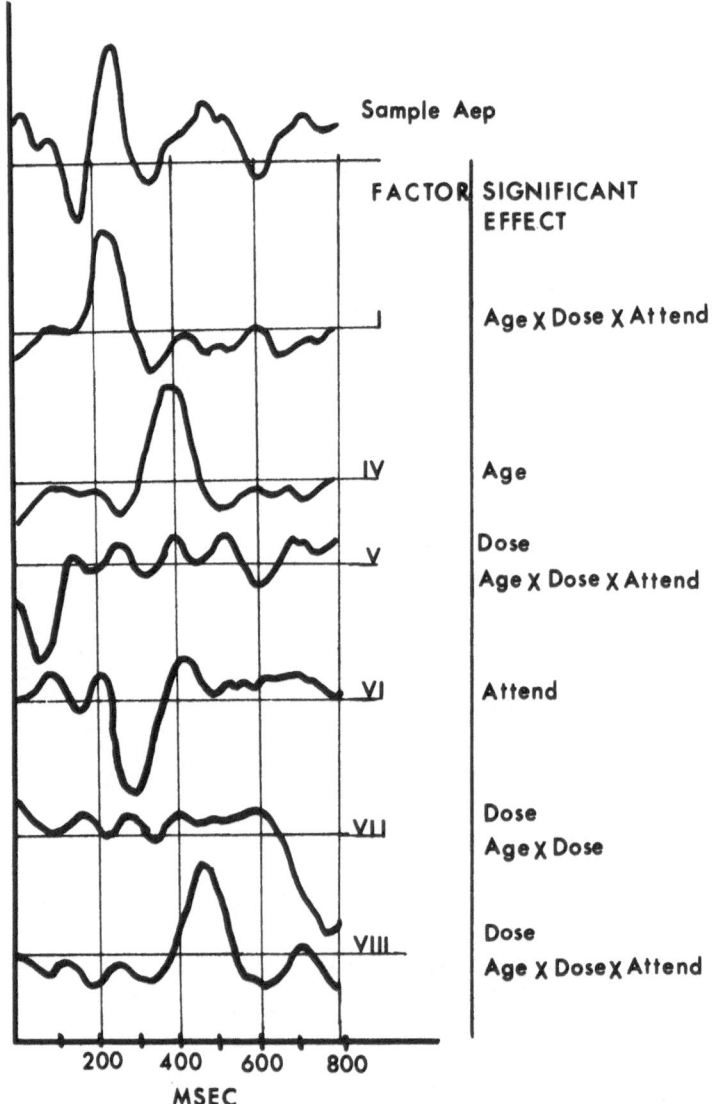

Fig. 6. Normalized ERP component loading functions and experimental conditions which yielded significant effects.


## Reaction Time

Reaction times to the dim flash were influenced both by age and by dose. They were also, as might be expected, significantly increased by replication, and reaction time tended to be faster in later trials than in earlier trials. In general, older children were faster (F = 6.5; df = 1,17) as would be expected. DOSE effects were significant (F = 13.3; df = 3,51) with significant linear and quadratic components. This is illustrated in Fig. 8.

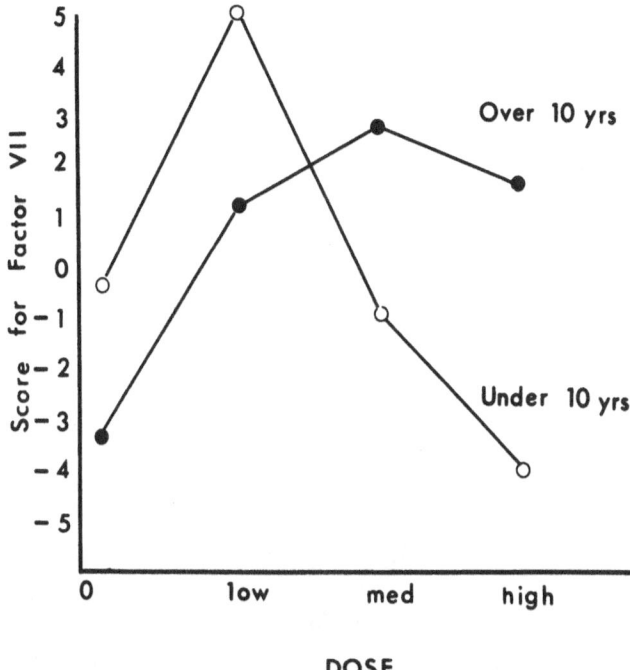

DOSE

Fig. 7.  Methylphenidate dose/response curves for factor loadings
on Factor #7 (450 msec) in two age groups of hyperactive children.

Higher dose produced a slight increment in speed for the older
children and a near significant slowing for the younger children.
Reaction time variability also decreased with DOSE (F = 3.8; df =
3,51) but showed neither AGE, nor AGE X DOSE effects.

DISCUSSION

In general, our findings suggest that the effects of methylphenidate to nonsignal stimuli are far more complicated than previously
realized.  In the analysis of conventional N1 and P2 components
of the ERP neither age, dose nor attention produce first order
effects.  Dose plays a role in all of the interactions, but dose
effects are different, depending upon the particular component being
analyzed and the method used to measure it.

The nonmonotonic increase in N159 amplitude during active-attending with increasing dosage has been previously reported (Elliott et
al., in press).  However, the inverted-U shape function appears to
be restricted to older children.  Younger children show a different
function in which dosage exerts its principal effect during the passive-observing task.  Latency also changed with dose and age.  With

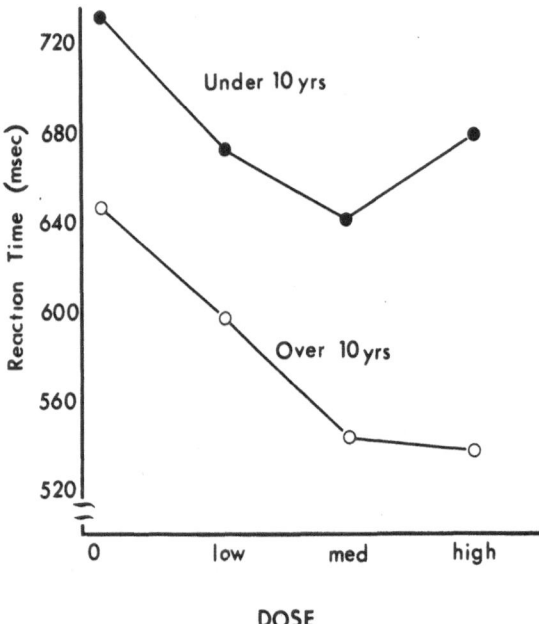

Fig. 8. Methylphenidate dosage effects on reaction time in two age groups of hyperactive children.

increasing dosage, the latency of younger children increased while older children showed a marked decrease. P2 (P228), however, did not show an age effect and the effect of dosage was to decrease the amplitude of this component in the attending condition. Thus, when N1 and P2 are measured independently, rather than peak-to-trough, the components are seen to respond differently to variations in the experimental paradigm.

In general, the principal components factor analysis produced components which appear reasonable. Most of the factor components were unimodal and occurred in the expected time bands. However, some of the factor analysis components did not show the same dose/ response functions as did the analogous components picked visually. Factor #9, for example, appeared to be the N159 component. Yet, this factor did not show a significant AGE X DOSE X ATTENTION interaction. It may well be that the effects of methylphenidate are obscured by a method that ignores individual differences in N1 latencies.

We had previously suggested that methylphenidate acted principally on the 100-200 msec portion of the ERP (Callaway et al., 1978). The present results, however, indicate that the effects are not as restricted as we had proposed. Dose interacted with age and attention in both the early (50 msec) component and the 450 msec late

component.  Additionally, a very late component (750 msec) was affected by age and dose.  While the effects of methylphenidate on
late ERP activity are consistent with the work of Klorman (1978),
the effects on the 50 msec component are surprising.  However, we
note that a recent study by Sohmer and Student (1978) has reported
delays in the central transmission time of far field potentials in
hyperactive children, thus opening up the possibility that early
cortical activity may be delayed and perhaps affected by stimulants.

The present findings reconcile some apparently discrepant reports in the literature.  For example, with low doses of stimulants
we find speeding of reaction time but very little effect on the
event related potential.  This confirms a report of Hink et al.
(1978) who obtained similar results in adults given 10 mg of methylphenidate.  By contrast, we find a reduction in P2 amplitude and a
shortening of N1 latency at very high doses.  This is confirmatory
of the findings reported by Velasco et al. (1977) who gave 40-50 mg
dextroamphetamine to adults and noticed a reduction in the P200
amplitude.

Age appears to be one of the most interesting factors.  Indeed,
had we not taken age into account, many of the effects noted would
have simply disappeared.  Satterfield and Braley (1977) have reported striking age differences in auditory ERPs of normals and
hyperactives.  They suggested that younger hyperactives may be
hyperaroused relative to older hyperactives.  This hypothesis predicts that increasing arousal with a stimulant would make the
older hyperactive child look increasingly like younger hyperactives
without stimulant.  This suggestion finds some confirmation in our
N159 data.  In particular, older hyperactive children show a decrease in N159 amplitude for the passive-observing task with stimulant, making their values approach those of young subjects without
drugs.  Stimulants also make the older subjects have shorter N159
latencies, again more like the younger drug-free subjects.  However,
their theory does not explain why increasing dosage should increase
the amplitude of the N159 component in younger children.  The only
other data published on age differences in hyperactive children was
by Buchsbaum and Wender (1973).  They found, as we did, that younger
children show faster N159 latencies.

Several other age related phenomena can also be cited as
playing a role in the differences observed in this report.  For
example, the diagnosis of hyperactivity is much easier to make at
age ten years than at age seven years and there is some evidence
that clinical response is somewhat better in older children (Loney
et al., 1978; Halliday et al., in press).  Thus, older hyperactives
may be a more homogeneous group than younger hyperactives with
respect to the primary underlying symptom of this disorder.  Finally,
developmental changes in cognitive skills may account for the age

effects noted. Hagen and Hale (1975), for example, have noted that
young children are more likely to attend to stimuli that are peripheral to a central task than older children. If stimulants act on
attentional capabilities, then age dependent responses to stimulants would be anticipated.

The present data suggests that N159 and P228 represent different levels of stimulus selection in the total attentive process.
N159 may reflect a channel selection or wide band filter, and P228
a narrower band process. Arousal and attention interact to narrow
the focus of both processes. Thus, with increasing stimulant, a
non-target stimulus in the relevant modality is quickly excluded by
the narrow process, while it continues to receive more energy from
the broader focused process. As focusing continues the broader
process also comes to exclude the non-target.

To be more graphic, consider the multidimensional field over
which selective attention operates as reduced to two dimensions.
The non-target stimulus is imagined as a light-sensitive device
slightly removed from the target stimulus itself, which is the focal
point of two spotlights. The two spotlights have a variable focus
and illuminate in sequence the spot that represents the stimulus.
The energy of the first light on the spot produces N1 - and that of
the second, P2. As stimulant dose increases and the focus narrows,
the N1 light is first concentrated on the spot, while the P2 light
begins to exclude it. So N1 increases and P2 falls. Then, as
focusing continues, the N1 light also begins to exclude the stimulus-
spot, and N1 also begins to fall.

This scheme is testable. One can use stimuli that are more
distant from the target as, for example, stimuli in a different
modality. We would then expect the N1 for the more remote stimulus
to show a nearly monotonic decrease like the P2 of the less distant
stimulus. P3 of the central stimulus would, however, show a nearly
monotonic increase.

This theory is sure to be wrong, at least in some details, but
provides a useful framework for a start. Such ERP dissection of
attention allows us to take a new look at concepts of arousal-
induced narrowed attention. Such ideas have been of some interest
in the past (Callaway and Stone, 1960; Easterbrook, 1959), but
could not be pursued effectively in the laboratory at that time.
This ERP dose/response paradigm promises to be a new and effective
tool for application to this problem.

SUMMARY

Visual event related potentials were examined in nineteen

hyperactive (HA) children under four different dosages of methylphenidate and two levels of attention.  Dosage had a significant
effect on the VERP but specific findings were found to depend on
the child's age, level of attention and the component measured.  In
HAs over ten years, N159 amplitude in the attending condition bore
an inverted-U shape relationship to dosage.  In HAs under ten years,
the amplitude of this component increased linearly with dosage but
this effect was only found in the passive-observing condition.  N159
latency increased with dosage in younger children but decreased in
older HAs.  P228 amplitude decreased linearly with dosage in the
attending condition but showed no significant age effects.

A principal components factor analysis was computed on normalized VERP waveforms.  Factor scores describing each of the experimental conditions were obtained and analyzed by ANOVA.  Nine factors
were extracted and five of these were affected by dosage in combination with either age or attention.  Dosage effects were found in both
early and later components.

The relevance of these findings to other studies was discussed.
A two stage modal of attention was proposed, and the use of VERP dose/
response curves as a method for untangling various attentional mechanisms was presented.

ACKNOWLEDGEMENTS

This research was supported by a National Institute of Mental
Health Research Grant MH-22149 and a gift from CIBA Pharmaceutical
Co.

REFERENCES

Barkley, R. A., A review of stimulant drug research with hyperactive
    children.  J.  Child Psychology and Psychiatry, 1977, 18,
    137-165.

Buchsbaum, M and Wender, P., Averaged evoked responses in normal and
    minimally brain dysfunctioned children treated with amphetamine.
    Arch. Gen. Psychiat., 1973, 29, 754-770.

Callaway, E. and Stone, G., Re-evaluating focus of attention, L. Uhr
    and J. G. Miller (Eds.), Drugs and Behavior, New York: John
    Wiley and Sons, 1960.

Callaway, E., Halliday, R., Naylor, H. and Rosenthal, J., Early
    attention defect in minimal brain dysfunction.  Presented at
    annual meeting of Biological Psychiatry, Atlanta, Georgia,
    May 3-7, 1978.

Cohen, M. N., McNutt, B. A. and Sprague, R. L., Dosage effects of methylphenidate in children. In, Sprague, R. L. and Werry, J. S., Final Report of Grant MH18909-March 1974, p. 120.

Conners, C. K., A teacher rating scale for use in drug studies with children. Amer. J. Psychiat., 1969, 126, 152-156.

Easterbrook, J. A., The effect of emotion on cue utilization and the organization of behavior. Psychol. Review, 1959, 66, 183-201.

Elliott, L. A., Halliday, R. A. and Callaway, E., Brain event related potentials: some contributions to research in learning disorders. In, H. Myklebust (Ed.), Progress in Learning Disabilities, New York: Grune and Stratton, in press.

Hagen, J. and Hale, G., The development of attention in children. In, A. D. Pick (Ed.), Minnesota Symposium on Child Psychology, Vol. 7, 1973.

Halliday, R., Rosenthal, J. H., Naylor, H. and Callaway, E., Averaged evoked potential predictors of clinical improvement in hyperactive children treated with methylphenidate: an initial study and replication. Psychophysiology, 1976, 13, 428-440.

Halliday, R. A., Gnauck, K., Rosenthal, J. H., McKibben, J. L. and Callaway, E. The effects of methylphenidate dosage on school and home behaviors of the hyperactive child. Paper presented at the 1978 NATO Conference on the Treatment of Learning Disabilities, Cantrakon, Canada.

Hink, R. F., Fenton, W. H. Jr., Tinklenberg, J. R., Pfefferbaum, A. and Kopell, B. S., Vigilance and human attention under conditions of methylphenidate and secobarbital intoxication: an assessment using brain potentials, Psychophysiology, March 1978, 15, No. 2, 116-125.

Klorman, R., Methylphenidate and hyperactives' evoked responses. Arch. Gen. Psychiat., in press.

Loney, J., Langhorne, J. E. and Paternite, C. E., An empirical basis for subgrouping the hyperkinetic/MBD syndrome. J. of Abnormal Psychology, 1978, 87, 431-441.

Satterfield, J. H., Braley, B. W., Evoked potentials and brain maturation in hyperactive and normal children. Electroenceph. Clin. Neurophysiol., 1977, 43, 43-51.

Sohmer, H. and Student, M., Auditory nerve and brain stem evoked
    responses in normal, autistic, minimal brain dysfunction and
    psychomotor retarded children.  Electroenceph. Clin. Neuro-
    physiol., 1978, 44, 380-388.

Velasco, M., Velasco, F., Almanea, Y., Munoz, J. and Olvera, A.,
    Effect of dextroamphetamine on somatic evoked potential com-
    ponents in man with special reference to task relevance and
    selective attention.  Neuropharmacology, 1977, 16, 819-825.

EVOKED POTENTIAL INDICANTS OF SIZE- AND ORIENTATION-SPECIFIC
INFORMATION PROCESSING:  FEATURE-SPECIFIC SENSORY CHANNELS
AND ATTENTION

M.R. Harter, F.H. Previc and V.L. Towle

University of North Carolina at Greensboro

Greensboro, North Carolina 27412

One advantage of evoked potentials (EPs) to transient stimuli
is that they contain information as to the time-course of the electrophysiological response to such stimuli.  This time course may be
presumed to reflect the temporal sequence in which information contained in the stimulus is processed.  The present paper is primarily
directed toward a better understanding of the time course of information processing specific to the size (spatial frequency) and
orientation of the elements of visual stimuli.  Such processing
will be considered both in relationship to sensory information
channels and selective attention.  The final section will be a
brief review of preliminary data on the potential applications of
these types of procedures to clinical problems.

EP MEASURES OF FEATURE-SPECIFIC SENSORY CHANNELS

Psychophysical data from man (Blakemore et al, 1973; Blake
and Levinson, 1977) and electrophysiological data from animals
(Wiesel and Hubel, 1966; Ikeda and Wright, 1972) indicate that
there are sensory channels selectively responsive to specific
spatial frequencies and orientations of pattern stimuli.  The bandwidths of spatial frequency and orientation channels vary between
1-2 octaves and 3-40° respectively, depending on the procedure used.

Interocular suppression of transient VEPs has been used as an
electrophysiological measure of spatial frequency (Harter et al.,
1976) and orientation (Harter, 1977; Harter et al., in prep.) channels in man.  In these studies high contrast patterns of different
check sizes or orientations were continuously presented to one eye

while VEPs were obtained to a pattern flashed to the other eye.  The
amplitude of particular VEP components progressively decreased as
the spatial frequency or orientation of the flashed and continuously
presented pattern was made more similar.  The bandwidths were about
2 octaves and $40^0$, respectively, for size- and orientation-specific
suppression.  These values correspond reasonably well to those based
on psychophysical measures obtained under comparable conditions.
Orientation-specific suppression had the greatest effect on components peaking between 75 and 110 msec poststimulus, whereas size
(spatial frequency)-specific suppression had the greatest effect
on components peaking between 125 and 160 msec poststimulus.  This
difference suggests that the orientation of the stimulus may be
processed before its spatial frequency.  On the other hand, however,
it simply could reflect the effects of the different experimental
conditions employed in the procedures of the two studies.


SELECTIVE ATTENTION AND SENSORY CHANNELS

There has been considerable discussion as to the nature of
mechanisms which might mediate the effects of selective attention
(see reviews by Tueting, in press; Hillyard, et al. in press;
Donchin et al., in press).  Harter and Previc (in press) hypothesized
that the specificity of selective attention, as reflected by VEPs,
may be determined by the specificity of sensory information channels.  To test this hypothesis subjects were presented checkerboard light flashes which varied randomly in check size.  One of the
check sizes was made task relevant (attended) and all others task-
irrelevant (ignored).  When subjects selectively attended a given
check size, the VEP to that check size contained a negative component which began at approximately 210 msec and peaked at about 160
msec poststimulus.  An inverted U-shaped function was obtained
between the amplitude of this negative component and the flashed
check size with the peak of this function associated with the
attended check size.  The fact that this size-specific attention
was reflected in the VEP as early as 160 msec poststimulus and has
a bandwidth comparable to sensory size channels (about 2 octaves)
supports the hypothesis that sensory channels are the functional
units that mediate the specificity of attention to check size.

A comparison of the results of the above studies of interocular
size and orientation suppression and of size-specific attention
suggests the following conclusions:  first, orientation-specific
suppression is of greater magnitude and occurs earlier in time than
size-specific suppression.  This suggests that orientation channels
may precede spatial frequency channels; secondly, the effects of
interocular suppression occur earlier in time than the effects of
selective attention.  This suggests that the earliest sensory
channels, as reflected by feature-specific interocular suppression,

may not be directly influenced by selective attention.  These conclusions, however, must be considered tentative since they were
based on a comparison between studies conducted under different
experimental conditions.

   In order to further substantiate these conclusions, two studies
of spatial frequency and orientation effect on VEPs were conducted
under virtually identical stimulus conditions:  Experiment A investigated the effects of intra- and interocular suppression (Towle
et al., in prep.), while Experiment B investigated the effects of
selective attention (Harter and Previc, in prep.).  In addition to
the question of the time course of the suppression and attention
effects, these experiments were concerned with the specificity of
these effects.  For example, if these effects are interdependent,
then grating of a given spatial frequency and orientation would
only influence the response to other gratings of that same spatial
frequency and orientation.  If, on the other hand, these effects
were independent, a grating of a given spatial frequency and orientation would influence other gratings of that same orientation but
of different spatial frequencies, and vice versa.  Interdependence
of effects would indicate "pattern-specific" type channels, whereas
independence of effects would indicate "feature-specific" type
channels.


                              Method

   The stimuli were four black and white square-wave grating transparencies consisting of 9 or 36 min bars (3.3 or 0.83 c/d) oriented
vertically or horizontally.  These four patterns will be referred to
as 9V, 9H, 36V and 36H, respectively.  Monocular (right eye) evoked
potentials were obtained only to the 9V and 36H gratings by back
illuminating these transparencies once every 780 msec with a 10
msec light flash.  The intensity of this flash was 2.5 log units
above threshold.  The visual fields viewed by the left and right eye
subtended $7^\circ$ and were binocularly fused by means of a haploscope
(Fig. 1).  The constant luminance of each field was 4 mL.

   Monopolar EEGs were obtained with Grass gold-cup scalp electrodes, the active electrode placed 2.5 cm above the inion on the
midline (Oz) and the reference electrode attached to the right earlobe (A2).  They were amplified with a Model 7WC Grass Polygraph
(1/2 amplitude high and low frequency filters set on 36 and 1 Hz,
respectively).  Evoked potentials to the 9V and 36H flashed gratings
were averaged (N=64) for 512 msec poststimulation.  Each experimental condition was replicated four times during the course of
the experiment.

   The purpose of Experiment A was to compare the time courses of

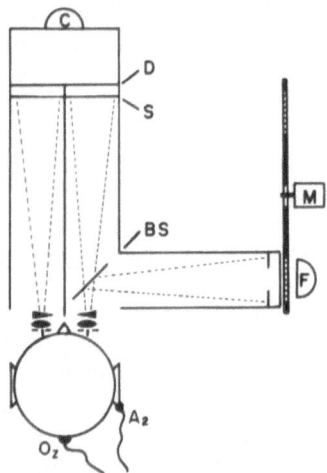

Fig. 1. Haploscope. Subjects continuously viewed dichoptically
presented suppressing stimuli (S) illuminated by an incandescent
light source (C) behind a diffusing screen (D). Gratings mounted
in a multistimulus projector (M) were flashed (F) through the
right channel. From Towle et al. (in prep.).

size- and orientation-specific suppression and to investigate the
interaction between them. Both interocular and intraocular suppression were investigated to assess the contribution of peripheral
and central mechanisms to such effects. In the interocular suppression conditions, the left eye continuously viewed either the 9V,
9H, 36V or 36H gratings (presented in counterbalanced order) while
VEPs were obtained to the 9V or 36H grating flashed to the right eye.
In the intraocular suppression conditions, both the flashed and continuously presented gratings were presented to the right eye.
Diffuse flashes were randomly intermixed among the sixty-four flashed
gratings. The subject's task was to give selectively an RT response
to the flashed gratings and not to the diffuse flashes. Performance
was measured in terms of d'. If the subject did not respond within
375 msec poststimulus, negative feedback was presented in the form
of a "click". Six subjects participated in Experiment A.

Experiment B was an investigation of the effects of directing
the subject's attention selectively toward either the 9V, 9H, 36V
or 36H grating while recording VEPs to the 9V and 36H flashed gratings. This experiment was identical to Experiment A with the
following exceptions: 1) both eyes continuously viewed diffuse
light; 2) the four different gratings were flashed in a random
sequence until both the 9V and 36H gratings had been flashed sixty-
four times; 3) the subject's task was to selectively give an RT

response to the attended or relevant grating and to withhold responses to the other three gratings. A negative feedback "click" was given if the subject did not respond within 375 msec following the relevant grating. The percentage of RT responses to all four stimuli were recorded, and once again a signal detection criterion was used with d' measuring how selectively subjects were responding to the relevant grating. Eight subjects participated in this experiment.

The changes in VEP amplitude as a function of the experimental conditions of both experiments were quantified by measuring amplitude at fixed or relatively fixed points in time after stimulation, in reference to a baseline (average voltage level of the first 45 msec). For Experiment A, these latencies were 75 msec, 100 msec, 125 msec, a negative peak between 125-195 msec (N150), a positive peak between 200-250 msec (P230), 275 msec, a positive peak between 280-380 msec (P320) and 425 msec. For Experiment B these latencies were 75, 125, 175, 200, 225, 250 and 375 msec. These latencies were selected either on the basis of measures used in previous studies, the peaks and troughs of the raw VEP waveform or the peaks and troughs of the difference potentials. These measures were analyzed statistically with repeated measures analyses of variance, and individual means were compared with either Newman-Keuls or Dune multiple range tests.


                                   Results


The psychophysical (d') data of Experiment A indicated subjects had more difficulty discriminating the grating from diffuse flashes when the 9V, as compared to the 36H, grating was flashed (p < .01). The suppressing effects of the other three continuous gratings and the effects due to intra- vs interocular presentation of the continuous stimulus did not differ significantly.

The d' values obtained in Experiment B indicated the four gratings differed in terms of how selectively subjects could respond to them (p < .01). The highest to lowest d' values were associated with attending to the 36V, 36H, 9V and 9H gratings, respectively. A greater number of false alarms were made to irrelevant stimuli of the same size, as compared to the same orientation, as the relevant grating.

The results will be represented in the form of difference potentials (bottom Fig. 2 and Fig. 3) which reflect the change in VEP amplitude and/or latency due to reducing the number of features of the continuous or relevant grating identical to those of the flashed grating. Any significant deviation from a flat difference potential indicates the change in the continuous or relevant grating influenced

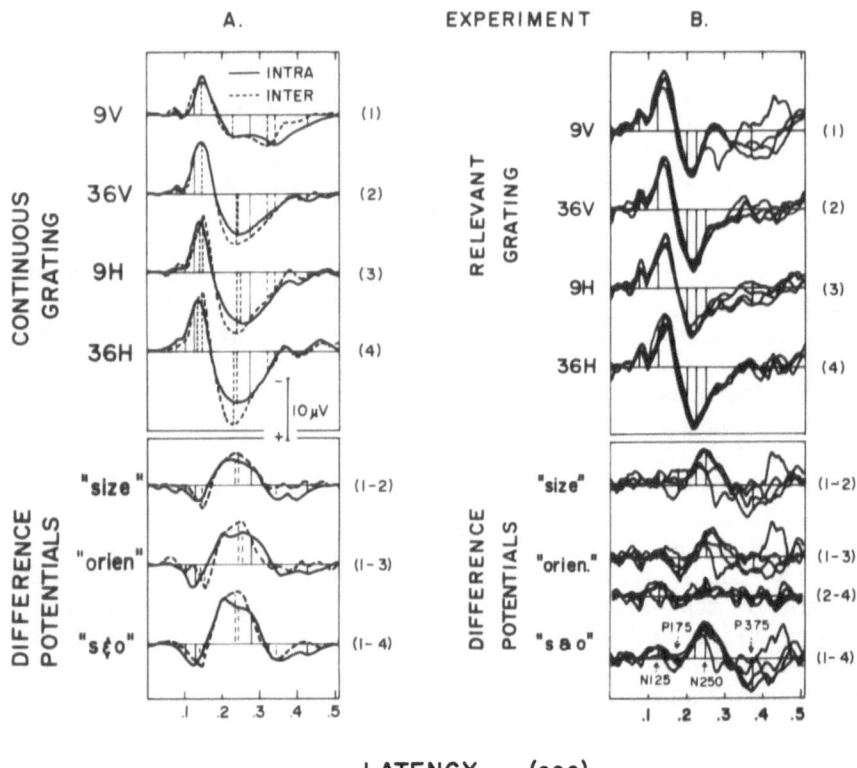

Fig. 2.  VEPs (top) and difference potentials (bottom) to the 9V
flashed grating.  Subject MRH.  Amplitude measures were made at peaks
and troughs of raw data (vertical dashed lines) and at fixed latencies (vertical solid lines).  <u>Left</u>.  (Experiment A)  Effects of a
continuous grating upon VEPs to the flashed grating when the two
gratings were viewed by the same eye (intraocular condition) or
different eyes (interocular condition).  <u>Right</u>.  (Experiment B)
Effects of attending one of the four gratings on VEPs to the 9V
grating.  The difference potentials indicate the change in VEPs when
one or more features of the continuous or relevant (attended) grating
were made identical to those of the flashed grating.  The numbers
(9 and 36) and letters (V and H) indicate the bar width (min) and
orientation of the gratings.

the VEP to the flashed grating.  Only VEPs to the 9V grating will be
discussed in the present paper.  The VEPs to the 36H gratings (Towle
et al., in prep.) confirm that the effects to be discussed were
feature- or pattern-specific, unless otherwise stated.

The results of Experiment A (left column Fig. 2) indicated
the time course of the effects of the continuous grating on VEPs to
the flashed grating was similar for both the inter- and intraocular
conditions, except that intraocular suppression was greater 100-150
msec post stimulus (p < .05). The grouped data, averaged across the
intra- and interocular suppression conditions, are shown in Fig.
3 (last column).

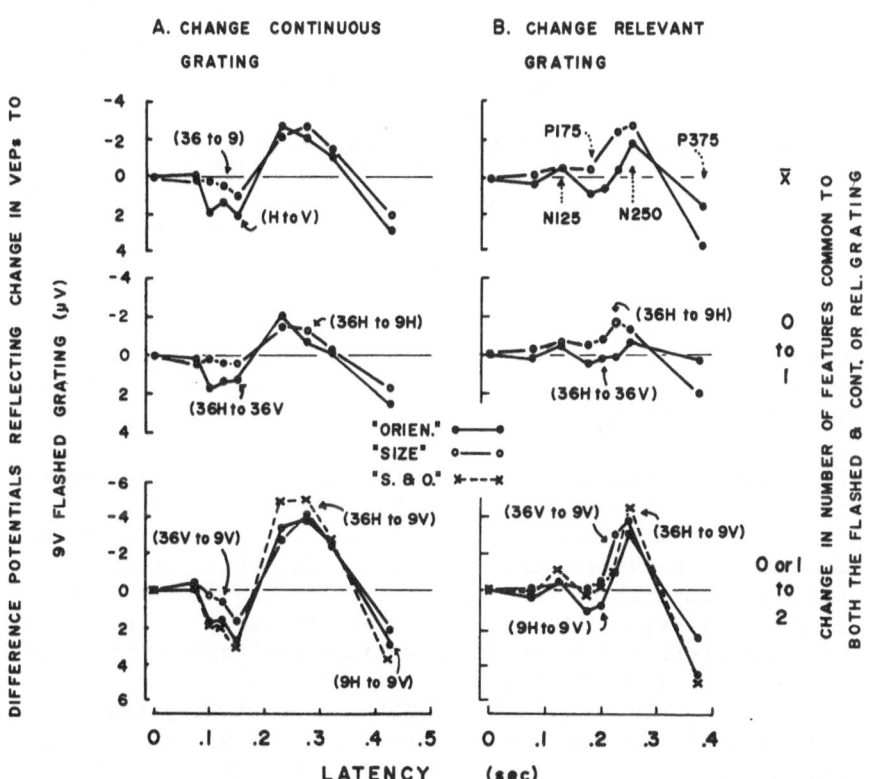

Fig. 3.  Quantified difference potentials averaged across subjects
and replication indicating the change in VEP amplitude due to making
a feature of the continuous grating (Experiment A) or relevant
grating (Experiment B) identical to that of the 9V flashed grating.
Top row are the means (X) reflecting the effects of a change from
0 to 1 and from 1 to 2 features in common.  Nine and 36 followed by
V and H indicate the bar width (min) and orientation of the gratings.

The changes in VEP amplitude from 100 to 150 msec poststimulus
indicated the following: a) greater orientation-specific than size-
specific suppression; b) orientation-specific suppression was
independent of spatial frequency--that is, the VEP to the 9V flashed
grating was suppressed by changing the continuous gratings from 36H
to 36V; c) spatial frequency-specific suppression was dependent
upon orientation--that is, the VEPs to the 9V flashed grating were
suppressed only by changing the continuous grating from 36V to 9V
and not by the change from 36H to 9H.

After about 150 msec poststimulus, the nature of suppression
to both bar size and orientation was similar. The two types of
suppression were of about the same magnitude and were reflected by
a negative shift in amplitude between 150 and 350 msec, followed
by a positive shift in amplitude between 350 and 450 msec. At all
latencies, the suppression effects were greatest when the continuous
grating had both features in common with the flashed grating.

The results of the selective attention experiment (Experiment
B, right column Figs. 2 and 3) indicated that which grating was task
relevant influenced VEP amplitude to the 9V grating, as measured 125,
200, 225, 250 and 375 msec poststimulus (p < .01 except 200 msec
where p < .05). The change in VEPs to the 9V flashed grating, due
to increasing the relevance of this grating, was characterized by
increased negativity between 100 and 150 msec (N125), increased
positivity between 150 and 200 msec (P175), increased negativity
between 200 and 300 msec (N250) and increased positivity between
200 and 400 msec (P350).

The effect of task relevance on N125 is of particular interest
in that such an early effect has not been reported in response to
visual stimuli in the previous literature. The influence of selective attention was evident only when the orientation of the relevant
stimulus was identical to that of the flashed grating (9V and 36V)
and was fairly independent of the spatial frequency of the relevant
grating. The average difference potentials reflecting this orientation attention effect (solid line top-right Fig. 3)--that is,
the increased negativity from 75 to 125 and positivity from 125 to
175 msec--were statistically significant (p < .025 and < .01, respectively). It should be noted that this effect was not evident in
VEPs to the 36H flashed gratings (data not shown).

In general the changes in N250 and P375 in Experiment B indicated considerable interdependence between the effects of the size
and orientation of the flashed and attended gratings. The effects
of attending a grating with only one feature in common with the
flashed grating had little influence upon the VEP amplitude. There
was a small effect of this type only when the flashed and attended
grating were of the same spatial frequency. A shift in attention

had the greatest effect when it was from a grating with neither
feature in common to a grating with both features in common with
the flashed grating (i.e., from 36H to 9V).


## DISCUSSION

The results will be discussed in regards to two interrelated
questions: What is the sequence in which the spatial frequency and
orientation of a pattern is processed, both in terms of the neural
representation of the pattern (presumably in sensory information
channels) and the effects of selective attention to the pattern?
And secondly, to what extent may the effects of selective attention
be related to the nature of activity in sensory information channels?
The series of studies reported above will be related to these two
questions by first summarizing how the changes in sensory channels
(induced by sensory suppression) and changes in attention (induced
by task relevance) affect the VEP. Then the interrelationship of
activity in sensory channels and mechanisms of selective attention
will be assessed by comparing these suppression and attention
effects both in terms of their time course and their specificity.


### Early VEP Components and Sensory Channels

For the purposes of discussion it will be assumed that VEP
components earlier than 200 msec poststimulus reflect sensory
activity and/or activity not directly associated with motor processes.
This assumption is based on the fact the VEP components occurring
earlier than 200 msec poststimulus are influenced by stimulus
parameters per se in passive subjects (Harter et al., 1976; Harter
et al., in prep.) and that RT latency is typically greater than 300
msec poststimulus in a choice RT task.

The size- and orientation-specific suppression of early VEP
components obtained in Experiment A may be interpreted within the
framework of feature-specific neural channels (Harter et al., 1976;
Harter, 1977; Towle et al., in prep.; Harter et al., in prep.).
The continuously presented grating is presumed to activate and
saturate those feature channels selectively sensitive to the features of the continuous grating. The response to a flashed grating
with similar features would, therefore, be suppressed since this
response would be mediated by the saturated channel. The response
to a flashed grating with different features than the continuous
grating would not be suppressed, because these different features
would be processed in different neural channels. The interocular
transfer of the suppression effects indicates they are mediated by
cortical neural channels.

Two findings support Campbell and Maffei's (1971) suggestion that orientation channels may precede spatial frequency channels. First, orientation-specific suppression was greater in magnitude earlier in time (100 msec poststimulus) than size-specific suppression. And second, orientation-specific suppression was, in part, independent of spatial frequency or bar width. Maffei and Fiorentini (1977) have proposed a cortical model of spatial frequency rows and orientation columns which provides one possible explanation of the difference between orientation and spatial frequency effects obtained in Experiment A.

It should be noted, however, that Smith and Jeffreys (1978) reported that the CI (75 msec) component was suppressed by both spatial frequency and orientation. This may bring the above interpretation into question. Their study differed from Experiment A in a number of respects in that they: a) used a masking paradigm, b) stimulated different portions of the visual field and recorded from different electrode positions, c) did not compare the magnitude of the effects of spatial frequency and orientation on CI; d) reported that gratings did not elicit a CII component (a component comparable to the 100 msec measure in Experiment A). These differences make it difficult to compare directly the spatial frequency and orientation effects in the two studies.

Selective attention to a grating of the same orientation as the flashed grating (9V or 36V) caused an increase in negativity of the VEP to the 9V flashed grating between 100 and 150 msec (N125). A number of factors indicate this effect might reflect the modulation of activity in orientation-specific sensory channels. First, the latency and polarity of N125 is comparable to that of the effects of pattern per se (Harter and Previc, 1978, and others). Second the continuous orientation suppression in Experiment A was reflected in increased positivity between 100 and 150 msec poststimulus which is as expected since suppression effects are presumably of opposite polarity as the facilitory effect due to selective attention. Finally it is unlikely that differential states of preparation for the relevant and irrelevant gratings can account for the N125 effect since these gratings were presented randomly. The N125 effect adds to previous data which indicate selective attention influences the amplitude of sensory VEPs (Eason et al., 1969; Harter and Salmon, 1972: Van Voorhis and Hillyard, 1977; Harter and Previc, 1978). It should be noted that this N125 attention effect appears to be uniquely related to attending vertical gratings.

## Late VEP Components and Cognitive Processes

The negativity peaking at about 250 msec and positivity peaking at about 350 msec in both Experiments A and B may be attributed to cognitive processes related to performing the RT task. These late effects have not been reported in previous studies of suppression where the subjects were not required to discriminate stimuli (Harter et al:, 1976; Harter, 1977; Smith and Jeffreys 1978; Harter et al., in prep.). In the case of Experiment A it is not clear just what cognitive processes might account for the change in amplitude of N250 and P350. The components have been attributed to either task relevance or subjective probabilities of stimuli (Donchin et al., in press). Yet in Experiment B these processes were not applicable since the evoking 9V grating was always task relevant and of the same probability (.5) as the irrelevant diffuse flashes. Visual inspection of the raw VEPs indicate the changes in N250 amplitude cannot be related to changes in latency of this component. Most likely these later components may be attributed to changes in difficulty in performing the choice RT task due to the suppressing effect of the continuous stimulus.

## APPLICATIONS

Preliminary data on the potential applications of the above procedures may be briefly summarized as follows:

1. Estimation of perceptual acuity. Towle and Harter (1977) reported that the smallest pattern element size that would elicit

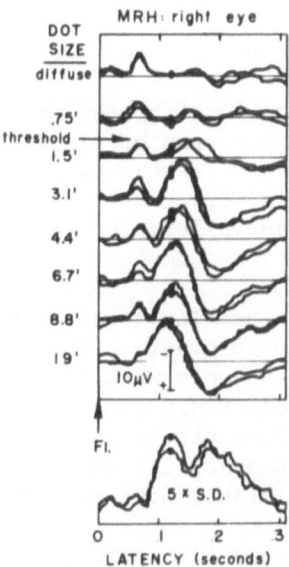

Fig. 4. Example of how differences in diffuse and pattern VEPs may be used to estimate visual acuity. The smallest dot-size eliciting a pattern VEP was 1.5' and was the smallest dot-size perceptible. Data from Towle and Harter (1977).

VEPS OF INFANT SUBJECT
(KW)

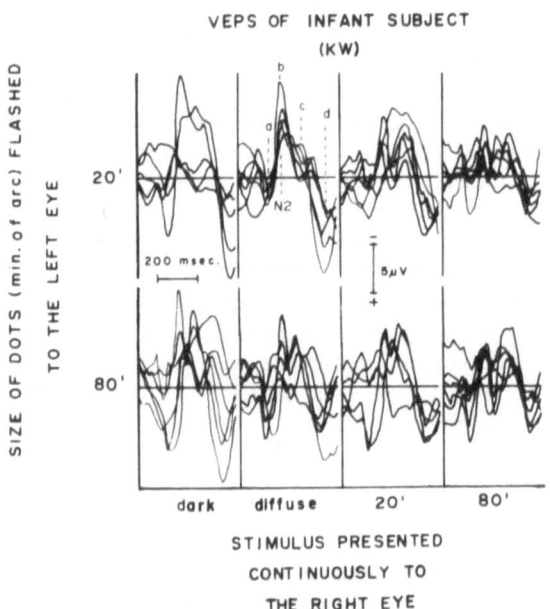

Fig. 5. Example of interocular suppression of VEPs in an infant
due to the presence and size of pattern in the contraocularly
presented continuous stimulus. From Odom and Harter (in prep.).

a pattern VEP--the VEP pattern threshold--was highly correlated
(r=.89) with perceptual measures of visual acuity. Perceptual
acuity could be estimated to within plus or minus .29 decimal units
on the basis of VEPs (Fig. 4). Harter et al. (1977a,b) and others
(see review by Dobson and Teller, in prep.) have used pattern VEPs
to estimate visual acuity in human infants.

     2.  Estimation of binocularity and depth perception ability.
Harter et al. (1977c) found greater size-specific interocular
suppression of VEPs in subjects with good stereopsis and depth
perception. Odom and Harter (in prep.) used the color separation
(anaglyphic) method to demonstrate interocular suppression of pattern VEPs in human infants (20-112 days of age)(Fig. 5). These
results indicate human infants have some degree of binocular vision.

     3.  VEP selective attention effects in learning disabled chil-
dren. Musso and Harter (in press) reported that the effects of
selective attention on VEP amplitude (N200 to P300) were significantly greater in reading disabled than normal children. This
finding was interpreted as indicating reading disabled children were
compensating for a deficit in processing visual information.

## CONCLUSION

The studies summarized here investigated how the visual system extracts, processes and selects relevant features from the visual image--specifically the features of size (spatial frequency) and orientation. Two types of paradigms were used in these studies. The first isolated feature-specific sensory channels by assessing the effects of continuously presented suppressing gratings on VEPs to a flashed grating. These studies demonstrated interocular suppression due to both spatial frequency and orientation. This suggests that such suppression is partially mediated by binocular cortical channels. The nature of feature-specific suppression of the early VEP components (100-200 msec poststimulus) was interpreted as indicating that orientation channels may be activated before size channels and are initially independent of size channels. In contrast, spatial frequency and orientation effects did not closely parallel the behavioral measure of suppression. Suppression of the later components (200-400 msec poststimulus) indicated size and orientation effects were approximately the same magnitude, were interdependent and were related to the behavioral measure of suppression.

The second experimental paradigm employed was designed to assess the effects of selective attention to a particular pattern on VEPs to patterns varying orthogonally in size and orientation. Of particular interest was the finding that an early component (N125) was influenced by selective attention. This early effect could reflect the modulation of activity in orientation channels since it was orientation-specific. Yet since it was to reflected in VEPs to the 36H grating when it was selectively attended, the origin of this component is uncertain. The effects of attention on later components (N250 and P357) (a) were specific to the size and orientation of the relevant grating, (b) were greater when the relevant and flashed grating had the same spatial frequency as compared to orientation and (c) indicated considerable interdependence of the processing of size and orientation as did the behavioral data. The changes in the later components appeared to reflect differential processing of information prior to initiation of the motor response but did not appear to reflect directly the modulation of activity in the earliest feature-specific sensory channels.

The time course of both the suppression and attention effects upon the VEPs reflected a temporal progression from relative independence to interdependence of spatial frequency and orientation channels (i.e., from feature-specific to pattern-specific processing).

Preliminary data were presented reflecting the potential application of these VEP measures as correlates of visual acuity and binocularity in adult and infant subjects and as correlates of attentional differences in reading disabled and normal children.

SUMMARY

   Visual evoked potentials were used to investigate the processing of information in spatial frequency and orientation channels.
Intra- and interocular suppression of early VEP components (100-200
msec poststimulus) indicated that there are spatial frequency and
orientation channels and that orientation channels are activated
before spatial frequency channels.  Suppression of later VEP components (200-400 msec poststimulus) indicated an additional type of
channel which was spatial frequency- and orientation-specific, and
which appeared to mediate the specificity of the behavioral measure
of suppression.  The effects of selective attention to a given grating on VEP amplitudes were specific to the size and orientation of
the relevant grating.  These effects appeared to be mediated by
the modulation of activity in cortical sensory channels.  The time
course of both the suppression and attention effects on VEP reflected a progressive increase in the specificity of information channels
- from feature-specific to pattern-specific - up to that point in
time when the behavioral response was initiated.

REFERENCES

Blake, R. and Levinson, E.  Spatial properties of binocular neurons
      in the human visual system.  Exp. Brain Res., 1977, 27, 221-232.

Blakemore, C., Muncey, J.P.J. and Ridley, R.M.  Stimulus specificity
      in the human visual system.  Vis. Res., 1973, 13, 1915-1931.

Campbell, F.W. and Maffei, L.  The tilt aftereffect: A fresh look.
      Vis. Res., 1971, 11, 833-840.

Dobson, V. and Teller, D.Y.  Visual acuity in human infants: A
      review and comparison of behavioral and electrophysiological
      studies. (In prep.)

Donchin, E., Ritter, W. and McCallum, W.C.  Cognitive psychophysio-
      logy: The endogenous components of the ERP.  In E. Callaway
      (Ed.), Event Related Brain Potentials in Man, New York: Aca-
      demic Press, in press.

Eason, R.G., Harter, M.R. and White, C.T.  Effects of attention
      and arousal on visual evoked cortical potentials and reaction
      time in man.  Physiol. Behav., 1969, 4, 283-289.

Harter, M.R.  Evoked potentials to flashed patterns:  Effects of
      element size and orientation.  In H. Spekreijse and L.H. van
      der Tweel (Eds.), Spatial Contrast, New York: North Holland
      Publishing Co., 1977.

Harter, M.R., Conder, E.S. and Towle, V.L.   Orientation-specific
    interocular suppression of visual evoked potentials in man.
    (In prep.)

Harter, M.R., Deaton, F.K. and Odom, J.V.   Maturation of evoked
    potentials and visual preference in 6-45 day old infants:
    Effects of check size, visual acuity and refractive error.
    Electroenceph. Clin. Neurophysiol., 1977a, 42, 595-607.

Harter, M.R., Deaton, F.K. and Odom, J.V.   Pattern visual evoked
    potentials in infants.  In J.E. Desmedt (Ed.), Visual Evoked
    Potentials in Man:  New Developments, Oxford: Clarendon, 1977b.

Harter, M.R. and Previc, F.H.   Size-specific information channels
    and selective attention:  Visual evoked potential and behavioral
    measures.  Electroenceph. Clin. Neurophysiol., in press.

Harter, M.R. and Previc, F.H.   Feature-specific selective attention:
    Spatial frequency and orientation. (In prep.)

Harter, M.R. and Salmon, L.E.   Intra-modality selective attention
    and evoked cortical potentials to randomly presented patterns.
    Electroenceph. Clin. Neurophysiol., 1972, 32, 605-613.

Harter, M.R., Towle, V.L. and Musso, M.F.   Size spedificity and
    interocular suppression:  Monocular evoked potentials and
    reaction times.  Vis. Res., 1976, 16, 1111-1117.

Harter, M.R., Towle, V.L., Zakrzewski, M. and Moyer, S.   An objec-
    tive indicant of binocular vision in humans:  Size-specific
    interocular suppression of visual evoked potentials.  Electro-
    enceph. Clin. Neurophysiol., 1977c, 43, 825-836.

Hillyard, S.A., Picton, T.W. and Regan, D.M.   Sensation, perception
    and attention: Analysis using ERPs.  In E. Callaway (Ed.)
    Event Related Brain Potentials in Man, Academic Press: New
    York, in press.

Ikeda, H. and Wright, M.J.   Differential effects of refractive
    errors and receptive field organization of central and peri-
    pheral ganglion cells.  Vis. Res., 1972, 12, 1465-1476.

Maffei, L. and Fiorentini, A.   Spatial frequency rows in the striate
    visual cortex.  Vis. Res., 1977, 17, 257-264.

Musso, M.F. and Harter, M.R.   Contingent negative variation, evoked
    potential and psychophysical measures of selective attention in
    children with learning disabilities.  In D. Otto (Ed.), Multi-
    disciplinary Perspectives in Event Related Brain Potential

Research, U.S. Government Printing Office: Washington, D.C.,
in press.

Odom, V. and Harter, M.R.   Young infants' binocular interaction:
Evoked potential measures. (In prep.)

Smith, A.T. and Jeffreys, D.A.   Size and orientation specificity
of transient visual evoked potentials in man.   Vis. Res.,
1978, 8, 651-655.

Towle, V.L. and Harter, M.R.   Objective determination of human
visual acuity: Pattern evoked potentials.   Invest. Ophthal.,
1977, 16, 1073-1076.

Towle, V.L., Harter, M.R. and Previc, F.   Binocular interaction of
size and orientation channels:  Evoked potentials and observer
sensitivity.   (In prep.)

Tueting, P.   Event related potentials, cognitive event and information processing.  In D. Otto (Ed.), Multidisciplinary Perspectives in Event Related Brain Potential Research.  U.S.
Government Publication Office: Washington, D.C., in press.

Van Voorhis, S. and Hillyard, S.A.   Visual evoked potentials and
selective attention to points in space.   Percept. Psychop.,
1977, 22, 54-62.

Wiesel, T.N. and Hubel, D.H.   Spatial and chromatic interactions
in the lateral geniculate body of the rhesus monkey.   J.
Neurophysiol., 1966, 29, 1115-1156.

# MATURATION AND TASK SPECIFICITY OF CORTICAL POTENTIALS ASSOCIATED WITH VISUAL SCANNING

Diane Kurtzberg and Herbert G. Vaughan, Jr.

Rose F. Kennedy Center for Research in Mental Retardation and Human Development, Albert Einstein College of Medicine, Bronx, New York

## INTRODUCTION

During normal vision the world is continuously scanned by a sequence of saccadic eye movements that shift the direction of gaze from two to six times each second. When viewing a stationary field, perceptual information is derived from the retinal images formed during fixational pauses. Eye position during fixation determines the portion of the visual scene that is available for processing and the duration of each fixation defines the time required for processing that information before the next saccade. Thus, the recording of eye movements provides an objective behavioral index of visual processing. Since visual scanning behavior is observed in the alert human subject from birth, oculomotor behavior provides a unique index of visual processing that can be observed throughout life.

It has been shown, both in free scanning and in controlled visual search tasks, that fixation duration (or intersaccade interval*) increases with field and task complexity (e.g., Gould and Schaffer, 1967; Gould and Peeples, 1970). Mean fixation duration also varies with age, progressively decreasing during childhood. There is a differential effect of task variables on these maturational changes, with the adult fixation duration being achieved by six years for picture scanning (Mackworth and Bruner, 1970), but not until 12-14 years of age for reading and numerical processing

---

*5% or less of visual scanning time is occupied by saccades, so that measurement of intersaccade interval provides a close approximation to fixation duration.

(Gilbert, 1953).  Thus, visual processing time as indexed by measurement of intersaccade interval shows both maturational and task
related variations that can in part be related to efficiency of
visual information processing.

Recordings of brain potentials concurrent with visual scanning
provide a direct probe of the cortical mechanisms underlying vision.
By averaging cortical activity in synchrony with saccades, eye movement potentials (EMP) are recorded that both precede and follow the
eye movements.  The antecedent potentials consist of activity that
begins approximately 200 msec before eye movement onset, culminating
in a sharp positive deflection that peaks during the saccade.  These
potentials are maximum in amplitude over the posterior parietal and
posterior frontal regions and are presumably implicated in the programming and initiation of saccades.  The potentials that follow the
eye movements, designated the lambda complex, are largest over the
occipital region and vary in morphology and timing as a function of
field characteristics and eye movement size.  As the amplitude and
duration of voluntary saccades are progressively increased, distinct
components that are temporally related to saccade onset and to the
subsequent fixational pause, become increasingly differentiated.
For eye movements less than 10° in amplitude, however, the lambda
complex comprises a composite of overlapping saccadic and fixational
components (Kurtzberg and Vaughan, 1977).

The recording of eye movements and the associated EMP during
visual scanning provide behavioral and electrophysiologic indices
of visual processing that could provide valuable information on
normal and deviant perceptual and cognitive development.  In order
to assess the potential value of these methods in developmental
studies of vision, we have surveyed the maturational changes in EMP
and fixation duration from birth to adulthood and have examined task
related differences in these measures in school-age children and
adults.

## METHODS

### Subjects

Thirty infants ranging from 34 weeks post-conception to 10
months of age, ten children 4 to 16 years of age and eight adults
from 20 to 48 years were studied.  All of the children and adults
were right handed.

### Visual Stimuli

The scanning targets differed with the age of the subject.

For preterm, newborn, and young infants, the targets were black
and white patterns (e.g., bullseye, schematic face) which elicit
robust scanning behavior. Older infants were shown simple colorful
pictures of animals mounted on a white background.

For preschool children, pictures were taken from children's
books that depicted events in the schoolroom, at a train station,
at the circus, etc. All of these materials subtended a total
visual angle of 30-40°.

School-age children and adults were presented with three kinds
of visual stimuli: 1) museum reproductions of paintings; this
condition was analogous to the target and picture scanning of the
younger children. 2) pencil mazes; this was considered to be a
non-verbal, purely spatial task. 3) reading selections taken from
the Houghton-Mifflin reading program; children were given selections to read from their grade level and from lower and higher
grades as well; adults were given selections from 6 grade levels
(2, 4, 6, 7, 8, 9). These stimuli subtended visual angles between
20 and 40°.


Recording Procedures

EEG was recorded from electrodes placed at 01,2; T5,6; P3,4;
C3,4; and F3,4 referred to the linked ears. Horizontal and vertical EOG were recorded from electrodes placed at the outer canthi
of both eyes, and above and below the orbit of one eye. EEG and
EOG were recorded on a Model 6, Grass EEG machine, with system
gain of 10K and frequency response down 3dB at 1 and 70 Hz. The
electrophysiologic signals were recorded on a 14-track FM tape recorder.


Data Analysis

The data were digitized off-line by a Nicolet Med 80 computer
programmed to average from the onset of each saccade over a specified epoch before and after each eye movement. The computer was
set to reject epochs in which potentials exceeded a designated
voltage so as to exclude blinks and other artifacts from the averaged EMP. EMP were averaged for each task separately and contained
a minimum of 150 epochs. The averaged EMP were written out on an
XY plotter. Peaks were identified visually and designated by polarity and peak latency. The duration of the principal lambda potential was also measured. This component was usually clearly defined in the occipital recordings either by a sharp departure and
return to the baseline or by small negative peaks that preceded
and followed it.

Intersaccade interval distributions for each task were obtained by measurements taken directly from the paper record. Intervals bounded by or interrupted by blinks or other artifacts were rejected. Mean intersaccade intervals were calculated and intersaccade interval histograms were constructed for each scanning task.

RESULTS

Maturation of Eye Movement Potentials

In the normal full term infant, brain potentials associated with the scanning of patterns precede and follow the eye movements (Figure 1A). The lambda response consists of a relatively simple positive wave most prominent over the occipital region, with mean peak latency from eye movement onset of $279 \pm 60$ msec and a mean duration of $259 \pm 82$ msec. The individual differences in the temporal characteristics of the lambda response are paralleled by variations in mean intersaccade interval. Mean intersaccade interval for these infants is $504 \pm 65$ msec. Pairwise correlation between lambda duration and mean intersaccade interval across infants is .87 (p<.005), indicating a close relationship between the behavioral and electrophysiological indices of visual processing time.

In premature infants, scanning of black and white targets was observed as early as 34 weeks post-conceptional age (i.e., 2 months before term). In these babies, the periods of active scanning are brief and the associated cortical potentials are often poorly defined. As infants approach term (i.e., 40 weeks post-conceptional age), scanning behavior is more consistently elicited. The eye movement potentials of the premature infants at term display similar morphology to that recorded from the full term infant but differ in the temporal characteristics of the lambda response. The mean peak latency of the lambda wave in the preterm infants is $437 \pm 135$ msec, and lambda duration is $353 \pm 177$ msec. The mean intersaccade interval for the group is $530 \pm 74$ msec. All of these measures of visual processing time are longer in the premature infant at 40 weeks than the full term baby at the same age. The correlation between mean intersaccade interval and lambda duration, .73 (p<.025), is somewhat lower than in the full term infants.

During the first four to six months of life, the lambda potential is similar in waveform to that of the newborn (Figure 16, 1B) but the large positive component peaks at progressively shorter latencies, being reduced to 200 msec by six months of age. Around this time, the potentials become more complex (Figure 1C) and except for a systematic decrease in latency with age, are similar in wave-

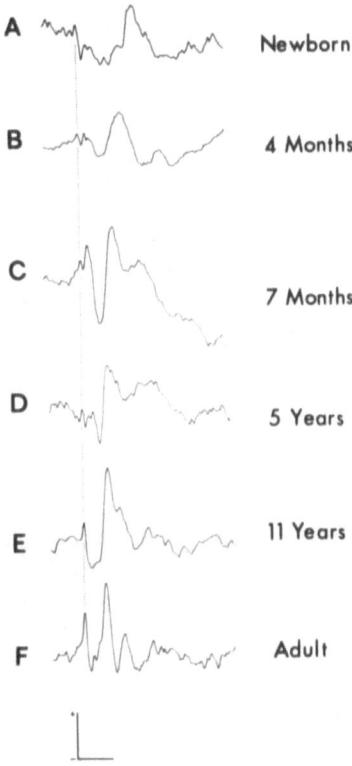

Figure 1.   Eye movement potentials associated with pattern or picture scanning in (A) a newborn (N=225);   (B) 4 month old (N=400);
(C) 7 month old (N=260);   (D) 5 year old (N=384);   (E) 11 year old
(N=185);   and (F) adult (N=242).   Dotted line indicates eye movement onset.   Recording site:   occipital.   Calibration:   10 uV for
A-E and 5 uV for F;   200 msec.   Note the progressively shorter peak
latency of the prominent positive lambda potential with maturation.

shape to the potentials associated with picture scanning in children and adults (Figure 1D, E and F).   The lambda complex comprises
a small negativity at 20-30 msec followed by a series of small and
variable positive wavelets at 35-80 msec seen at these latencies
both in children and adults.   There is however, a decrease in latency of the later components from children to adults.   A negative
wave peaks at a mean latency of 89 ± 15 msec for the children and
79 ± 14 msec for the adults and is followed by a positivity at
141 ± 24 msec (children) and 121 ± 11 msec (adults).   These negative and positive components are the largest and most consistent

portions of the lambda complex during picture scanning.  Later components are smaller and more variable: a negativity peaking at
256 + 76 msec (children) and 186 + 20 msec (adults), followed by a
positive wave at 403 + 59 msec (children) and 239 + 13 msec (adults).

   The duration of the main positive wave of the lambda complex
differs substantially between the children and adults, being 201 +
59 msec in children and 108 + 17 msec in adults.

   Although the mean intersaccade interval is substantially reduced in children and adults as compared to the values observed in
the infant subjects, the relation of lambda response latency and
duration to mean intersaccade interval differs across these age
groups.  Whereas the lambda wave duration is reduced by an average
value of 58 msec between the infants and children and a further 93
msec between the children and adults, the mean intersaccade interval diminishes 220 msec from infants to children (504 to 284 + 28
msec), but the adult mean intersaccade interval (298 + 31 msec)
does not change significantly from the children's value.  Despite
this discrepancy across age groups, the correlations between lambda
duration within each group remains fairly high, .78 (p<.005) for
children and .68 (p<.05) for adults.  These findings indicate that
the duration of the occipital lambda wave, while related to processing time as indexed by the mean intersaccade interval, does not
fully depict the mechanisms underlying the determination of fixation
duration.

   The foregoing description of maturational changes applies to
the occipital lambda response.  EMP are also recorded over other
portions of the scalp, usually at lower amplitude and most consistently in the posterior temporal and parietal regions (Figure 2).
Some of the temporoparietal activity possesses the same latency and
waveshape as the occipital response but is generally smaller.  These
potentials are considered to be volume conducted from the occipital
cortex.  Other activity is seen at longer latencies than the corresponding occipital components.  Distinct differences in the timing
of temporal and parietal potentials are seen principally in components that peak more than 80 msec after eye movement onset and
the largest difference is in the main positive wave that peaks between 125 and 200 msec in the children and adults and the negativity
that follows it between 200 and 300 msec.  During the first few
months of life, distinct temporoparietal potentials are inconstant.
After six months, however, prolonged posterior temporal potentials
become evident that are also prominent in the younger children.
Most of the school-age children and adults show a sequence of temporal
and parietal potentials that differ in latency from the occipital
lambda response.  In children and adults, the largest positive lambda
component is 50 msec longer in latency in the temporal region on the
average, than in the occipital region.  The parietal positive wave
lags the occipital by an average of only 10 msec.

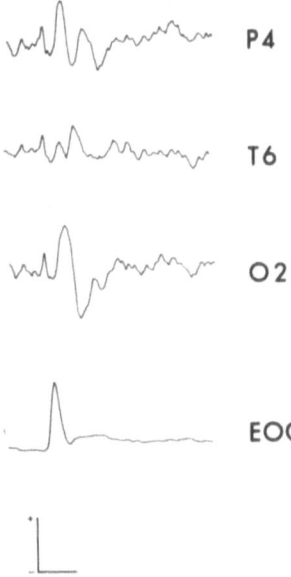

P4

T6

O2

EOG

Figure 2.  Eye movement potentials associated with picture scanning
recorded from an adult subject.  N=280.  Calibration:  5 uV, 200
msec.  Note the prominent positive lambda potential recorded at
maximum amplitude over the occipital region.  Potentials that differ in timing are also seen at both the parietal and temporal sites.


EMP During Reading and Maze Tracing

     EMP recorded during reading and maze tracing in school-age
children and adults differ in morphology and temporal characteristics from those recorded during picture scanning.  Typical waveforms for the reading and maze conditions recorded from the right
and left occipital and temporal electrodes are depicted in Figure
3 for one subject.  It can be seen that there are differences in
the timing of both the occipital and temporal lambda components
in the two tasks.  In general, the components are longer in duration or latency in the maze task as compared to reading.  The peak
latencies of the occipital and temporal lambda components are summarized in Table I.  Latency differences between occipital and parietal
components are small.  In each condition, latencies for all but the
first two lambda components are longer in children than in adults.
With only one exception, the latencies are greater for picture scanning and maze tracing than for reading.  Occipital lambda wave duration also manifests similar changes, being briefer in the adults for
all conditions and shortest for reading in both age groups.  Inter-

D. KURTZBERG AND H.G. VAUGHAN, JR.

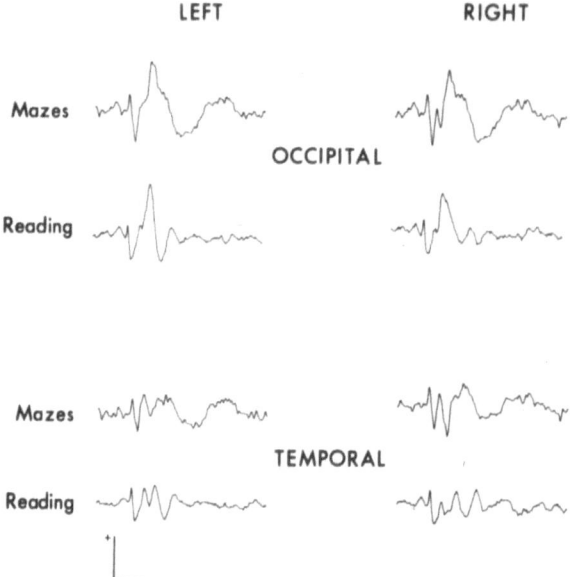

Figure 3.  Eye movement potentials associated with maze tracing
(N=290) and reading (N=432) recorded from an 11 year old child.
Calibration: 10 μV, 200 msec.  Note the shorter latencies of the
potentials associated with reading compared with those recorded
during maze tracing and the relative amplitude differences between
the occipital and temporal electrode pairs for the two tasks.


saccade intervals show similar effects of task, but are essentially
the same within each task across age groups.  It should be recalled
that this reduction in lambda wave duration without a corresponding
decrease in intersaccade interval was also found between the children
and adults in picture scanning.  In that condition, however, the correlations between lambda duration and intersaccade interval within
each age group were substantial, r=.78 for children and r=.68 for
adults.  In reading the correlations were smaller, .51 in children
and .42 in adults.  No relationship between occipital lambda duration and intersaccade interval was found (r=.25 for children and
r=.15 for adults) in the maze tracing tasks.  It appears, therefore,
that the occipital lambda duration is most closely related to intersaccade interval in picture scanning.  The potentials recorded
in the temporal region appear to show a relationship to fixation
duration in reading and maze tracing inasmuch as the mean differences in intersaccade interval between these tasks are similar to
the differences in mean peak latency of the late positive temporal
lambda components.  Furthermore, in reading the intragroup correlations between the temporal lambda peak latency and intersaccade
interval are substantial, being .75 (p<.005) for children and .65
(p<.005) for adults.  However, the correlations for maze tracing
are relatively low:  .16 for children and .48 for adults.  The

Table 1.   Latency of EMP peaks.

LATENCY SUMMARY

| | N | P | N | P | N | P |
|---|---|---|---|---|---|---|
| **OCCIPITAL** | | | | | | |
| **Pictures** | | | | | | |
| Children | 21 ± 4 | 32 ± 4 / 68 ± 5 | 89 ± 15 | 141 ± 24 | 256 ± 76 | 403 ± 59 |
| Adults | 28 ± 9 | 36 ± 11 / 65 ± 13 | 79 ± 14 | 121 ± 11 | 186 ± 20 | 239 ± 13 |
| **Mazes** | | | | | | |
| Children | 26 ± 5 | 40 ± 6 / 68 ± 4 | 84 ± 10 | 130 ± 14 | 274 ± 26 | 385 ± 74 |
| Adults | 28 ± 7 | 41 ± 10 / 70 ± 7 | 77 ± 16 | 111 ± 11 | 170 ± 21 | 224 ± 36 |
| **Reading** | | | | | | |
| Children | 25 ± 5 | 39 ± 10 / 69 ± 18 | 81 ± 17 | 122 ± 13 | 225 ± 24 | 300 ± 55 |
| Adults | 22 ± 5 | 34 ± 8 / 60 ± 9 | 70 ± 15 | 109 ± 12 | 168 ± 22 | 234 ± 38 |
| **TEMPORAL** | | | | | | |
| **Pictures** | | | | | | |
| Children | 26 ± 11 | 27 ± 6 / 68 ± 12 | 105 ± 10 | 199 ± 25 | 288 ± 21 | 390 ± 70 |
| Adults | 20 ± 0 | 35 ± 8 / 66 ± 13 | 95 ± 13 | 128 ± 8 / 174 ± 33 | 195 ± 7 | |
| **Mazes** | | | | | | |
| Children | 26 ± 5 | 38 ± 10 / 77 ± 18 | 112 ± 16 | 166 ± 42 / 225 ± 64 | 330 ± 27 | 453 ± 75 |
| Adults | 23 ± 7 | 33 ± 8 / 72 ± 8 | 99 ± 10 | 130 ± 12 / 203 ± 23 | 260 ± 14 | |
| **Reading** | | | | | | |
| Children | 24 ± 8 | 60 ± 14 | 92 ± 21 | 126 ± 26 / 172 ± 25 | 248 ± 40 | 324 ± 63 |
| Adults | 20 ± 0 | 35 ± 8 / 69 ± 8 | 89 ± 8 | 118 ± 13 / 150 ± 22 | 180 ± 10 | 222 ± 36 |

only significant correlation between parietal lambda peak latency
and intersaccade interval, r=.68 (p<.005), was found in the adult
subjects during reading.

     In order to assess possible interhemispheral differences in
amplitude of the lambda response in relation to the verbal or non-
verbal nature of the visual task, amplitude ratios for the main
positive lambda component were computed between homologous electrode
pairs in each stimulus condition.  There was a small mean right
hemispheral amplitude preponderance for the maze task in the occipital, posterior temporal and parietal lambda for both children and
adults.  Among the fifteen individual subjects for whom interhemispheral ratios were calculated, ten manifest a right sided lambda
preponderance at the occipital and parietal sites and nine at the
posterior temporal.  Two subjects at the parietal and one at the
occipital and temporal electrodes show no interhemispheral asymmetry,
whereas the remaining subjects have responses that are larger on the
left side.  During reading, by contrast, ten subjects show a left
occipital preponderance, thirteen a left temporal preponderance,
but only in eight is the left parietal response larger than the
right.  A particularly instructive comparison between the tasks
is depicted in Figure 4.

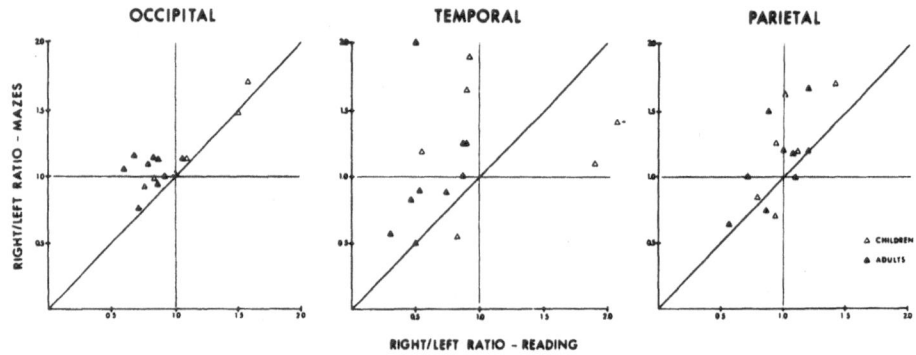

Figure 4.  Scatterplots depicting the right-left ratios of lambda
potential amplitude for the occipital, temporal and parietal
electrode pairs in maze tracing and reading.  The dotted lines
represent ratios of 1 which indicate no amplitude asymmetry.
Points to the left of 1.0 on the abscissa represent subjects who
displayed a left-sided predominance during reading.  Points above
1.0 on the ordinate are subjects who showed a right-sided preponderance for maze tracing.  The diagonal line represents equal interhemispheral ratios for each task.  Points above and to the left
indicate a left-sided shift in amplitude for reading compared with
maze tracing; below the line, a right-sided shift.

In the graph, the subjects who manifest a shift toward amplitude ratios favoring the left hemisphere for reading as contrasted
to maze tracing, appear above and to the left of the diagonal.  At
the occipital electrode, only one subject, a six year old child,
fails to show change in amplitude ratio favoring the left hemisphere
during reading.  At the temporal site, the three youngest subjects
shift toward the right, an eight year old shows no shift, whereas
the children over eight years of age and all of the adults shift
toward the left.  The amplitude ratios at the parietal location
also shift to the left during reading in eleven of fiteen subjects.
Here, however, two adults and one child show a right sided shift and
one child shows no task related shift.  These data, therefore, show
a strong tendency for the occipital and parietal lambda response
amplitude to manifest a relative amplitude increase in the dominant
hemisphere during reading in comparison with a non-verbal task.  A
similar shift is seen over the posterior temporal region, but this
is age related, with only the adults and older children manifesting
the tendency toward relative increase in left hemispheral activity.


DISCUSSION


Before commenting on these findings, attention must be drawn
to the unique features of the EMP associated with active scanning.
Alone among the various event related cerebral potentials, these
EMP index cortical processes that reflect the active exploration
of the environment by the subject.  In contrast to the repetitive
presentation of brief stimuli required in conventional evoked potential recording, the changes in visual input required to elicit
brain responses are produced by the saccadic shifts in eye position
actively generated by the subject as he processes the information
contained in a given visual scene.  Although the saccadic system
is partially under volitional control, the eye movements of active
scanning are largely involuntary, being defined jointly by the
nature of the visual field and the cognitive requirements of the
viewer.  With the sole exception of the rapid eye movements of
paradoxical sleep, saccadic scanning occurs only in alert subjects
presented with a patterned visual stimulus focused on the retina.
Under these conditions scanning appears to be virtually obligatory,
a fact that permits EMP to be sttudied in infants, young children
and others who may be incapable of making reliable behavioral responses to significant stimuli.  The occurrence of scanning behavior
implies that visual information is being processed to the extent
required to program the sequence of fixations and saccades.

It is important to recognized that the visual processing during
a given fixation necessarily occupies only the time required to
transmit and extract information needed to program the following

saccadic vector.  This may not correspond to the total amount of.
time during which information of cognitive significance is derived
from that fixational input.  Thus, brain activity related to cognitive processing of the visual input might continue after the initiation of the succeeding saccade.  An analogous situation is found
with  event related potentials recorded during discriminative tasks
that require a motor response.  Often, the response precedes the
late ERP components that are presumed to reflect some aspect of
cognitive processing (Ritter et al., 1972).  Despite the possibility that cortical processing of input from each fixation might out-
last the fixational pause, the major lambda response components
were all shorter in latency than the mean intersaccade interval.
This is consistent with the supposition that processing of information derived from each fixation is essentially completed before the
next saccade is generated.

One objective of the present study was to evaluate the extent
to which intersaccade interval is correlated with the timing of EMP
components.  Since it has been shown that the EMP comprises several
components, some associated with saccade onset and others with onset of fixation (Kurtzberg and Vaughan, 1977), it was anticipated
that the timing of some portions of the EMP would not be related
to fixation duration.  Furthermore, variations in the nature of
the visual processing requirements would be expected not only to
affect processing time, but should engage different cerebral mechanisms, so that associated variations in EMP configuration and topography  are to be anticipated.

It is noteworthy that newborn infants who manifested the simplest lambda response, a single positive wave, showed the highest
correlation between mean intersaccade interval and lambda duration.
The strength of the relation between mean intersaccade interval and
occipital lambda duration in picture scanning diminished somewhat
in children and adults whose potentials manifested greater spatial
and temporal complexity than the newborns.  Yet, even in adults
the duration of the main occipital peak accounted for approximately
50% of the variance in mean intersaccade interval  across subjects.
It seems reasonable to conclude, therefore, that the neural processes reflected in the principal occipital lambda component may be
involved in determining the duration of fixation during picture
scanning.

It is also likely that the maturational decrease in both intersaccade interval and lambda wave duration reflects increasing efficiency of visual processing with age.  It is of interest that
within each age group there was a considerable spread in the measures
of visual processing time, indicative of substantial individual
differences in efficiency of visual processing.  The study of individual differences in visual scanning and EMP may prove of con-

siderable value, not only for investigating variations in visual
processing in normal subjects, but also for detecting and probing
the mechanisms of deviant visual processing in infants and children.

In the present investigation we found that premature infants
often manifested prolonged cortical lambda potentials and mean
intersaccade intervals at 40 weeks conceptional age, in comparison
with normal full term newborns. In view of the fact that a number
of these infants also have impaired visual orienting behavior
(Kurtzberg et al., submitted for publication), analysis of the
maturation of visual scanning in infants at risk for deviant neuro-
behavioral development may provide a useful tool for early detection of higher visual processing disorders.

The functional correlates of task-related differences in lambda
response morphology and topography remain to be established, but the
present study provides some tentative indications. The high correlation between occipital lambda duration and intersaccade interval
in all age groups during picture scanning, and the relatively low
correlations at the occipital site for reading and maze tracing,
suggest that the neural processes related to control of fixation
duration are reflected in the occipital response only for picture
scanning. Reading, however, is associated with enhanced temporal
and parietal lambda responses that manifest a moderately high
correlation between their timing and the mean intersaccade interval.
It seems reasonable to conclude that these temporoparietal potentials index some aspect of the information processing specific to
this task. Only maze tracing failed to show significant correlations
between the behavioral and electrophysiologic indices of processing
time at any of the electrode sites. Thus, cortical potentials
specifically related to the control of fixation duration remain to
be identified in the latter task.

Despite this failure to detect activity related to fixation
duration in the spatial task, the analyses of interhemispheral
differences between reading and maze tracing revealed rather consistent asymmetries in relative lambda amplitude that conformed
to the presumptive lateral specialization for verbal versus non-
verbal processing. These findings encourage the use of EMP recording in the investigation of lateral specialization of cortical
visual mechanisms. The study of children with developmental dyslexia
and other learning disorders may also be a fruitful application of
these methods.

These developmental studies of EMP during active visual scanning are still in progress, incorporating improvements designed to
enhance the spatial and temporal resolution of individual components
that may reflect specific aspects of visual processing mechanisms.
It is anticipated that these investigations will yield useful

information on cortical processes associated with normal and
deviant perceptual and cognitive development.

## SUMMARY

EMP associated with scanning of patterns in infants below four
to six to six months of age are rather simple, with a single
positive occipital lambda wave predominating.  Around six months
the occipital lambda potentials become more complex in form.  Temporal and parietal components emerge that are distinguishable from
the occipital potentials on the basis of differences in waveshape
and timing.  After six months, the waveform of the lambda complex
undergoes little change except for systematic decreases in latency
during childhood.  There is a significant relation between the mean
intersaccade interval and the occipital lambda duration for individual subjects within each age group, with correlations of .87
for full term infants, .78 for children and .68 for adults.
Visual scanning and the associated EMP are influenced by both the
characteristics of the visual field and the nature of cognitive
processing requirements, intersaccade intervals increasing with
field and task complexity.  EMP recorded in school age children
and adults during reading and the performance of non-verbal spatial
tasks, manifest characteristic differences in timing and topography
as a function of stimulus and task variables.  The potentials recorded during reading are shorter in duration than those associated
with non-verbal tasks in both children and adults.  It also appears
that differences in visual processing may be reflected in differential topographic features, especially in the later lambda components.  There is a relative left-sided preponderance in lambda
amplitude during reading as compared to a non-verbal task in right-
handed subjects.  This left preponderance is most marked in the
posterior temporal region of adults, whereas the children's
lateralization is more consistent in the occipital recordings.

## ACKNOWLEDGMENTS

The authors wish to thank Judith A. Kreuzer and Maria Spam-
pinato for their invaluable experimental assistance and Linda
Peterson for preparation of the manuscript.  This research was
supported by USPHS Grants MH 06723, HD 01799 and HD 11562.

## REFERENCES

Gilbert, L. C., Functional motor efficiency of the eyes and its
     relation to reading.  Univ. Calif. Publications in Educ.,
     1953, 11, 159-232.

Gould, J. D. and Peeples, D. R., Eye movements during visual search
    and discrimination of meaningless, symbol and object patterns.
    J. Exp. Psychol., 1970, 85, 51-55.

Gould, J. D. and Schaffer, A., Eye-movement parameters in pattern
    recognition.  J. Exp. Psychol., 1967, 74, 225-229.

Kurtzberg, D. and Vaughan, H. G., Jr., Electrophysiological observa-
    tions on the visuomotor system and visual neurosensorium.  In,
    J. E. Desmedt (Ed.), Visual Evoked Potentials in Man: New
    Developments.  Oxford: Clarendon Press, 1977, Pp. 314-331.

Kurtzberg, D., Vaughan, H. G., Jr., Daum, C., Grellong, B. A.,
    Albin, S. and Rotkin, L., Neurobehavioral performance of low
    birth weight infants at 40 weeks conceptional age: Comparison
    with normal full term infants.  Developmental Medicine and
    Child Neurology, submitted for publication.

Mackworth, N. H. and Bruner, J. S., How adults and children search
    and recognize pictures. Human Development, 1970, 13, 149-177.

Ritter, W., Simson, R. and Vaughan, H. G., Jr., Association cortex
    potentials and reaction time in auditory discrimination.
    Electroenceph. Clin. Neurophysiol., 1972, 33, 547-555.

MULTICHANNEL MAPPING OF SPATIAL DISTRIBUTIONS OF SCALP POTENTIAL

FIELDS EVOKED BY CHECKERBOARD REVERSAL TO DIFFERENT RETINAL AREAS

D. Lehmann and W. Skrandies

Deparment of Neurology, University Hospitals

Zurich, Switzerland

This paper will examine the components of potentials evoked by checkerboard reversal. The components will be defined in terms of latency and scalp location, and we will show changes of components as a function of retinal stimulus site. A considerable problem in conventional evoked potential assessment is the different potential waveshapes which are recorded from different electrode sites on the head (see Fig. 1). In addition, waveshapes at given electrode sites may change when a different reference is used. An example is shown in Fig. 1 where a set of simultaneously recorded evoked potential data from forty-seven electrodes is illustrated as waveforms using two different reference points, the mean of the ears or an anterior midline electrode (Fig. 1A and B). Of course, any one of the forty-seven channels could have been used as a reference, creating an immense number of different waveshapes out of the same data set.

However, this data set can easily be reviewed when it is presented in the simple form of a sequence of equipotential line maps which illustrate the distribution of the evoked scalp field at different times after the stimulus onset. Fig. 2 gives examples constructed from the same data as Fig. 1. The maximal response (i.e., the maximal voltage within the field) can be located in the maps quite easily. The structure of the field distributions, and thus the locations of maximal field values, is independent of a reference point; only the labelling of the equipotential lines changes with a change of reference (Lehmann, 1977).

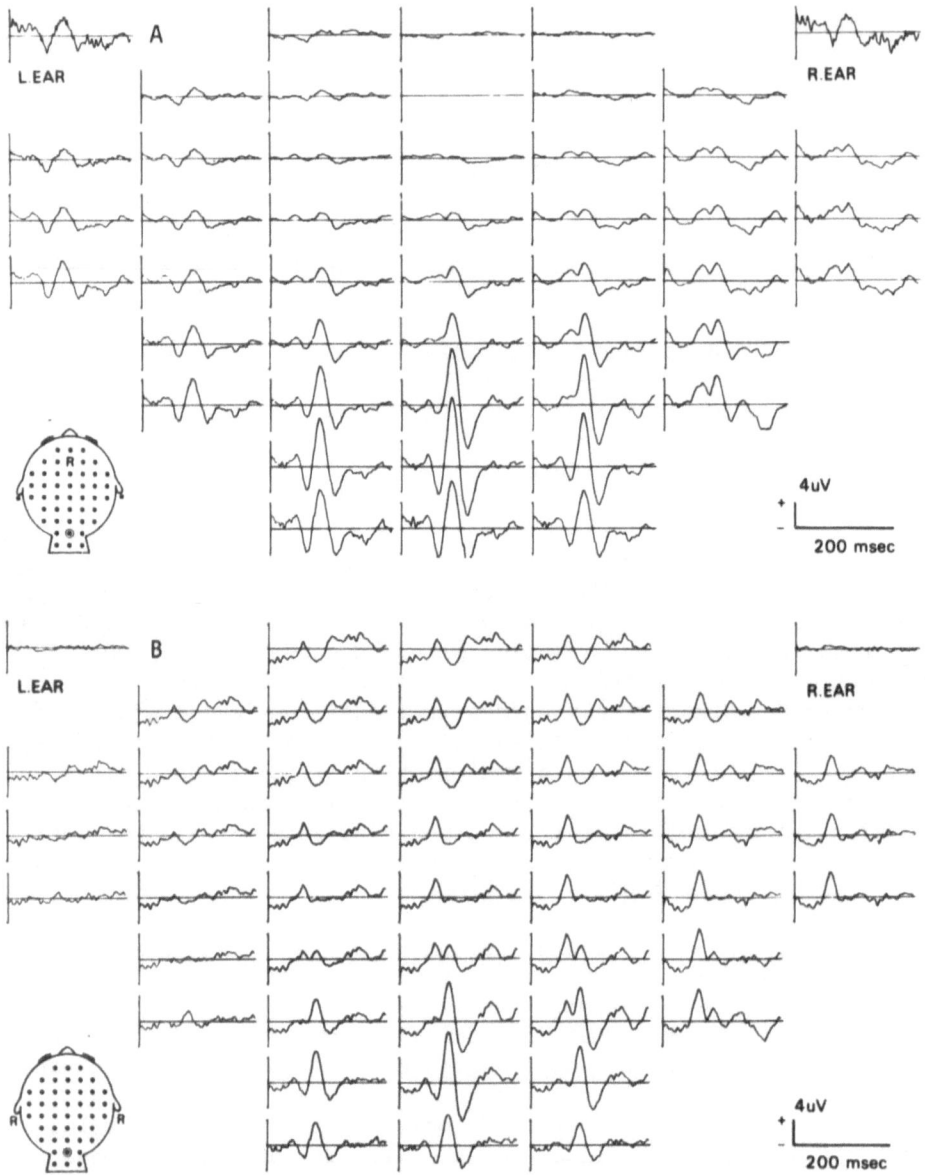

Fig. 1.    Average (N=110) potential waveforms evoked by 2/sec checkerboard reversal (circular 26° field, checks 40', right eye, fixation
upper target edge) and recorded simultaneously from forty-seven
electrodes as indicated in inset.    Head seen from above, nose up,
circled electrode=inion.    Waveforms in A referred to an anterior midline reference (R), in B to mean of both ears.    Both sets of waveforms and Fig. 2 were computed from same data set.    (From Lehmann
and Skrandies, in prep.)

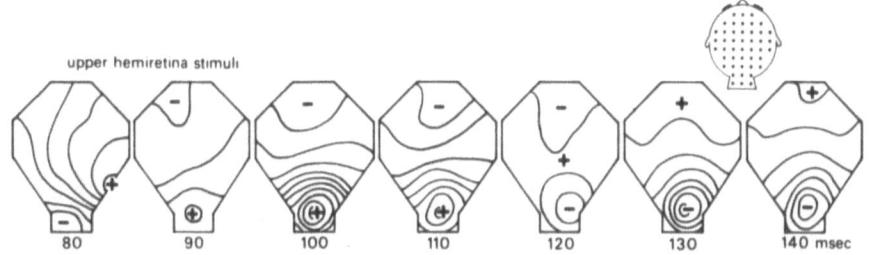

Fig. 2.  Scalp field equipotential line maps, constructed from same
data set as Fig. 1 (47 channel recording), for different times after
stimulus reversal onset.  The potential step between two adjacent
lines is 1 µV.  Electrode array see inset.  (From Lehmann and Skrandies, in prep.)

## METHODS

All data were collected from healthy volunteers (20-45 years
of age).  The checkerboard (checks of 40 or 50 min arc) was back-
projected as a circular field onto a translucent screen (white:
1.8 log fL, 96% contrast ratio) and reversed at 2 changes per
second using a feedback controlled mirror (General Scanning CCX-101,
3 msec reversal time, no overshoot).  Data were collected from Grass
gold cup electrodes attached with Grass electrode cream, using up
to forty-seven preamplifiers (constructed by J. Madey, 0.5 - 100 Hz
at 6 dB).  The data were simultaneously A/D converted at 512 s/sec/
channel, stored and sequentially read via a 64 channel converter
and formatter (B. Fricker, H.P. Meles and V. Croti, Inst. Tech.
Physics, ETH Zurich, and Neurology Dept., University of Zurich) and
via DMA into a PDP-11/10 for further analysis.

### Determination of the Time of Maximal EEG Response

It is reasonable to assume that the maximal response of the
brain is reflected on the scalp as a maximal voltage difference
between two recording points.  Since it cannot be known in advance
which two sites on the scalp will show a maximal voltage difference,
all recording points must be compared.  This procedure will determine two recording points at every analysis time, one for the
maximal and one for the minimal voltage of the field.  Using this
approach, the size of the maximal voltage difference within the
recorded area can be plotted as a function of time (Fig. 3B for
upper hemiretina stimulation) and indicates times of maximal response.  A global assessment of the amount of all voltage differ-

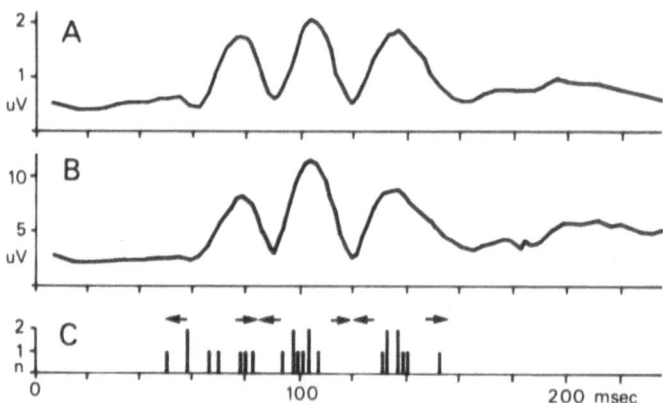

Fig. 3.   A:   Amount of relief of the evoked field distribution as a
function of time ("hilliness curve"); B:  Maximal voltage difference
between any two electrodes within the field as a function of time.
A and B during upper hemiretina stimulation, same data as Figs. 1A
and 2.  C:  Times of peaks of hilliness curves obtained from eight
subjects during upper hemiretina stimulation.  Peaks determined for
three analysis periods (arrowheads).  (From Lehmann and Skrandies,
in prep.)

ences between all electrodes in the scalp field is the computation
of the average, absolute deviation of voltage per electrode from
the mean of all instantaneous voltages (average reference).  This
mean of the absolute voltage deviation per electrode is a measure
of the amount of relief or "hilliness" of the scalp field.  The
hilliness (Lehmann 1971) is a measure of the relative power of the
evoked field distribution.  The values can be plotted against time
(Fig. 3A), and typically the resulting curve for a given subject is
similar, although not identical, to the curve of the maximal voltage differences between any two electrodes in the field, as Fig. 3A
shows.  Both curves show three distinct peaks as 77, 102 and 135
msec.  We now may go back to Fig. 2 and examine the scalp field
distributions which exist at about the occurrence time of the peak
values of the hillimess curve.  We note that the distributions at
100 and 130 msec are quite distinct and show occipital maximal values
of inverted polarity at the two times.  These occipital extreme
values are, or course, also seen in conventional waveshape recordings.

     We collected scalp field data from eight subjects using upper
hemiretina checkerboard stimulation (15-26 deg. arc field).  The
hilliness curves were constructed for each subject and searched
for peak values during the three peak periods of 50-85 msec, 85-120

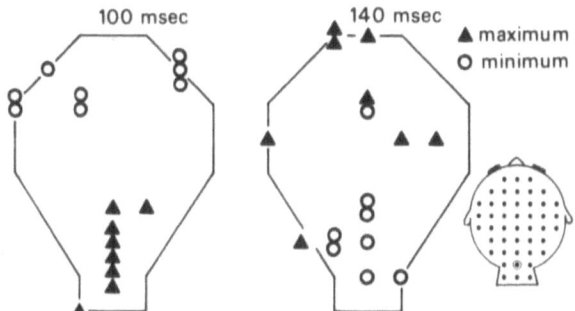

Fig. 4.  Scalp electrode locations of maximal (triangles) and minimal (circles) field values at two peak times (about 100 and 140 msec) of the individual hilliness curves (see Fig. 3C) of eight subjects. Upper hemiretina stimuli.  Head with electrode array seen from above; outline of plots indicates array.  (From Lehmann and Skrandies, in prep.)

msec and 120-155 msec latency.  The resulting distribution of peak times is illustrated in Fig. 3C.  There is considerable scatter for the peaks during the earliest analysis period, but the two later hilliness peaks show a satisfying consistency of latencies across subjects.  Thus these two moments in time after the stimulus may be used as times of maximal response for the subject population. In order to determine the spatial distribution of the peaks we now plot the scalp locations of the maximal and minimal field values at the subjects' individual peak latencies of their hilliness curves (Fig. 4).  It is evident that the group data show an occipital posi- tivity at about 100 msec and an occipital negativity at about 140 msec.  Thus this method determines objectively time and scalp loca- tion of the major components of the brain response to checkerboard reversal stimuli.

## Right Versus Left Hemiretina

Several papers investigated the shapes of potentials evoked by right or left half field stimulation (Cobb and Morton, 1970; Lesevre, 1972; Barrett et al., 1976; Blumhardt et al., 1977).  The results were contradictory as to correct lateralization of the evoked responses on the scalp.  We suggested (Europ. EEG Meeting, Venice, 1976) that the degree of "wrong" lateralization may increase with target size.  If we inspect a subject's scalp fields which were evoked by hemiretinal stimulation (Fig. 5), things turn out to be somewhat more complicated (the fields of Fig. 5 were con-

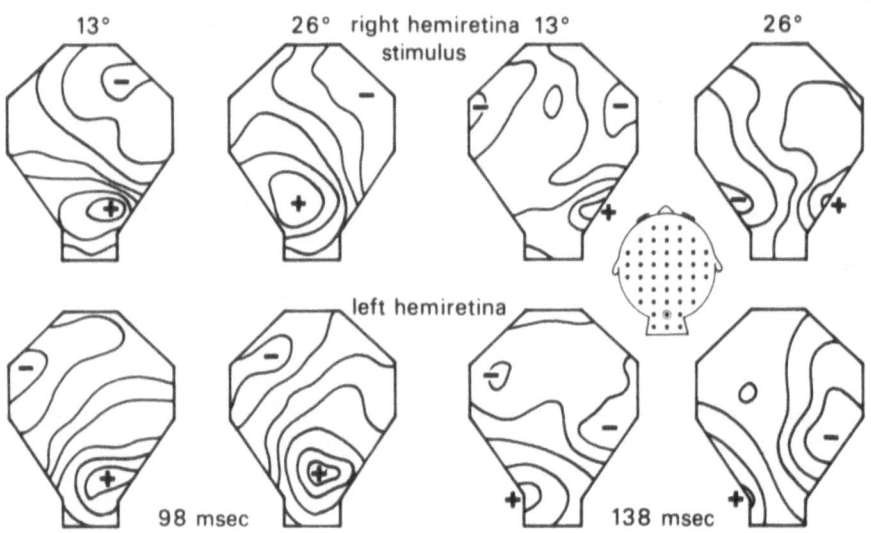

Fig. 5. Scalp field distributions (equipotential-line maps) for
right and left hemiretina stimulation at the peak times of the subject's hilliness curve. Each equipotential line = voltage step of
1 μV. (+) and (-) indicate extrema areas, not exact electrode locations.

structed at times of maximal hilliness of the evoked potential
field; these times were identical for upper, right and left hemiretinal stimulation). We note that for small target size, the field
at 98 msec is lateralized over the right occiput for both right and
left hemiretina stimuli. However, the positive portion of the field
which was evoked by right hemiretinal stimuli has a steeper gradient
to the right side, whereas that for left hemiretina stimuli is
steeper to the left side. In other words, for these small targets
thère is at 98 msec a lateralization of the occipital field distribution towards the "correct" side, ipsilateral to the stimulated
hemiretina. At the same latency for 26 deg. arc targets, the opposite shift of the occipitally evoked, positive portion of the field
towards the "wrong" side, contralateral to the stimulated hemiretina,
is seen in Fig. 5. The fields at 138 msec appear to be largely
similar for small and large targets with the maximum over the "correct" side in the occipital area and the minimum more anterior over
the "wrong" side.

The relative shift of location can be expressed as a vector
whose origin is, say, at the electrode that detects the maximal
field value for right hemiretinal stimuli and whose head is at the
electrode which detects the maximal field value for left hemiretina

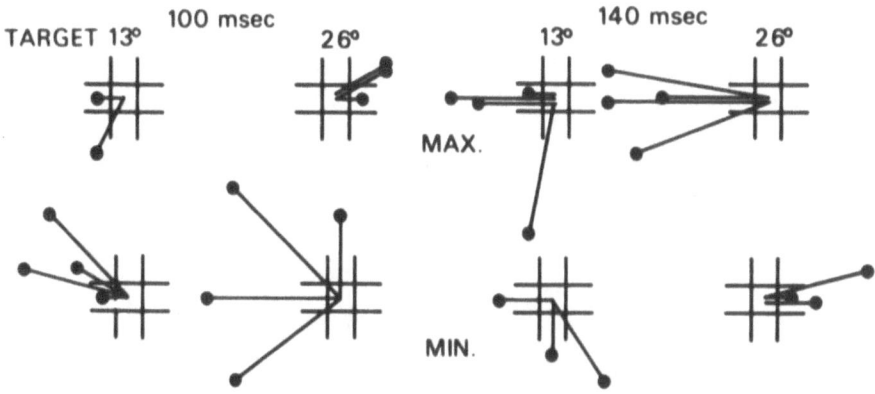

Fig. 6.  Vectors indicating direction and amount of change of location of the evoked maximal (MAX) and minimal (MIN) field values of
four subjects with change of the stimulation from right to left hemiretina, for the two target sizes and for the two hilliness peak times.
Center of reference grid is the location of maximal (minimal) value
for right hemiretina stimuli; dots give relative location of the
same value for left hemiretinal stimuli; dots give relative location
of the same value for left hemiretinal stimuli in the different subjects; no dot = case of no change; one square = one interelectrode
distance.  Head seen from above, nose up.  Two of the subjects showed
no change for maximal value location with 13° targets at 100 msec,
but there was a change of the field distribution in the same direction as in the other two subjects (see Fig. 5 for example).


stimuli.  We examined four subjects (including the subject of Fig.
5) with 13 and 26 deg. arc checkerboard stimuli using lateralized
retinal stimulation.  We plotted the shifts of the maximal and minimal field values at the respective peak times of the subjects'
hilliness curves.  Fig. 6 shows that at 100 msec the maximal field
values shift towards the "correct" side for 13 deg. arc targets
(two of four subjects) and to the "wrong" side for 26 deg. arc targets (three of four subjects); cases without shift of the maximal
values showed displacements of the field distributions similar to
the other subjects (Fig. 5 shows an example).  The minimal field
values at 100 msec (i.e., the anterior field troughs) shift towards
the "correct" side for both small and large targets.  The later
(140 msec) components show clear results for the maximal field
value but less consistent results for the negative extreme value.
Fig. 5 illustrates this observation inasmuch as the maximal field
value is centered occipitally over the "correct" hemisphere, whereas the minimal value typically is more anterior over the "wrong"
hemisphere.  The occipital response at 140 msec is expected to be

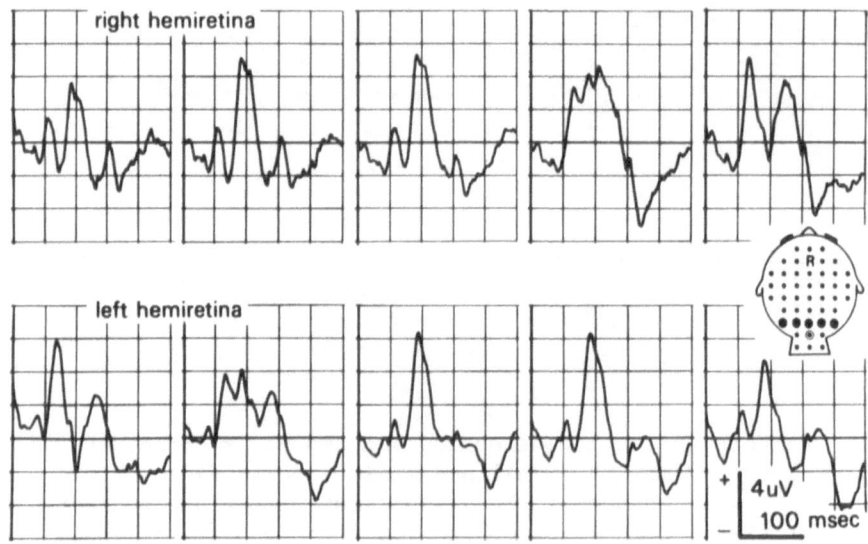

Fig. 7. Evoked potential waveshapes reconstructed from multichannel data of one subject, for right (upper row) and left (lower row) hemi-retina stimulation (26$^{\circ}$ target), between an anterior midline elec-trode (R) and a left to right transverse row of five electrodes 3.5 cm above the inion (heavy dots in inset). Note the positive compo-nent at 100 msec over the "correct" hemisphere. Same data as in Fig. 5.

negative, as was demonstrated with centered retinal stimulation (Figs. 2 and 4). With lateralized retinal stimuli we observe that this minimum appears over the "wrong" hemisphere in line with the "wrong" localization of the positive extreme value at 100 msec. But at 140 msec the occipitally dominating field characteristic which is evoked by lateralized stimuli is the positive extreme value over the "correct" hemisphere. This result is easily picked up and quite impressive in conventional waveshape recordings against an anterior reference (Fig. 7; see also Fig. 1 in Blumhardt et al., 1977) which show a late positive response over the "correct" occi-put.

One may argue that since the response to small targets proba-bly is generated by the foveal projection area around the occipital pole of the hemisphere, the maximal field value tends towards the "correct" side. On the other hand, since peripheral retinal areas are projected to cortical regions on the medial brain surface, the maximal scalp field value then tends to appear over the "wrong"

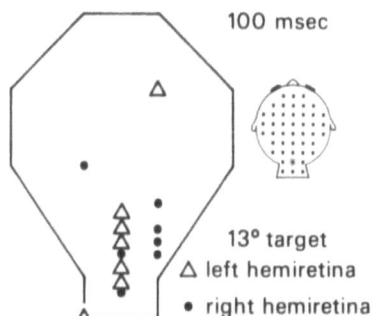

Fig. 8.  Absolute scalp locations of positive extreme field values
at peak times of individual hilliness curves (seven subjects) at
about 100 msec for right and left hemiretina stimulation with 13°
target.  (From Lehmann and Skrandies, in prep.)


side (see also Barrett et al., 1976) for larger targets.

The observation that the response at 100 msec shows an occipital maximum for lateralized stimuli, as well as for centered stimuli,
whereas the 140 msec response shows an occipital maximum for lateralized stimuli but an occipital minimum for centered stimuli, is
indicative of activity of two different neural generator populations.

The described group characteristics of relative location change
of extreme field values do not imply consistency of the absolute
locations across subjects.  Fig. 8 demonstrates the absolute scalp
locations at individual hilliness peak times around 100 msec for
seven subjects using left and right hemiretinal, 13 deg. arc targets.  Obviously there is a considerable scatter of the absolute
locations between subjects, although the population shows the
general tendency for field shifts towards the "correct" hemisphere
when the stimulation is changed from one to the other retinal half.


Upper Versus Lower Hemiretina

When the upper hemiretina is stimulated selectively, field
distributions are observed with maximal values at a more anterior
location than when the lower hemiretina is stimulated (Lesevre,
1973).  Fig. 9 illustrates such scalp field series (15 deg. arc
targets).  These scalp fields reach maximal values at an earlier
time for upper than for lower hemiretinal stimuli.  These latency
differences might be critical when potentials evoked by checkerboard
reversal are used for clinical MS diagnosis (Halliday et al., 1973).

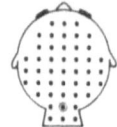

## UPPER HEMI-RETINA

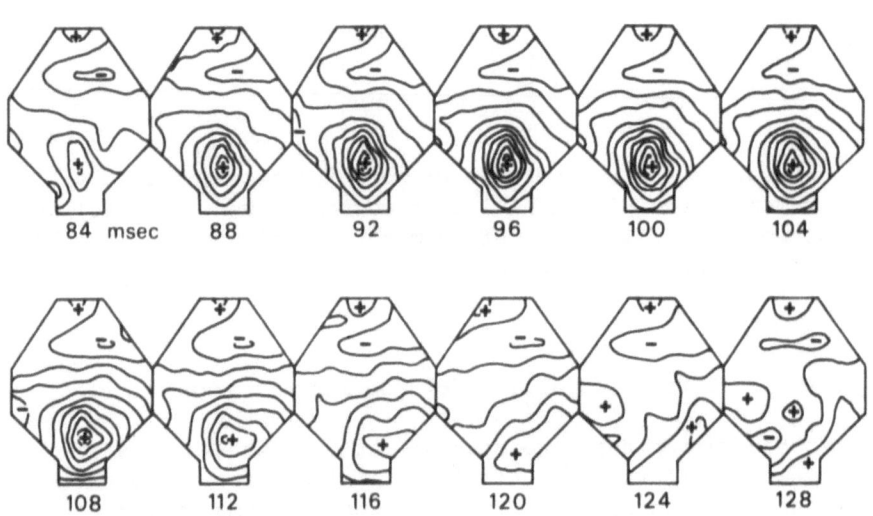

## LOWER HEMI-RETINA

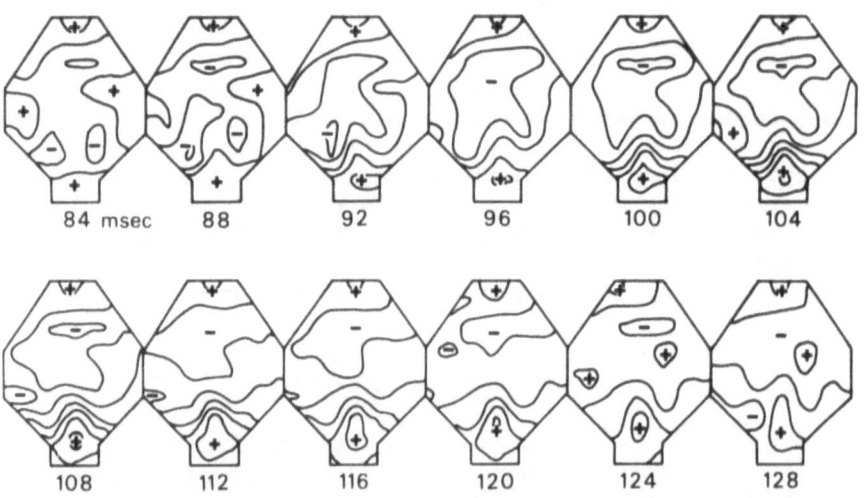

Fig. 9. Equipotential-line maps of average scalp field distributions evoked by stimulation of the upper and lower hemiretina (15° field, 50' checks). Head seen from above, nose up. Each equipotential-line represents a step of 2.2 μV. (From Lehmann and Skrandies, in prep.)

In an earlier paper on this problem (Lehmann et al., 1977) we had
shown that scalp field latency differences may look like waveform
inversions in conventional recordings.  We had demonstrated scalp
fields evoked by lower hemiretina stimuli where the occipital field
peak was at the border of the recorded area, and accordingly field
peak migration towards the recording area was not excluded as a
possible cause of the latency differences.

   To settle the latency question we will have to use subjects
whose field peaks remain in the recorded area during the crucial
time.  Since the scalp fields are centered at the occiput around
the sagittal midline and since the anterior distribution is flat
in these stimulus conditions, we need only to search a midline row
of electrodes in order to (a) construct a curve of potential differences over time between any two of the eight midline electrodes
and (b) make certain that the maximal values are neighbored by non-
extreme field values so as to rule out peak migration.  Out of
twenty-five subjects, only five fulfilled this latter restriction.
Profiles of the instantaneous voltages at the eight electrodes
along the midline were constructed and searched for maximal potential differences at each analysis time (plotted vertically in the
example of Fig. 10).  The time of the largest value of the voltage
differences between any two electrodes determined the response
latency.  Median latencies of the five subjects for upper and lower
hemiretina stimuli are given in Table I; the difference is significant at $p < .031$ in Walsh Tests.

   These latency differences between upper and lower hemiretina
evoked potentials are in line with a number of anatomical (e.g.,
Osterberg, 1935) and behavioral observations in man, amongst them
reports on a longer reaction time for lower hemiretinal stimuli
(e.g., Payne, 1967).

Table I.  Median response latencies of five subjects, in msec, at
1.6 checkerboard reversals/sec ($15^\circ$, 40').

| Stimulated hemiretina | | upper | lower |
|---|---|---|---|
| subject | 1 | 98.0 | 110.0 |
| " | 2 | 96.5 | 116.0 |
| " | 3 | 99.0 | 116.0 |
| " | 4 | 94.0 | 106.0 |
| " | 5 | 104.0 | 115.0 |

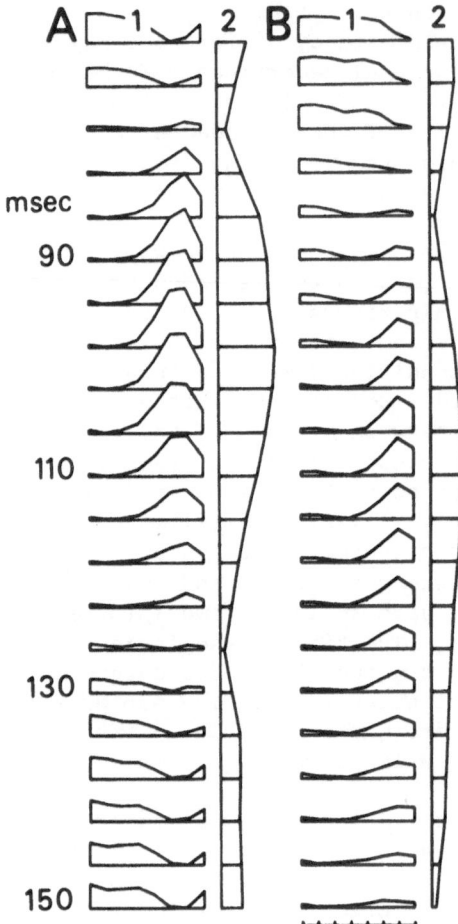

Fig. 10.  Profiles of average evoked potential fields (column 1)
from an anterior to posterior midline row of eight electrodes (left
to right, horizontal bar with marks at bottom).  A upper, B lower
hemiretinal stimuli.  The lowest voltage determines baseline of each
profile.  The maximal voltage difference between any two electrodes
in a given profile is shown by a horizontal bar in column 2.  (From
Lehmann and Skrandies, in prep.)


SUMMARY

    Using multichannel recordings, the latencies of components of
potentials evoked by checkerboard reversal were defined by (a) the
maximal voltage difference between any two electrodes in the field
or by the more general term (b), the maximal value of the mean voltage deviation per electrode from the mean voltage of all electrodes

(hilliness, or relative power). Scalp location of the components
was defined as point of maximal (or minimal) voltage on the scalp.
Two response times were found in the subject population: 100 and
140 msec. For centered stimuli, there was an occipital maximum at
100 msec and an occipital minimum at 140 msec. With lateralized
hemiretinal stimuli, the lateralization of the evoked fields depended on target size: at 100 msec, 13 deg. arc targets evoked maxima
which tended towards the "correct" side ipsilateral to the stimulated hemiretina, whereas with 26 deg. arc targets, maxima were
found over the "wrong" side. The 140 msec response for lateralized
stimuli was occipitally positive (as opposed to negative for central
fixation) and lateralized over the "correct" side for small and
large targets. The occipital polarity for the late response changes
to lateralized in comparison to centered stimuli. This is not true
for earlier responses and indicates two different neural generators.
Upper hemiretina stimuli produced shorter (mdn:12 msec) response
latencies than lower hemiretina stimuli. Scalp field migration was
excluded as possible cause of this difference. Several behavioral
and anatomical observations are in agreement with this difference.
For clinical applications it appears advisable to test hemisphere
functions with larger size stimuli and to consider the latency differences between upper and lower hemiretinae.

## ACKNOWLEDGEMENTS

This work was supported by the Swiss National Science Foundation; EMDO Foundation, Zurich; Hartmann-Muller Foundation, Zurich;
Smith-Kettlewell Eye Research Foundation, San Francisco; Roche
Studienstiftung, Basel. We thank Mr. H.P. Meles for programming
assistance.

## REFERENCES

Barrett, G., Blumhardt, D.L., Halliday, E. and Kriss, A. A paradox
    in the lateralization of the visual evoked response. Nature,
    1976, 261, 253-255.

Blumhardt, L.D., Barrett, G. and Halliday, A.M. The asymmetrical
    visual evoked potential to pattern reversal in one half field
    and its significance for the analysis of visual field defects.
    Brit. J. Ophthalmol., 1977, 61, 454-461.

Cobb, W.A. and Morton, H.B. Evoked potentials from the human scalp
    to visual half field stimulation. J. Physiol., 1970, 208,
    39-40.

Halliday, A.M., McDonald, W.I. and Mushin, J. Visual evoked response in diagnosis of multiple sclerosis.  Brit. Med. J., 1973, 4, 661-664.

Lehmann, D.  Multichannel topography of human alpha EEG fields. Electroenceph. Clin. Neurophysiol., 1971, 31, 439-449.

Lehmann, D.  The EEG as scalp field distribution.  In A. Remond (Ed.), EEG Informatics: A Didactic Review of Methods and Application of EEG Data Processing, Amsterdam: Elsevier, 1977.

Lehmann, D., Meles, H.P. and Mir, Z.  Average multichannel EEG potential fields evoked from upper and lower hemiretina: Latency differences.  Electroenceph. Clin. Neurophysiol., 1977, 43, 725-731.

Lesevre, N.  Potentiels evoques par des patterns chez l'homme: Influence de variables caracterisant le stimulus et sa position dans le champ visuel.  In A. Fessard and G. Lelord (Eds.), Activites Evoques  et Leurs Conditionnement, Paris: INSERM, 1973.

Osterberg, G.  Topography of the layer of rods and cones in the human retina.  Acta Ophthal. (Kbh.), 1935, Suppl. 6, 1-102.

Payne, W.H.  Visual reaction times on a circle about the fovea. Science, 1967, 155, 481-482.

SPONTANEOUS AND EVOKED CEREBRAL ELECTRICAL ACTIVITY AND LOCALIZATION

OF LANGUAGE FUNCTION IN CHILDREN WITH MINIMAL CEREBRAL DYSFUNCTION

M.D. Low, L.J. Rogers, S.J. Purves and H.G. Dunn

University of British Columbia and Vancouver General

Hospital

## INTRODUCTION

One of the major theoretical constructs in the field of cognitive science holds that higher order cerebral tasks are performed in so-called association areas of the cortex, or at least in brain regions different from those serving primary sensorimotor functions. An important element in this concept is that these higher order tasks may also be performed differentially and preferentially by the left and right hemispheres. Most of the evidence for such localization of function has been indirect, derived from clinical-behavioral observations and either post-mortem or ante-mortem diagnostic procedures demonstrating alterations in brain structure.

Neuropsychological experiments (Kimura, 1961; Dimond and Beaumont, 1974; Gazzaniga, 1974; Milner, 1974), cerebral bloodflow studies (Ingvar, 1974) and recording and analysis of brain electrical activity (Harnad et al., 1977; Desmedt, 1977) have all been used in attempts to obtain direct evidence of higher order processing and the distribution or location of such activity within and between the hemispheres in the intact brain. The rationale for such investigations is not only to seek evidence of normal brain mechanisms subserving cognition, language, etc., but also to respond to the powerful motivation of clinical need. At present clinical problems involving higher order dysfunction are extremely difficult to evaluate in objective, quantifiable terms.

Neuropsychological experiments with split brain patients and employing hemisphere directed stimuli have provided unequivocal evidence of differential activity of the left and right hemispheres,

but the applicability of these findings to the intact, integrating
brain is uncertain.  Cerebral bloodflow recording has also provided
direct and definite evidence not only for lateralization of function
but for intrahemispheric localization of function as well.  However,
such experimental procedures are extremely specialized and expensive.
They can be accomplished only in very few centers, and the necessity
for injection of a radioisotope would limit the ethical application
of such studies to cases with real medical need.

    Electrophysiological studies of cognitive and conative function
have been broadly used, and it is generally accepted that high level
processing of sensory input and the cerebral activity involved in
preparing for and carrying out action will influence brain electrical patterns.  Beyond this point there is very little agreement.
The hypothesis that the brain events critical for the appropriate
processing of sensory input, formation of percepts and concepts,
memory retrieval, association, evaluation, volition and action will
be signalled by specific and identifiable changes in the electrical
patterns recordable from the scalp is intuitively appealing.  But
while the literature abounds with reports of changes in or the
appearance of brain waves which are supposedly correlates of some
specific higher order process, for virtually none of these is there
general agreement both about the true cerebral origin of the activity
recorded and the specific brain process giving rise to the activity.
The relevant literature has recently been extensively and critically
reviewed (Donchin et al., 1977; Donald, 1978) and will not be reported here.  But with the possible exception of the early segment
of the Bereitschaftspotential (BSP) or motor potential complex, it
is clear that there is as yet no universally accepted electrophysiological evidence of localization (or, for that matter, lateralization) of higher cerebral function that even approaches in precision
the details of the constructs derived from clinical studies.

    Our own experience in this area began with a search for a motor
speech analog of the contingent negative variation (CNV or slow
component of the BSP; some investigators consider them to be equivalent), the results of which have been published elsewhere (Low
et al., 1973; Low et al., 1976; Low and Fox, 1977).  The motivation
was primarily clinical need.  We are frequently required to assess
patients for possible brain surgery, and for whom an unequivocal
determination of hemisphere dominance for language is essential.
The carotid Amytal test of language dominance is considered reliable,
but it is not without risk and cannot be used at all in young children.  A noninvasive substitute, applicable to children, would be
very valuable.

    Our data, now from more than 125 recording sessions with normal
subjects and patients, led us to conclude that there is a slow potential recordable from the posterior and inferior frontal regions

prior to speech in a manner analogous to the vertex CNV in the usual
cued reaction time paradigm, and that these speech CNVs do show asymmetries which in grouped data can be related to cerebral dominance
for language.  However, the procedures involved present serious methodological difficulties as several investigators, including ourselves,
have documented (Szirtes and Vaughan, 1977; Grozinger et al., 1977;
Low and Fox, 1977).  Furthermore, we were unable to achieve better
than 80% accuracy in prediction of hemisphere dominance (as finally
determined by the carotid Amytal test) when using speech CNV criteria alone.

Because a number of reports in the literature have suggested
that other measures of cerebral electrical activity are related to
language dominance (Cornil and Gastaut, 1947; Galin and Ornstein,
1972; Callaway and Harris, 1974; Butler and Glass, 1974; Beck et
al., 1975; Donchin et al., 1977), we reasoned that some of these
could be used either to strengthen the evidence of lateralization
in the presence of a consistently asymmetrical CNV or to provide
definitive lateralizing information when the CNV asymmetry was variable or inconsistent (as is often the case).

Consequently, we developed a comprehensive test "battery" including a number of neurophysiological measures (i.e., visual evoked
potentials to words and pattern reversal, the CNV, EEG power and
coherence spectra) which we anticipated would assist both in the
assessment of hemisphere dominance and the demonstration of regional
changes in brain electrical activity during reading, speech and
other activities presumed to engage primarily the left or the right
hemisphere.  We have applied our neurophysiological test battery in
recordings from fifty-one children who are participants in a study
being conducted by the U.B.C. Division of Pediatric Neurology.  The
study is a prospective one of children born prematurely and/or with
low birth weight compared to a group of age-matched full birth weight
children.  We have, therefore, had access to a very highly selected
group of subjects with very detailed gestation, birth, neurological,
neurophysiological and developmental histories, all of whom have
been followed clinically for up to 15 years.

Data analysis was intended to provide answers to primarily two
questions:  (1) Are there consistent relationships between the different electrophysiological measures, functional laterality and
hemisphere dominance for language so that one may be reliably predicted from another in a given individual? (2) Are there consistent
electrophysiological correlates of minimal cerebral dysfunction?


METHOD

Subjects for the study were all children between the ages of
12-1/2 and 15 years.  They included twenty-nine normal controls

(seventeen male and twelve female) and sixteen with the MCD syndrome
(eleven male and five female).  All were proven dextrals by laterality testing (handedness, footedness, eyedness).  Data from an additional six sinistrals (four MCD and two normal) are not included in
this report.

     To obtain the diagnostic criteria for the MCD syndrome, clinical
assessments were made in four major areas, i.e., neurological signs,
organic behavioral syndrome signs, routine electroencephalogram
findings (including hyperventilation, photic stimulation and sleep)
and psychometric testing (Table I).  Subjects were given a score of
0 for normal, 1 for abnormal or 1/2 for borderline in each area.
The original clinical diagnostic classification was based upon the

TABLE I

DIAGNOSTIC CRITERIA - MCD

I.    Organic Behavior Syndrome

      Excessive motor activity, impulsiveness, destructiveness, short
      attention span, distractibility, irritability, mood swings,
      perseveration, unpredictability, sleep disturbance.

II.   Neurological Abnormalities

      Eye - Squint, nystagmus, etc.
      Motor - Dystonia, abnormal reflexes, involuntary movements,
           poor gross or fine coordination, cross-laterality.
      Sensory - Finger agnosia, astereognosis, lack of R-L distinction
      Congenital Stigmata - Hypertelorism, abnormal palm prints,
           multiple cafe au lait spots.

III.  Psychometric Abnormalities

      WISC - Full scale IQ assumed 80 +
           - Significant (15+) difference verbal/performance
           - Subtest scatter
      Good Enough - Harris man/woman average IQ
      Knox Cube
      Vocal Encoding

IV.   EEG Abnormalities

      Routine 16-channel recording; awake, asleep, hyperventilation
           and photic stimulation.

total of the four scores with 0 - 1.5 considered normal and 2 - 4 considered MCD.

All electrophysiological recordings were done in an electrically shielded, sound-deadened room with the subjects seated in a reclining chair. Word stimuli were displayed via a 24 cm monochrome TV monitor placed 1 meter in front of the subject's face. The center of the screen was marked for visual fixation. The stimulator for pattern reversal VEPs was a grid of red light-emitting diodes.

Recordings were done with a Beckman Type "R" Dynograph. The recording system bandwidth was 0.025 Hz to 100 Hz (3 dB points) and preamplified EEG signals were led directly to the A/D converters of a PDP 11/20 computer which controlled all of the stimulus presentation and data acquisition. During all recording sessions an automatic artifact rejection routine was used which excluded a trial from the average if the voltage in the electro-oculogram (EOG) channel exceeded a preset limit empirically determined at the beginning of the session (Low, 1977).

The neurophysiological test battery included:

(a)  Power spectral analysis.  This was obtained for four electrode positions (F3, F4, P3, P4 - paired ear reference) during four conditions - resting with eyes open, resting with eyes closed, performance of a right hemisphere dependent task (Street Gestalt completion) and performance of a left hemisphere dependent task (WAIS Similarities Subtest for Children).  For each condition the power in the four canonical EEG frequency bands was measured during ten 4 sec sampling periods.

(b)  Coherence functions.  Coherence in the alpha band was calculated for F3/F4, P3/P4, F3/P3, F4/P4 during the above four conditions.

(c)  Speech CNVs.  The speech CNV was recorded from eight temporal and posterior frontal scalp locations as illustrated in Fig. 1 using the contralateral ear as reference.  The computer controlled paradigm presented a 3-5 letter word as S1 on the video screen.  The word was displayed for 50 msec, and 1.5 sec later a tone pip occurred as S2.  Subjects were instructed to watch the center of the screen, read the word as it appeared and to say the word aloud as soon as the tone sounded.  Up to thirty different words were presented, and averages of blocks of fifteen or thirty trials were obtained in 2.3 sec epochs each beginning 0.5 sec prior to the appearance of the word on the screen.

CNV measures were derived as integrations over time of the negative and positive voltage in each of the two successive 500 msec intervals preceding the onset of S2 as illustrated in Fig. 2.  The

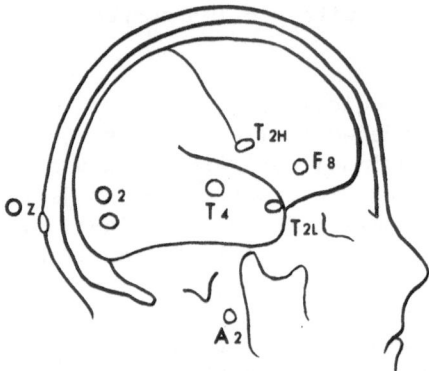

Fig. 1. Electrode placements for recording speech CNVs, WEPs and
pattern reversal VEPs. TH and TL are 2 cm above and 2 cm below a
point midway between the midtemporal (T3,T4) and posterior-frontal
(F7,F8) electrodes.

data from the second interval was later excluded from the analysis
because of possible artifact contamination.

(d) Visual evoked potentials to words (WEPs). From the same eight
scalp locations, four amplitude measurements of the WEP to the word
presented as S1 in the CNV paradigm were made as shown in Fig. 2,
i.e., a-b, b-c, c-d, d-e.

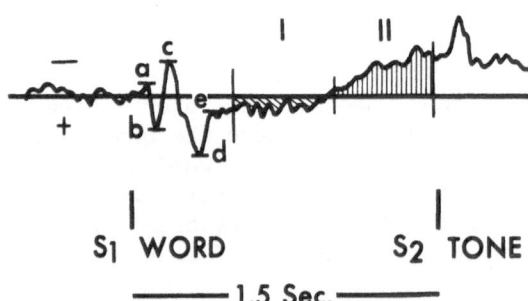

Fig. 2. Illustration of the WEP peak-to-peak amplitude measurements
(a-b, b-c, c-d, d-e) and speech CNV voltage integrations (a positive
and a negative value are possible in each time segment 1 and 11).

(e)  Pattern visual evoked potentials.  Using the reversing red light
pattern stimulator, VEPs were recorded from three electrode locations
(O1, Oz and O2 - paired ear reference).  Stimuli were delivered to
the left and right eyes independently, and responses were recorded
and averaged in blocks of 100.

Measures of patterned visual evoked potential parameters were
derived as the latencies of P100 and N200 components at the Oz
electrode position with left and right eye stimulation and the amplitude (peak-to-peak) of the P100 - N200 segment at the O1 and O2
electrode positions with left and right stimulation.

Due to the length of time required to accomplish all of the
above and to avoid subject fatigue the procedures were divided into
two parts, and the subjects completed the two recording sessions on
different days separated by as much as several weeks.  Specific
test items included in a given day's recording were variable, but
usually the power spectra, coherence functions, speech CNVs and
evoked potentials to words were obtained during a single session.


## RESULTS

From the 156 separate neurophysiological-dichotic listening
measures we have derived an additional 300 variables including inter-
and intrahemispheric ratios of the measures listed above.  This
extremely large data base presents many analytical possibilities,
and while a number are being pursued, this report is only concerned
with the question of correlations between electrophysiological
measures of differences between left and right hemisphere activity
(termed interhemispheric ratio variables) and with the differences
between all of the measures in the normal and MCD subject groups.


### Covariance in Electrophysiological Measures

The neurophysiological data from the twenty-nine normal subjects
(all dextrals) were taken separately and analyzed for possible co-
variances between interhemispheric measures made of speech CNV,
evoked potential and EEG power spectra at rest and during differential task engagement.  A complete search for the dependencies between
these variables was impossible because of the relatively small number
of subjects.

As an initial step a correlation matrix was calculated for all
of the interhemispheric (left-right) ratio variables.  This showed
no significant correlations.  Principal components (Bio-Med "P"
series, program P4R; Dixon, 1977) were then calculated for each of
the three sets of variables, i.e., CNVs, WEPs and EEG excluding

only the intrahemispheric ratio variables.  The first principal
component of the CNV data measured left-right differences in a way
analogous to the second principal component of the whole data set
(see below, Table IV).  The other two data sets did not yield similar left-right principal components.  The CNV first principal component was then used as the dependent variables in separate stepwise
regression calculations (Bio-Med "P" series, program P2R) with each
of the two other data sets' (word evoked potential and EEG) prin-
·cipal components as independent variables.  Two further stepwise
regression runs were made, again with the CNV first principal component as the dependent variable and each of the two other data
sets' untransformed variables as independent variables.  Although
a few of the resulting correlations might have been considered significant, no interpretable or consistent pattern emerged, and it was
concluded that these scattered correlations arose by chance.


Between Groups Differences in Electrophysiological Measures

     In considering the possible separation of the normal and MCD
subject groups a preliminary analysis of the effect of combining
the four separate diagnostic scores (neurological exam, O.B.S.,
psychological testing and routine EEG findings) into a single score
was undertaken.  It was found that the psychological and EEG scores
were less reliably related to the other two (see Table II which
shows the correlation the correlation matrix of all four scores)
and had higher variances.  Consequently it was decided to use as
a final diagnostic score a weighted sum of the four subscores with
the EEG and psychological testing carrying one-half the weight of


TABLE II

CORRELATION ANALYSIS OF FOUR DIAGNOSTIC VARIABLES

|        | NEURO | OBS | EEG | PSYCH | MEAN | ST.DEV. | $R^2$* |
|--------|-------|-----|-----|-------|------|---------|--------|
| NEURO | 1.000 | | | | 0.3222 | 0.356 | 0.384 |
| OBS | 0.568 | 1.000 | | | 0.278 | 0.362 | 0.351 |
| EEG | 0.328 | 0.187 | 1.000 | | 0.300 | 0.418 | 0.108 |
| PSYCH | 0.287 | 0.325 | 0.075 | 1.000 | 0.400 | 0.434 | 0.121 |

*   Squared multiple correlation of each variable with the other
    three.

the other two.  This resulted in a better regression (more significant) analysis of the CNV variábles against diagnostic score.

Since the diagnostic score did not have an obvious bimodal
distribution, for further analysis the data were treated in a single
group, and multivariate regression analysis with the diagnostic score
as the dependent variable was undertaken.  The speech CNV measurements yielded forty-eight variables grouped into three categories:
a) integrated amplitude of speech CNV, b) interhemispheric ratios
of these integrated amplitudes and c) intrahemispheric ratios of
the integrated amplitudes.  Since there were forty-eight variables
and only forty-four subjects, considerable data reduction was
necessary, and two methods were used.  (One further subject was
eliminated.  The regression analysis indicated that this subject
was an outlier, and this clinical diagnosis carried a special note
indicating possible serious neurological problems.)  The first was
stepwise multivariate linear regression (from UCLA Bio-Med "P"
series, program P2R) used to select from the forty-eight variables
the subset best related to the MCD diagnostic score.  The initial
(step 0) partial correlations are listed in Table III.  The criterion chosen for entering variables was to maximize the change in the
residuals (called F method by P2R).

An intrahemispheric ratio (F8/F8+T4, speech CNV, early segment
negative integration) was entered first.  Examination of Table III
shows that the category of right intrahemispheric ratios contains
much information related to MCD, with temporal interhemispheric
ratios and temporal right hemispheric positive integrations nearly
as significant.  The F-to-enter values for the second step of the
stepwise regression program show that most of the negative integration variables were sufficiently correlated with the chosen variable
that their F-to-enter values dropped.  Many of the positive integration values, however, had increased F-to-enter values for the second
step, and the entry of the T4 positive integration variable increased the significance of the regression over that of the first step.
The F ratio at this point was highly significant $[F(2,41)-24.77,p]$.
The variables entered in the next several steps decreased the significance of the F ratio.

A closer examination of the data for the intrahemispheric
ratios indicated that minimal cerebral dysfunction is indicated by
large ratios while normal ratios are more likely to be near 0.5
(the ratio F8/F8+T4 equals 0.5 if F8 equals T4).  In the case of
F8/F8+T4, one half of the subjects with the original diagnosis of
normal had ratios below 0.5 and one-half above (Fig. 3).  Thirteen
of the fifteen subjects diagnosed as having MCD had ratios above
0.5.  In fact eleven of the fifteen had ratios above 0.7.

The second method of data reduction was to calculate the principal components of the standardized CNV variable data matrix (using

TABLE III

CORRELATIONS OF THE SPEECH CNV VARIABLES WITH THE DIAGNOSTIC
VARIABLE DETERMINED BY STEPWISE REGRESSION ANALYSIS

| Left Hemisphere Measurements | | | Left Intrahemispheric Ratios | | |
|---|---|---|---|---|---|
| | Negative | Positive | | Negative | Positive |
| | Integrations | | | Integrations | |
| F7 | 0.348 | -0.278 | F7/F7+T1H | 0.005 | -0.157 |
| T1H | 0.226 | -0.064 | F7/F7+T1L | 0.283 | 0.008 |
| T1L | 0.290 | 0.019 | F7/F7+T3 | 0.397 | -0.092 |
| T3 | 0.074 | 0.117 | T1H/T1H+T1L | 0.011 | 0.202 |
| | | | T1H/T1H+T3 | 0.284 | 0.022 |
| | | | T1L/T1L+T3 | 0.325 | -0.134 |

| Interhemispheric Ratios | | |
|---|---|---|
| | Negative | Positive |
| | Integrations | |
| F8/F8+F7 | 0.371 | -0.126 |
| T2H/T2H+T1H | 0.351 | -0.255 |
| T2L/T2L+T1L | 0.491 | -0.474 |
| T4/T3+T4 | 0.559 | -0.366 |

| Right Intrahemispheric Ratios | | |
|---|---|---|
| | Negative | Positive |
| | Integrations | |
| F8/F8+T2H | 0.342 | -0.201 |
| F8/F8+T2L | 0.448 | -0.393 |
| F8/F8+T4 | 0.584 | -0.372 |
| T2H/T2H+T2L | 0.197 | -0.239 |
| T2H/T2H+T3 | 0.411 | -0.329 |
| T2L/T2L+T4 | 0.361 | -0.099 |

| Right Hemisphere Measurements | | |
|---|---|---|
| | Negative | Positive |
| | Integrations | |
| F8 | -0.003 | 0.026 |
| T2H | -0.169 | 0.177 |
| T2L | -0.325 | 0.454 |
| T4 | -0.418 | 0.504 |

Bio-Med, program P2R). The second principal component was the most
highly correlated {correlation - 0.58552, F ratio for the regression
21.91 [F(1,42)]} with the diagnostic score and was comparable to
F8/F8+T4 in this respect. No other principal component in combination with the second supplied sufficiently different information to
increase the significance of the F ratio.

The second principal component (Table IV) can be interpreted
as indicating a difference between the left and right hemispheric

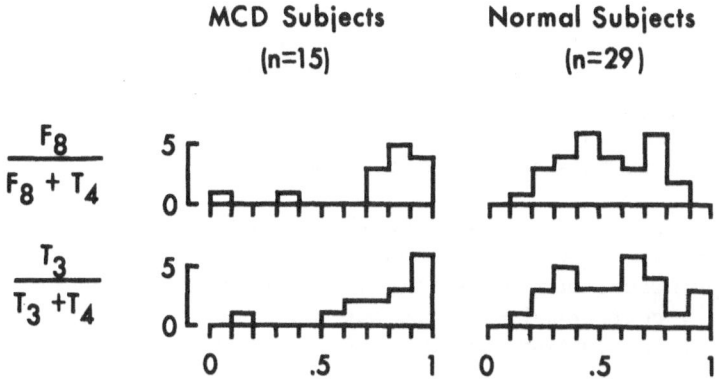

Fig. 3. Histogram of the distribution of the early segment speech CNV ratio values (intra- and interhemispheric) in normal and MCD children.


TABLE IV

SECOND PRINCIPAL COMPONENT OF SPEECH CNV DATA

This table lists the second eigenvector values for the 24 positive integration variables of the speech CNV data. The eigenvector values for the 24 negative integration variables are not included because they provided essentially the same information.

| Left Hemisphere Measurements | | Interhemispheric Ratios | | Right Hemisphere Measurements | |
|---|---|---|---|---|---|
| F7 | -0.12* | F8/F8+F7 | -0.23** | F8 | 0.13* |
| T1H | -0.09 | T2H/T2H+T1H | -0.24** | T2H | 0.17* |
| T1L | -0.14* | T2L/T2L+T1L | -0.28** | T2L | 0.24** |
| T3 | -0.07 | T4/T4+T3 | -0.29** | T4 | 0.25** |

| Left Intrahemispheric Ratios | | | Right Intrahemispheric Ratios | |
|---|---|---|---|---|
| F7/F7+T1H | -0.06 | | F8/F8+T2H | -0.13* |
| F7/F7+T1L | -0.04 | | F8/F8+T2L | -0.18* |
| F7/F7+T3 | -0.07 | | F8/F8+T4 | -0.17 |
| T1H/T1H+T1L | 0.02 | | T2H/T2H+T2L | -0.09 |
| T1H/T1H+T3 | -0.04 | | T2H/T2H+T4 | -0.09 |
| T1L/T1L+T3 | -0.07 | | T2L/T2L+T4 | -0.04 |

*   Emphasis of values greater than 0.10
**  Emphasis of values greater than 0.20

CNV measures. The largest contributions to the principal component
are almost exclusively from the left-right interhemispheric ratios,
and the left hemisphere negative integrations are negatively weighted while the right hemisphere negative integrations are positively
weighted. It should be noted that the intrahemispheric ratios contribute little to this principal component.

Examination of Table IV shows that relatively larger left hemisphere negative integration measures result in a smaller (more
negative) principal component value. Since the principal component
is negatively correlated with the MCD diagnostic variable, relatively larger left hemisphere integrations are positively associated
with MCD.

The interhemispheric ratio with the highest principal component
coefficient was T3/T3+T4. For this variable (Fig. 3B) fourteen
normals had values below 0.5, and sixteen above, while fourteen of
the fifteen MCDs had ratios above 0.5 (eleven above 0.7).

The word evoked potential variable most significantly related
to the MCD diagnostic variable, according to stepwise regression,
was an intrahemispheric ratio (F8/F8+T4) for the N100 peak [p = 0.41,
$F(1,42) = 8.59$]. The second most significant was an intrahemispheric
ratio (T2L/T2L+T4) for P300 [p = 0.40, $F(1,42) = 7.77$]. All other
groups of variables were clearly less related. For the N100 variable
eighteen of twenty-nine normals had values above 0.5, but only six
of these were above 0.6 while eleven of fifteen MCDs had values above
0.6. For P300 thirteen of sixteen normals had ratio values above 0.5,
with six having values above 0.6, while ten of fifteen MCDs had values above 0.6. Some components of the word evoked potential, like
the early segment speech CNV, were therefore more asymmetrical (or
less evenly distributed within one hemisphere) in MCD children than
in normals.

Principal components were calculated separately for the variables derived from each of the four evoked potential peak measurements. The third principal component for the N100 variables was
significantly related to the MCD diagnostic variable [p = -0.464,
$F(1,42) = 11.53$]. The N100 principal component coefficients are
presented in Table V. The right intrahemispheric ratios contribute
most heavily to this principal component and, consistent with the
speech CNV data, a negative principle component score (higher intrahemispheric ratios) indicates minimal cerebral dysfunction.

In a similar fashion, multivariate linear regression and stepwise regression were utilized in analysis of the ten pattern visual
evoked potential variables. This analysis demonstrated that the
children with the highest degree of minimal cerebral dysfunction
tended to have the lowest amplitude visual evoked potentials at O1,
the shortest N160 latencies and highest pattern evoked potential
amplitude at O2.

TABLE V

PRINCIPAL COMPONENT OF WORD EVOKED POTENTIAL PEAK N100
Numbers are the eigenvalues of the variables listed

| Left Hemisphere Measurements | | Interhemispheric Ratios | | Right Hemisphere Measurements | |
|---|---|---|---|---|---|
| F7 | -0.07 | F7/F7+F8 | 0.04 | F8 | -0.10 |
| T1H | 0.06 | T1H/T1H+T2H | 0.06 | T2H | 0.05 |
| T1L | 0.01 | T1L/T1L+T2L | -0.09 | T2L | 0.09 |
| T3 | 0.13 | T3/T3+T4 | -0.14 | T4 | 0.33 |

| Left Intrahemispheric Ratios | | Right Intrahemispheric Ratios | |
|---|---|---|---|
| F7/F7+T1H | -0.22 | F8/F8+T2H | -0.26 |
| F7/F7+T1L | -0.09 | F8/F8+T2L | -0.30 |
| F7/F7+T3 | -0.27 | F8/F8+T4 | -0.45 |
| T1H/T1H+T1L | 0.12 | T2H/T2H+T2L | -0.10 |
| T1H/T1H+T3 | -0.06 | T2H/T2H+T4 | -0.36 |
| T1L/T1L+T3 | -0.20 | T2L/T2L+T4 | -0.35 |

The EEG variable first chosen by the stepwise regression procedure was intensity in the Delta (0-4 Hz) frequency band from electrode placement F3, eyes open condition [$p = 0.32$, $F(1,42) = 4.81$]. In general minimal cerebral dysfunction was positively related to delta and theta intensity and negatively related to alpha intensity. The second best variable [$p = 0.32$, $F(1,42) = 4.81$] was an intrahemispheric ratio, F3/F3+P3, of average intensities in the alpha band for the similarities condition. The frontal interhemispheric ratios and left hemisphere intrahemispheric ratios for each condition were nearly as significant. The variation in these variables was too great, however, to ascertain their distribution with respect to the symmetric ratio value of 0.5.

None of the EEG principal components was significantly related to the MCD diagnostic variable.

DISCUSSION

There are two main conclusions which follow from these experiments. The first is that we have failed to demonstrate a consistent correlation between electrophysiological measures presumed to reflect or to be affected by different activity in the two hemispheres

related to hemisphere dominance (at least as far as such dominance
is indicated by functional laterality). This is disappointing in
that we hoped to be able to show that combinations of such measures
would provide strong corroborative evidence of language dominance
in clinical situations.

One important reason for the lack of statistically significant
correlations among our event related and ongoing EEG potential measures is their marked variability within and between subjects. There
were left-right hemisphere differences in several measures both at
rest and during specific tasks presumed to depend primarily upon
one hemisphere or the other, and these differences were in the
expected directions in grouped data, but in a given subject could
show even opposing asymmetries on repeated measures. In these
studies the most consistent grouped data left-right hemisphere difference measures were those related to the speech CNV and the peak
amplitudes of word evoked potential components in the 100 to 200
msec latency range. Inspection of the raw data, however, revealed
that even these showed marked variability in left-right amplitude
ratios from sample to sample.

There is almost no information in the available literature on
the subject of correlations between slow potential phenomena such
as the CNV, other event related potential parameters and the ongoing
EEG. Curry (1977) examined the relationships between scalp recorded
slow potential fluctuations and event related potentials in an auditory discrimination task but found that there were very few consistent relationships among the measures. The correlations which he
did find were between CNV measures and evoked potential amplitudes.

Our failure to demonstrate any significant interrelatedness
among our various electrophysiological measures, many of which have
been shown to vary in left-right symmetry as a function either of
presumed cerebral dominance for language or verbal vs. nonverbal
task requirements, underscores a problem encountered by all researchers in the general field of cognitive science, and particularly by
those employing electrophysiological parameters as indicators of
higher order cerebral processes: in experiments with human subjects
it is extremely difficult, if not impossible at a given moment in
time, to specify and isolate a single cerebral process.

It appears to us that different electrophysiological parameters
reflect different aspects of the left-right and within-hemisphere
organization of the two halves of the brain. The data obtained in
this work support the concept that the normally functioning integrating brain participates in a more broadly based and less stereo-
typed fashion (in the processes indexed by our electrophysiological
measures) than either anatomical (Geschwind and Levitsky, 1968; Wada
and Davis, 1977) or clinical dysfunction evidence (Milner, 1974) has
been taken to suggest.

The second main conclusion is that as a group children with the minimal cerebral dysfunction syndrome do differ significantly from age-matched normal controls with respect to certain electrophysiological measures.

A similar general observation has been made by several other investigators including Low and Stoilen, 1973; Kinsbourne, 1973; Satterfield and Braley, 1977; John et al., 1977; Fuller, 1977 and Rebert et al., 1978, based upon demonstration of frequency, latency or amplitude abnormalities in either the EEG or event related potential parameters in groups of children with learning disorders or the MCD syndrome.  While there are scattered references in the existing literature to differences in EEG L/R symmetry measures between normal and learning disordered children, only one other group of investigators (John et al., 1977) has systematically explored intrahemispheric differences in cerebral electrical activity in this context.

In an ongoing study which now includes a large number of subjects, John and his colleagues have used a form of cluster analysis to differentiate not only abnormal (MCD or learning disabled) children from normals, but to distinguish between different kinds of learning disability.  However, their methods of data acquisition and analysis preclude any direct comparison with the regional differences we have found between our normal and MCD subjects.  It should be noted that while John et al. depend very heavily upon psychometric testing for diagnostic classification, we have found that psychological data is less reliably related to an overall diagnosis than either neurological examination or elements of an organic behavior syndrome.

The work that we are reporting here has shown that the single most potent measure discriminating MCD from normal children is the difference in magnitude of the early segment speech CNV between anterior and midtemporal sites in the right hemisphere, with the MCD children having greater differences (or more localized potential distribution over the scalp) than normal children.  The same kind of intrahemispheric differences were shown for mid-latency components of evoked responses to visually presented word stimuli while both speech CNVs and pattern reversal visual evoked potentials were more asymmetrical between homologous brain regions in MCD than in normal children.  All of these event related potential measures were better "indicators" of the MCD diagnosis than EEG frequency analysis although our finding of greater slow activity in MCD children than normals is consistent with the observations of many other investigators.  Some other very recent evidence (Shagass et al., 1978; Neville et al., 1978; Kurtzberg and Vaughan, 1978) has also demonstrated that differences in scalp distribution of event related potential measurements can provide significant diagnostic or discriminating information when comparing normal and abnormal subjects.

The possibility of artifact contamination must be considered in any explanation of our findings. Szirtes and Vaughan (1977), while admitting that the CNV paradigm might be the one possible way to avoid extra-cerebral artifact in such experimental studies, have argued that slow potential asymmetries preceding speech are most likely due to variations in the glosso-kinetic potential. Grozinger et al. (1977), in turn, have categorically stated that Szirtes and Vaughan were recording skin potentials or galvanic skin responses rather than glosso-kinetic, palate or pharyngeal muscle activity. While we always monitor the electro-oculogram (our computer controlled system automatically discards any trial from the average which is contaminated by even the slightest eye movement) we have only intermittently used recording of glosso-kinetic potentials to determine their possible contribution to the electrical activity recorded from anterior head regions. While we cannot agree with Grozinger et al. that the slow potentials observed by Szirtes and Vaughan must all be generated in the skin, neither can we agree with Szirtes and Vaughan that glosso-kinetic potentials account for most or all of the slow potential asymmetries which we have observed. In the absence of any physiological or anatomical evidence, we find it very difficult to credit their argument that asymmetrical tongue movements are related to language dominance. When we have employed glosso-kinetic potential recording we have found these potentials to be much shorter in duration and closer to the time of articulation than our early segment speech CNV, and furthermore they were almost never asymmetrical. We believe that the most parsimonious explanation of our data is that the early segment speech CNV is in fact a cerebrally generated potential.

Another possible source of contamination of our data, particularly with the electrode placements used, is lateral eye movement. It is well known that reading, as required by our speech CNV paradigm, may be associated with saccadic eye movements which, in turn, are associated with event related potentials in the brain. As indicated above, we have very carefully controlled for EOG artifact in our recording procedures. Close inspection of individual word evoked responses reveal that while they are often asymmetrical with higher amplitude on the right side than on the left, their various components are in phase over the two hemispheres. If these were being generated by or significantly influenced by lateral saccades (since we employed a contralateral ear reference), the potentials would often or always appear to be more or less equal in amplitude but up to 180° out of phase over the two sides. The possibility remains that what we are recording as word evoked potentials may be brain potentials related to very small saccadic eye movements.

Whatever the final explanation for the asymmetries and localization differences observed, these studies have clearly demonstrated that MCD children as a group show greater lateralization/localization over the scalp as compared to normals. This appears to be

particularly true for potentials presumably related to visual function, reading and language generation.  It is possible that these
findings are a reflection of less than normal cerebral integration
in the minimal cerebral dysfunction syndrome, and this may be one
reflection of the as yet completely unknown pathophysiology of this
disorder.

## SUMMARY

A comprehensive test battery including a number of neurophysiological measures for assessment of hemisphere activity during reading, speech and other tasks presumed to engage primarily in the left
or right hemisphere has been applied in a study of twenty-nine normal children and sixteen with the minimal cerebral dysfunction syndrome.  The electrophysiological measures included the speech CNV,
evoked potentials to visually presented word stimuli, alpha frequency
power spectra at rest and during left and right hemisphere tasks and
pattern reversal visual evoked potentials.  Correlations and multivariate analysis of the data (including stepwise regression and
principal component analysis) showed no consistent intrahemispheric
correlations among the different measures.  MCD children showed
significantly greater intrahemispheric and interhemispheric ratios
than normal children.

## ACKNOWLEDGEMENTS

The authors thank Jan Galloway and Mike Baker for technical
assistance and Louise Stevenson for manuscript preparation.  This
work was supported by Medical Research Council of Canada Grant MA3313.

## REFERENCES

Beck, E.C., Dustman, R.E. and Lewis, E.G.  The use of the
    averaged evoked potential in the evaluation of central nervous
    system disorders.  Int. J. Neurol., 1975, 9, 212-232.

Butler, S.R. and Glass, A.  Asymmetries in the CNV over left and
    right hemispheres while subjects await numeric information.
    Biol Psychol., 1974, 2, 1-16.

Callaway, E. and Harris, P.R.  Coupling between cortical potentials
    from different areas.  Science, 1974, 183, 873-875.

Cornil, L. and Gastaut, H.  Etude electroencephalographique de la
    dominance sensorielle d'un hemisphere cerebral.  Presse Med.
    1974, 37, 421-422.

Curry, S.H.  An examination of the relationship between scalp re-
    corded steady potential fluctuations and event related
    potentials in an auditory discrimination task. Thesis,
    Simon Fraser University, Vancouver, 1976.

Desmedt, J.E. (Ed.) Language and hemispheric specialization in man:
    cerebral event related potentials.  Prog. Clin. Neurophysiol.
    Vol. 3, Basel: Karger, 1977.

Dixon, W.J.  Biomedical Computer Programs 'P' Series.  University of
    California Press, 1977.

Dimond, S.J. and Beaumont, J.G. (Eds.)  Hemisphere Function in the
    Human Brain,  London: Elek, 1974.

Donald, M.W.  Limits on current theories of transient evoked poten-
    tials.  In J.E. Desmedt (Ed.), Cognitive Components in Cerebral
    Event Related Potentials and Selective Attention.  Prog. Clin.
    Neurophysiol., Vol. 6, Basel: Karger, in press.

Donchin, E., McCarthy, G. and Kutas, M.  Electroencephalographic
    investigations of hemispheric specialization.  In J.E. Desmedt
    (Ed.), Language and Hemispheric Specialization in Man.  Prog.
    Clin. Neurophysiol., Vol. 3, Basel: Karger, 1977.

Fuller, P.W.  Computer estimated alpha attenuation during problem
    solving in children with learning disabilities.  Electroenceph.
    Clin. Neurophysiol., 1977, 42, 149-156.

Galin, D. and Ornstein, R.  Lateral specialization and cognitive
    mode: An EEG study.  Psychophysiol., 1972, 9, 412-418.

Gazzaniga, M.S.  Cerebral dominance viewed as a decision system. In
    S.J. Dimond and J.G. Beaumont (Eds.), Hemisphere Function in
    the Human Brain, London: Elek, 1974.

Geschwind, N. and Levitsky, W.  Human brain: left-right asymmetries
    in temporal speech region.  Science, 1968, 161, 186-187.

Grozinger, B., Kornhuber, H.H. and Kriebel, J.  Human cerebral
    potentials preceding speech production, phonation and movements
    of the mouth and tongue, with reference to respiratory and
    extracerebral potentials.  In J.E. Desmedt (Ed.), Language and
    Hemispheric Specialization in Man.  Prog. Clin. Neurophysiol.,
    Vol. 3, Basel: Karger, 1977.

Harnad, S.R., Doty, R.W., Goldstein, L., Jaynes, J. and Krauthamer,
    G. (Eds.), Lateralization in the Nervous System, New York:
    Academic Press, 1977.

Ingvar, D.  Studies of cerebral blood flow during speech and reading. Electroenceph. Clin. Neurophysiol., 1974, 36, 561-576.

John, E.R., Karmel, B.Z., Cornig, W.C., Easton, P., Brown, D., Alm, M., John, M., Harmony, T., Prichep, L., Toro, A., Gershon, I., Bartlett, F., Thatcher, R., Kay, H., Valdes, P. and Swartz, E. Neurometrics, Science, 1977, 196, 1393-1410.

Kimura, D.  Cerebral dominance and the perception of verbal stimuli. Can. J. Psychol., 1961, 15, 166-171.

Kinsbourne, M.  Minimal brain dysfunction as a neurodevelopmental lag.  Ann. N.Y. Acad. Sci., 1973, 205, 268-273.

Kurtzberg, D. and Vaughan, H.G., this volume.

Low, M.D.  Event related potentials and the CNV.  In A. Remond (Ed.), EEG Informatics: A Didactic Review of Methods and Applications of EEG Data Processing, Amsterdam: Elsevier, 1977.

Low, M.D., Wada, J.A. and Fox, M.  Electroencephalographic localization of conative aspects of language production in the human brain.  Trans. Am. Neurol. Assn., 1973, 98, 129-133.

Low, M.D., Wada, J.A. and Fox, M.  Electroencephalographic localization of the conative aspects of language production in the human brain.  In W. C. McCallum and J. Knott (Eds.), The Responsive Brain, Bristol: Wright, 1976.

Low, M.D. and Fox, M.  Scalp recorded slow potential asymmetries preceding speech in man.  In J.E. Desmedt (Ed.), Language and Hemispheric Specialization in Man: Cerebral ERPs.  Prog. Clin. Neurophysiol., Vol. 3, Basel: Karger, 1977.

Low, M.D. and Stoilen, L.  CNV and EEG in children: Maturational characteristics and findings in the MCD syndrome.  Electroenceph. Clin. Neurophysiol., Suppl. 3, 1973, 139-143.

Milner, B.  Hemispheric specialization: Scope and limits.  In F.O. Schmitt and F.G. Worden (Eds.), The Neurosciences: Third Study Program, MIT Press, Cambridge, 1974.

Nelville, H.J., Snyder, E., Knight, R., Schulman-Galambos, C. and Galambos, R., this volume.

Rebert, C.S., Wexler, B.N. and Sproul, A.  EEG asymmetry in educationally handicapped children.  Electroenceph. Clin. Neurophysiol., 1978, 45, 436-442.

Satterfield, J.H. and Braley, B.W.  Evoked potentials and brain
    maturation in hyperactive and normal children.  Electroenceph.
    Clin. Neurophysiol., 1977, 43, 43-51.

Shagass, C., Roemer, R.E., Straumanis, J.J., Amadeo, M., this volume.

Szirtes, J. and Vaughan, J.R.  Characteristics of cranial and facial
    potentials associated with speech production.  Electroenceph.
    Clin. Neurophysiol., 1977, 43, 386-396.

Wada, J.A. and Davis, A.E.  Fundamental nature of human infants'
    brain asymmetries.  Can. J. Neurol. Sci., 1977, 4, 203-207.

HEMISPHERE DIFFERENCES IN EVENT RELATED POTENTIALS AND CNV'S

ASSOCIATED WITH MONAURAL STIMULI AND LATERALIZED MOTOR RESPONSES

W.C. McCallum and S.H. Curry

Burden Neurological Institute, Bristol BS16 1QT,

England

## INTRODUCTION

Hemispheric lateralization of cerebral processing of various kinds is well established, but the electrophysiological concomitants of such lateralization have proved more difficult to demonstrate. In the auditory system the principal projection is accepted as being to the temporal cortex contralateral to the stimulated ear, but with secondary projection to the ipsilateral temporal cortex. Lateralized motor resposes are, of course, even more clearly a function of the motor cortex contralateral to the responding limb.

Lateral evoked potential differences to auditory stimuli have been studied primarily with respect to the N1 or N1/P2 components. The N1 component has been generally accepted as the peak negative deflection occurring in the period 80 to 140 msec after an auditory stimulus and as reflecting the processes of selective attention. Its amplitude, either with respect to baseline or to the following P2, is largest at or near the vertex and diminishes progressively in all directions from that point (Vaughan and Ritter, 1970; Kooi et al., 1971; Picton et al., 1974). However, Vaughan and Ritter have suggested that its real origins are from dipole sources located in the temporal lobes and that the apparently larger amplitude seen at the vertex is merely the effect of summation there of volume conducted signals from the two temporal sources. They also noted in four subjects that N1 showed a slight contralateral predominance to monaural stimulation. Similarly increased contralateral amplitudes for N1 were reported by Tanguay et al. (1977); Hink et al. (1978); Wolpaw and Penry (1975; 1977). The last named authors noted that, in addition to the usual vertex N1 component at 105 msec, there was a second biphasic component at T3 and T4 which was more

asymmetric than the first and had a latency of 105-110 msec for the
initial positive wave and of 150-160 msec for the following negative
wave. A number of reports suggest that apart from the contralateral
effect there is also a tendency for there to be a right hemisphere
amplitude predominance (Peronnet et al., 1974; Tanguay et al., 1977;
Mononen and Seitz, 1976). However, not all studies confirm the
contralateral effect. Picton et al. (1974) report that N1-P2 distribution is the same whether stimulation is monaural or binaural,
and Hasland (1974) and Mononen and Seitz (1976) report no lateral
predominance to monaural stimuli. There have also been several
studies which have reported shorter N1 latencies over the contralateral hemisphere (Wolpaw and Penry, 1975; Butler et al., 1969;
Spreng, 1971).

Lateralized electrical changes associated with motor tasks
have been a little better established. A clearly lateralized motor
cortex potential accompanies movement of a contralateral limb and
the slow Bereitschaftspotential which precedes voluntary movements
is found to be slightly larger over the hemisphere contralateral to
the responding limb. On the other hand the CNV, which occurs during
warned foreperiods, has not shown consistent asymmetries although
there have been one or two reports of minor asymmetries over central
regions, the larger amplitudes being held to occur either over the
hemisphere contralateral to the responding hand or over the speech
dominant hemisphere when an appropriate task was employed (Butler
and Glass, 1971, 1974; Otto and Leifer, 1973; Low et al., 1976;
Rohrbaugh et al., 1976; Curry et al., 1978).

The present study investigates hemisphere involvement in auditory processing and in preparation for motor response. It was
hypothesized that asymmetries would be found in EP and slow potential components depending on the ear of stimulation and the lateralization of motor responses and that the relatively long latency
range normally allocated to evoked potentials referred to as N1
might be concealing the fact that more than one component was occurring during this period. Given that the existence of two or more
components could be established it was hoped, by studying their
relative distributions, to shed more light on the systems involved
and their functions.

METHOD

Evoked Potential-CNV Paradigm

Eighteen subjects, seven male and eleven female, were tested.
Twelve subjects classed themselves as right-handed and six as left.
Each subject was required to listen to a series of trials in which
a 30 msec warning tone was followed 1.5 sec later by a 500 msec

1000 Hz tone.  The warning tone could be either high (1600 Hz) or
low (600 Hz), and all stimulus pairs were delivered monaurally.
The high and low warning tones and the ear of stimulation were varied according to a pseudo-random sequence which was the same for
all subjects.  Subjects were instructed that if the warning signal
was high they were to terminate the following 1000 Hz tone as rapidly as possible by pressing a button with the hand ipsilateral to
the stimulated ear.  If the warning signal was low they were to use
the button in the hand contralateral to the stimulated ear to terminate the 1000 Hz tone.  Stimuli were delivered at approximately
60 dB to each ear.  All subjects had normal hearing in the frequency
ranges used and all reported that the intensity of stimuli was subjectively equal in both ears.

During the task, evoked potentials and slow potential changes
were recorded from Ag/AgCl electrodes located at positions Fpz, T3,
T4, T5, T6, C3, C4 and Cz of the international 10:20 system.  Lateral
electrodes were referred to the contralateral mastoid process; Fpz
was referred to the right mastoid, and Cz was referred separately
to both left and right mastoids.  Further pairs of electrodes on
the forearms recorded the EMG to button pressing.

Primary recording was by a modified 16 channel Elema-Schonander
Mingograph using 5 sec time constants and 70 Hz filters.  Two second
epochs of time, starting 100 msec before each warning tone, were
sampled for all channels and stored by a PDP-12 computer on digital
tape at a resolution of 8 msec per point.  Subsequently averages
were computed for twenty trials of each of the following four conditions:  (1) Left ear stimulation - left hand press; (2) Right ear
stimulation - right hand press; (3) Left ear stimulation - right
hand press; (4) Right ear stimulation - left hand press.  Reaction
time (RT) was recorded on each trial, and mean RT values were calculated for each of the four conditions.  Trials on which there was
excessive eye movement or other artifact were rejected on-line.

The same experimental paradigm was also presented to one patient
in whom intracerebral gold electrodes had been implanted for thera-
peutic purposes.  The presence of high amplitude, infra-slow activity
at these electrodes necessitated the use of a relatively short (0.6
sec) time constant in this case.  Recording was from an anterior-
posterior array of electrodes located subdurally over the fronto-
temporal regions of the right hemisphere and from selected electrodes
in the depths of the frontal lobes.  Each electrode was 150 microns
in diameter and 4 mm long.

Subjects' lateral preferences were assessed using the Edinburgh
Inventory (Oldfield, 1971), and measures of auditory lateralization
were made using a dichotic listening task which required them to
listen to sequences of six digits presented in pairs from pre-

recorded tape.  The two digits of a pair were presented simultaneously, one to each ear.  The task was to repeat as many as possible of the six digits after each sequence.  Two balanced sets, each
of twenty-five groups of six digits were presented.  The headphones
were reversed between the two sets to control for any possible
intensity differences or instrumental inequalities.  Three measures
were used:  (1) a percentage difference of correctly reported digits
for each ear; (2) a measure of ear reported first; (3) a measure
of absolute performance (i.e., percent correct irrespective of ear).

## Evoked Potential Paradigm

     Based on the results of the experiment already described, a
further ten subjects were tested in various auditory paradigms to
determine more precisely the latency and distribution of the auditory EP components seen and the validity of using the contralateral
mastoids as reference.  Each subject received minimally two series
of 30 msec, 1000 Hz 60 dB tone pips delivered irregularly at a mean
rate of one every 4 sec to left, right or both ears in a pseudo-
random sequence.  To one series he listened without responding, and
to the other he pressed immediately a button with the hand ipsilateral to the stimulated ear, making no press if the stimuli were
binaural.  In one subgroup of five subjects electrodes were located
at C3, C4, T3, T4, A1 and A2 and were referred (a) to a balanced
noncephalic reference as described by Stephenson and Gibbs, 1951;
Lehtonen and Koivikko, 1971; Wolpaw and Penry, 1975), (b) to the tip
of the nose, and (c) to contralateral mastoids.  Oculograms were
recorded from electrodes at the nasion and right outer canthus.  In
the remaining subjects further electrodes were added to give a complete coronal chain with 10% interaural spacing, plus left and right
neck electrodes 10% below the pre-auricular level, together with
Fp1, Fp2, F7, Fz, F8, T5 and T6.  Recording conditions were otherwise as described for the first experiment.

## RESULTS

## Measures and Analysis

     Preliminary analysis of the time interval normally attributed
to the N1 response revealed three negative components with differing distributions which we have defined as peak negative values in
the following latency brackets:  N1a (60-90 msec), N1b (95-115 msec)
and N1c (116-150 msec).  Latency and amplitude measures were made
for each of these components together with N2 and P3.  Three measures
of CNV amplitude were made:  early CNV - from 400 to 950 msec after
S1; late CNV - from 950 to 1500 msec after S1; 'standard' CNV -

from 1300 to 1500 msec after S1.  Each measure was expressed as a
mean value for the period concerned.  Difference measures were calculated for each component measure at homologous electrode sites
(e.g., T3-T4).  Additionally a more general hemisphere asymmetry
score was calculated by summing the difference scores for all homologous electrode pairs.  All amplitudes were measured with respect to
a baseline calculated as the mean amplitude level over the 1.0 sec
prior to S1.

All primary measures were initally analyzed using a four-way
ANOVA (sex X hand X electrode X condition).  Where permissible
separate one-way ANOVAs were performed to illuminate the main effects.
A posteriori contrasts were made using a Duncan multiple range test.
Significance levels for these and all subsequent procedures were
$p < 0.05$.  Pearson product moment correlations were performed on
selected pairs of variables.  The CNV measures were subjected to a
stepwise discriminant analysis (SPSS Version 7) in an attempt to
discriminate the experimental conditions.


## EP-CNV Paradigm

Evoked potentials.  N1a appeared primarily at the temporal
electrodes and at Fpz with a mean latency to peak over all electrodes of 75 msec.  Its mean latency diminished anteriorly, being
shortest at Fpz and longest over central regions where it was only
measurable on about half of the averages, usually as a slight inflection on the ascending part of the second negative-going component (N1b).  N1a was larger in the left hemisphere of right-handed
subjects and in the right hemisphere of left-handed subjects.  Its
amplitude was approximately -5 to -7 µV in anterior and temporal
areas, but was, when measurable, more variable over central regions
where it could range from -4 to more than -15 µV.

N1b had a mean latency of 106 msec and was distinguished as a
separate component both on the basis of its later occurrence and its
distribution.  It was measurable most consistently over central
electrodes where its mean amplitude was -16µV.  At temporal electrodes it was measurable on less than half the averages and at Fpz
on only one sixth.  At C3 and C4, amplitudes were larger over the
hemisphere contralateral to the stimulated ear, but this difference
failed to reach significance.  However, amplitude asymmetries were
significantly related to handedness, larger values being associated
with the hemisphere contralateral to the preferred hand, particularly in the left-handers.  Latencies showed no clear distribution
pattern but were significantly shorter in the hemisphere contralateral to the preferred hand.  At C3 and C4 there was also a significant relationship between N1b latency and the hand used for response; the shorter latency was at the contralateral electrode.

The third negative component (N1c) had a mean latency of 129 msec and was significantly larger over the hemisphere contralateral to the stimulated ear.  It was measurable on 82% of the averages from temporal electrodes and 75% of averages from Ppz, but on only 50% of the averages from central electrodes, where it could appear either as an extension of N1b or as a separate peak.  N1a amplitudes were also significantly larger and latencies significantly shorter in the hemisphere ipsilateral to the preferred hand.  Although this component was seen most consistently over temporal regions its mean amplitude at temporal electrodes was approximately $-8\mu V$ compared with -13 to -16 $\mu V$ at central electrodes.  At first it seemed possible that N1b might be the result of a fusion of the N1a and N1c components, but this proved to be unlikely as in many instances all three negative peaks could be separately distinguished at the same electrode.

The N1 series of components was followed by the usual P2, N2, P3 complex, the mean latencies being 182, 226 and 302 msec, respectively.  No significant hemisphere effect was found for N2; P3 showed a slight predominance contralateral to the ear of stimulation, but this did not reach significance.  P2 showed consistently higher mean amplitudes contralateral to the ear of stimulation. Mean hemisphere differences were in the order of 1-2 $\mu V$, but we are at this stage unable to say whether this difference is significant.

In addition to the condition and hand effects, some sex differences emerged.  Males showed significantly larger amplitudes for components N1B, N1C and N2 and females for P3.  Females also showed significantly shorter latencies for N1A.

Fig. 1 a-d illustrates averages across all subjects of the waveforms elicited by the four conditions.  Fig. 2 gives in histogram form the amplitude values for each of the components measured in each of the experimental conditions, including amplitude differences between homologous electrode pairs.


CNV


The group as a whole produced "normal" CNVs, the mean vertex amplitude for the late and standard CNV measures being -15 $\mu V$. Asymmetries of late and standard CNV measures were noted between homologous electrode pairs, these being highly significant between C3 and C4.  The larger amplitudes were found over the hemisphere contralateral to the responding hand.  Examination of subgroups showed that asymmetries were significantly larger when subjects used their preferred hand, particularly in left-handers and in the ipsilateral press condition.  Late CNVs were significantly larger in females than males.

The early component of the CNV was seen prominently at Fpz.
It was present, and relatively symmetrical over central and temporal
regions, diminishing posteriorly to -1 µV at T5 and T6.  Early CNV
amplitude showed no consistent relationship to the hand used for
pressing but showed a similar relationship to handedness as that
displayed by the late CNV.

Performance.  Mean reaction times (RT) for the four conditions
were:  (1) Stim. left/Press left: 186 msec; (2) Stim. right/Press
right: 190 msec; (3) Stim. left/Press right: 203 msec; (4) Stim.
right/Press left: 195 msec.  RT in condition 3 was significantly
different from that in the other conditions, but overall RT showed
no significant correlations with any of the CNV or EP measures.

Lateral preferences.  The mean Laterality Quotient (LQ) for
the right-handers, assessed by their scores on the Edinburgh Inventory, was +85, and for the six left-handers the mean LQ was -64 and
confirmed subjects' self-reports of handedness.

The first dichotic listening test measure was based on a percentage difference between reported digits in the right and left
ears.  The mean score for the group was -29 indicating a moderate
right ear advantage.  It was, however, only possible to administer
the test to twelve subjects, of whom eight showed a right ear advantage, two a left ear advantage and for two the difference was
zero.  The second measure indicated that right ear digits were reported first by nine subjects and left ear digits by three subjects.
No clear relationship to handedness emerged.  The mean level of
correctly reported digits was 77%, males performing significantly
better than females in the ratio of 91%: 70%.  Neither of the ear
advantage measures was significantly related to any of the other
experimental variables.


                              EP Paradigm


The results from the second phase of the experiment confirmed
the contralateral predominance of Nlb and Nlc and the distributions
of components as seen in the first phase of the experiment (see Fig.
3).  The improved resolution (2 msec per point) permitted more accurate measurement of latencies of the three principal negative
components which emerged as : -Nla: 60-78 msec; Nlb: 90-104 msec;
Nlc: 118 msec.  The additional electrodes at Fpl; Fp2; F7 and F8
also confirmed the frontal, as well as temporal, distribution of
Nla.

The three different references used in this study produced
very similar results.  From Fig. 3 it can be seen that the noncephalic and contralateral mastoid references produce the closest correspondence in both waveform and amplitude.  Reference to the nose

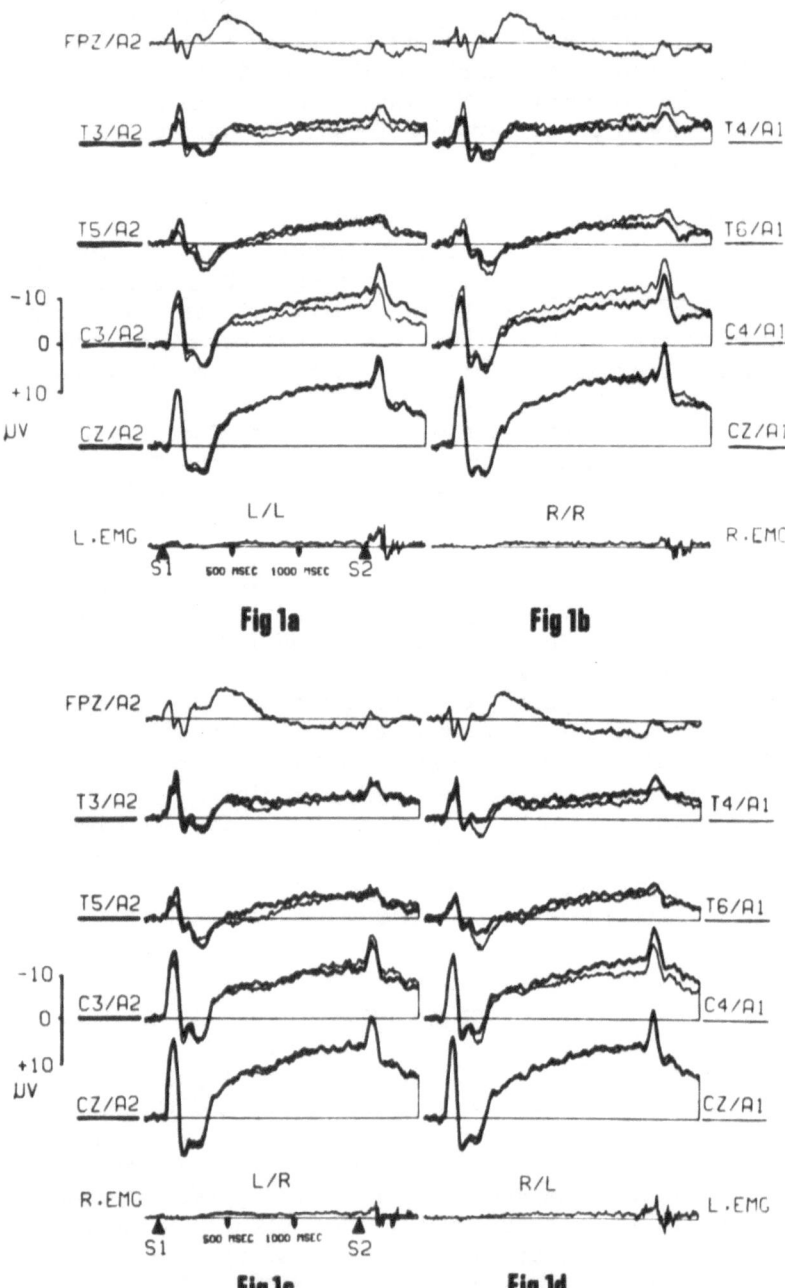

Fig. 1.   Averages across all subjects and all conditions.   Thickness
of line indicates the electrode from which each trace of a pair is
derived.   The ear of stimulation followed by the hand of response
are indicated immediately above the EMG trace for each of the four
conditions.

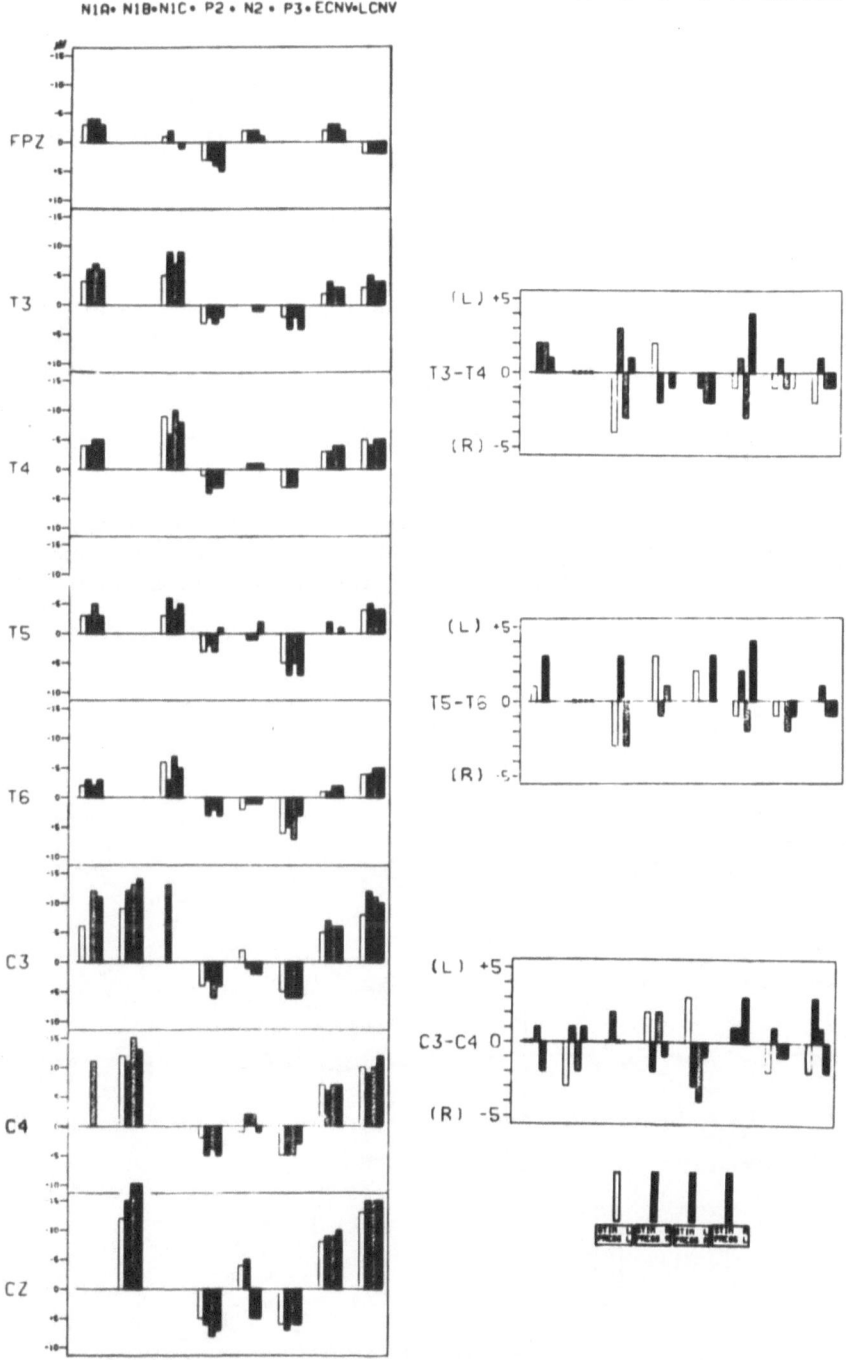

Fig. 2.   Histogram bars show mean amplitude of each component for each condition across all subjects.   On right are amplitude differences between homologous pairs of electrodes.

resulted in very slightly lower amplitudes and a tendency for the
N1a component to disappear.

The coronal chain of electrodes used showed no reversal of the
N1 series of components below the level of the Sylvian fissure as
reported by Vaughan and Ritter (1970).


### Intracerebral Evidence

Recordings were made from the patient with intracerebral gold
electrodes using both the original paradigm and the later higher
resolution EP paradigm.  The electrodes displaying the most prominent auditory EPs were those on the cortical surface of the right
hemisphere and five electrodes close to the orbital surface of the
right frontal lobe.

Although CNVs could be discerned at a number of sites in the
EP-CNV paradigm, the relatively short time constant used and the
presence of infra-slow activity made their evaluation uncertain.

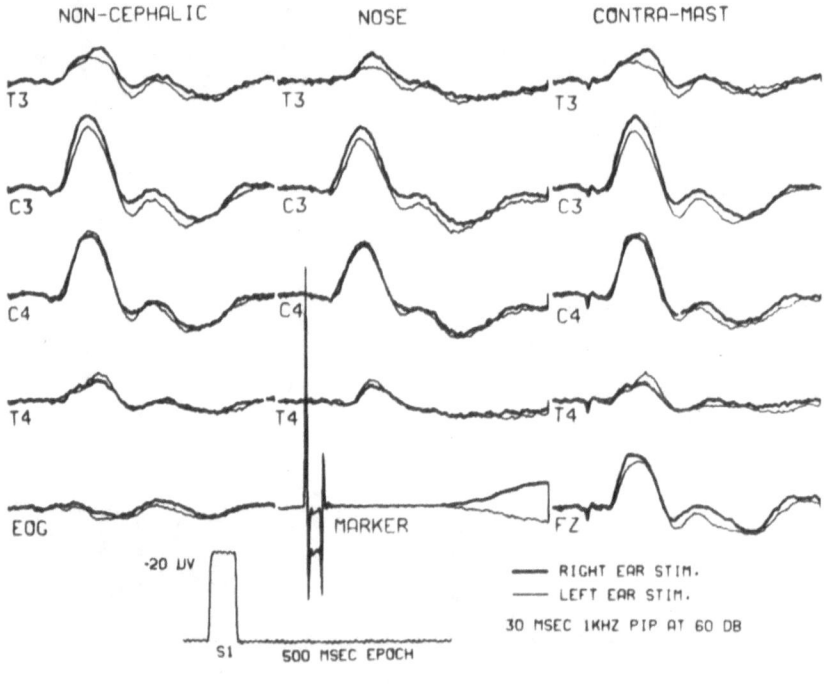

Fig. 3.  Comparison of balanced noncephalic, nose and contralateral
mastoid references for simultaneously recorded averages across five
subjects.

EPs at the cortical electrodes displayed a positive component
with peak latency at 84 msec, a prominent negative component peaking at 136 msec and a later positive complex with a peak latency of
188 msec.  In the EP-CNV paradigm the negative peak tended to be
larger in amplitude to left ear (i.e., contralateral) than to right
ear stimulation.  In the orbital regions of the frontal lobe the
most medial electrode, 64, showed an EP complex generally similar
in form and latency to that seen at the superior cortical electrodes.
Other evidence suggested that this electrode was in orbital gray
matter.  The four other electrodes examined showed a waveform which
was virtually phase reversed with respect to those at the cortex.
These electrodes were thought to be adjacent to the lower orbital
cortical layers, probably in white matter.  The latencies of the
principal components were approximately 16 msec shorter to left
than to right ear stimulation (see Fig. 4).


DISCUSSION

The first of the hypotheses tested, namely that longer latency
evoked potentials to monaurally presented stimuli would show an
amplitude predominance over the contralateral hemisphere has received clear support from the study.  Both the Nlb and Nlc components show this asymmetry, and there are indications that it may be
present to a lesser extent for P2 and P3.  There have, however, been
indications in some of our pilot and ancilliary studies that this
asymmetry can vary substantially with rate of stimulus presentation,
and stimulus characteristics and is influenced by the inclusion of
a motor response.

The second hypothesis tested, namely that the component frequently referred to as Nl is not a simple discrete entity but is
composed of at least two separate elements, received support.  Three
relatively independent components have emerged: the fronto-temporal
Nla with a predominance over the hemisphere contralateral to the
preferred hand, the central Nlb which seems to approximate most
closely to what is usually regarded as the vertex auditory response
and Nlc which is prominent temporally.

What function is reflected by the Nla component is difficult
to determine.  The slight predominance in the left hemisphere of
right-handers and in the right hemisphere of left-handers suggests
that it may be sensitive to lateral preference.  It is of particular
interest that it is one of the few late EP components to have a
frontal rather than a centro-parietal distribution.  In their outline of the scalp topography of auditory EPs, Goff et al. (1977),
using binaural stimulation, distinguished a negative component at
75 msec the distribution of which was similar in many respects to
that of Nla.  They speculated that this component might be myogenic

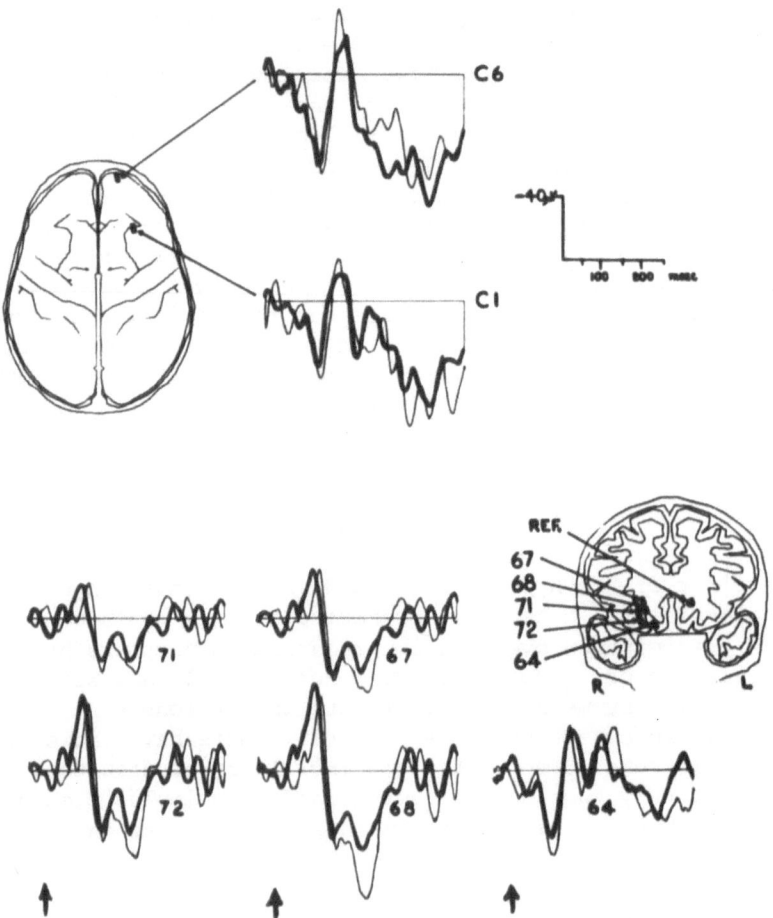

Fig. 4. Evoked potentials recorded intracerebrally to 60 dB monaural
tone pips in one female patient. Dark trace indicates right ear
stimulation, light trace left ear stimulation. Each trace is an
average of forty trials.

in origin. However, all our evidence points to the fact that Nla
has cerebral origins. There are some early indications that it
appears most consistently when stimuli contain information about the
side of response - whether immediate or delayed. Another feature
linking it with the selection of the side of response is the fact
that it is significantly larger in amplitude in the hemisphere crossover conditions (3) and (4).

The distribution and amplitude of Nlb indicated a central
predominance, although the relatively constant latency pattern
suggested its dependence upon more general activation from lower

systems.  Like N1a it tended to increase in amplitude in the crossover conditions (3) and (4).  Its amplitude predominance in the
hemisphere contralateral to the stimulated ear and its shorter
latency in the hemisphere contralateral to the hand selected for
response might suggest that it plays a key processing role between
stimulus and response.

N1c is probably the same component as that identified by Wolpaw
and Penry (1970) as the Tb component of their T complex.  Its
latency is slightly shorter than that originally attributed to Tb,
but Wolpaw and Penry regarded this as lengthened by the filters used
in the early experiment.  They report that recording with a different filter decreased latencies by 10-15 msec.  We discerned no consistent positive component at T3 and T4 which could be equated with
their Ta component.  However, we noted that in subjects with a
prominent blink potential the positive peak of that potential had a
latency of about 95 msec and could be seen in an attenuated form at
T3 and T4.  It would seem that in any experiments in which Ta is
to be studied as one of the variables, adequate control for eye
movements should be a prerequisite.  The origins and distribution of
N1C are still far from clear.  We would wish to view it as predominantly temporal by virtue of its higher incidence in those regions
and its significantly larger amplitudes and shorter latencies contralateral to the stimulated ear.  However, on those occasions when it
could be recorded over central regions the mean amplitudes there
were larger and the mean latencies shorter than elsewhere.  It is
possible that this apparent anomaly could be explained by a strong
sequential dependency upon the immediately preceding large N1b component almost invariably seen in such cases.  This is to some extent
a measurement problem which will require resolution in future experi-
mentation.

The previously reported general tendency for a right hemisphere
amplitude predominance of N1 was not confirmed by this study.  The
only consistent pattern across homologous electrode pairs was for N1a
to be slightly larger in the left hemisphere, the mean value of this
asymmetry being 0.8 µV.  N1b was the only component to show a mean
asymmetry favoring the right hemisphere, but this occurred at temporal electrodes only;  C3-C4, where the component was largest,
showed a slight left hemisphere predominance (0.5 µV).

The study provides no support for the Vaughan and Ritter (1970)
view that the vertex auditory response is a simple summation of
volume conducted signals from dipole sources in the temporal lobes.
The principal temporal component is of a longer latency than the
principal vertex component, and we failed to find any convincing
evidence of polarity reversals occurring below the level of the
Sylvian fissure.  Our evidence suggests that in some subjects the
nose constitutes an active electrode and that this is the most

likely explanation of those cases in which reversals have previously
been reported.

The experimental paradigm used produced the most consistent,
if relatively small, lateralization of the CNV that we have so far
encountered.  Both the "standard" and "late" CNV amplitude measures
showed this asymmetry, the higher amplitude being over the hemisphere
contralateral to the responding hand.  This was most prominent over
the central electrodes but could also be seen to a smaller degree
over temporal locations.  In this respect it contrasts with the
asymmetries seen in the Bereitschaftspotential (BP) which precedes
voluntary movement.  Although lateralized over central and motor
areas in conditions of unilateral pressing, BP asymmetries are not
generally reported over temporal areas.  The results of the stepwise
discriminant analysis produced a discriminant function based primarily on central CNV measures which were particularly effective in
identifying conditions by hand of response, but less effective in
identifying them by ear of stimulation.

In a subsequent analysis in which the four conditions were
reduced to two, based only on hand of response, the discriminant
function obtained successfully classified 80% of the cases.

The paradigm chosen for the experiment emerged as a useful one
for distinguishing those electrophysiological phenomena associated
with processing the auditory warning signal from those concerned
with preparation for the motor response.  The amplitude picture would
suggest that up to and including the P300 the system is evaluating
the information contained in the warning signal and that processing
predominates in the hemisphere more directly connected with the sensory organ, i.e., the hemisphere contralateral to the stimulated ear.
Thereafter the hemisphere concerned with the motor response tends to
predominate.  When the hand ipsilateral to the stimulated ear is to
be used both kinds of processing remain in the same, contralateral
hemisphere.  When the hand contralateral to the stimulated ear is to
be used the transfer from the sensory to the motor hemisphere is reflected in a crossover of the rising negative shift such that it ul-
timately predominates in the hemisphere contralateral to the hand to
be used.  Nevertheless the latency pattern of N1b, and its ability to
indicate the hand due to be used for pressing, argue against taking
too simplistic a view of the stage at which the major responsibility
for processing passes from one hemisphere to the other.

SUMMARY

Eighteen subjects with scalp electrodes and one patient with
intracerebral electrodes were tested in a warned foreperiod reaction
time paradigm in which S1 was a high or low monaural tone pip which
indicated whether the ipsilateral or contralateral hand was to be

used to respond to S2, a tone of intermediate frequency presented 1.5 sec after S1.

A further group of subjects was tested with monaural and binaural stimuli in both passive listening and immediate response situations recording from a coronal chain of electrodes with three different references.

The evoked potentials to S1 in the latency bracket of 60-140 msec were found to consist of three distinct components: an early fronto-temporal component, a middle latency central component and a later, essentially temporal component, the last two predominating over the hemisphere contralateral to the stimulated ear. No support was found for the view that vertex auditory responses are simple summations of temporal lobe responses.

The CNV which developed between S1 and S2 was of significantly higher amplitude over the hemisphere contralateral to the hand required for response.

## REFERENCES

Butler, R.A., Keidel, W.D. and Spreng, M. An investigation of the human cortical evoked potential under conditions of monaural and binaural stimulation. Acta. Otolaryngol., 1969, 68, 317-326.

Butler, S.R. and Glass, A. Interhemispheric asymmetry of contingent negative variation during numeric operations. Electroenceph. Clin. Neurophysiol., 1971, 30, 366.

Butler, S.R. and Glass, A. Asymmetries in the CNV over left and right hemispheres while subjects await numeric information. Biol. Psychol., 1974, 2, 1-16.

Curry, S.H., Peters, J.F. and Weinberg, H. Choice of active electrode site and recording montage as variables affecting CNV amplitude preceding speech. In D. Otto (Ed.), Multidisciplinary Perspectives in Event Related Brain Potential Research, EPA-600/9-77-043, Washington, D.C.: U.S. Government Printing Office, in press.

Goff, G.D., Matsumiya, Y., Allison, T. and Goff, W.R. The scalp topography of human somatosensory and auditory evoked potentials. Electroenceph. Clin. Neurophysiol., 1977, 42, 57-76.

Hink, R.F., Hillyard, S.A. and Benson, P.J. Event related brain potentials and selective attention to acoustic and phonetic cues. Biol. Psychol., 1978, 6, 1-16.

Kooi, K.A., Tipton, A.C. and Marshall, R.E. Polarities and field
    configurations of the vertex components of the human auditory
    evoked response: A reinterpretation. Electroenceph. Clin.
    Neurophysiol., 1971, 31, 166-169.

Low, M.D., Wada, J.A. and Fox, M. Electroencephalographic localiza-
    tion of conative aspects of language production in the human
    brain. In W.C. McCallum and J.R. Knott (Eds.), The Responsive
    Brain, Bristol: J. Wright and Sons Ltd., 1978.

Mononen, L.J. and Seitz, M.R. An AER analysis of contralateral
    advantage in the transmission of auditory information. Neuro-
    psychologia, 1977, 15, 165-173.

Oldfield, R.C. The assessment and analysis of handedness: The
    Edinburgh Inventory. Neuropsychologia, 1971, 9, 97-113.

Otto, D.A. and Leifer, L.J. The effect of modifying response and
    performance feedback parameters on the CNV in humans. In W.C.
    McCallum and J.R. Knott (Eds.), Event Related Slow Potentials
    of the Brain: Their Relations to Behavior., Electroenceph.
    Clin. Neurophysiol. Suppl. 33, 1973, 29-37.

Peronnet, F., Michel, F., Echallier, J.F. and Girod, J. Coronal
    topography of human auditory evoked responses. Electroenceph.
    Clin. Neurophysiol., 1974, 37, 225-230.

Picton, T.W., Hillyard, S.A., Krausz, H.I. and Galambos, R. Human
    auditory evoked potentials. I: Evaluation of components.
    Electroenceph. Clin. Neurophysiol., 1974, 36, 179-190.

Rohrbaugh, J.W., Syndulko, K. and Lindsley, D.B. Brain wave com-
    ponents of the contingent negative variation in humans.
    Science, 1976, 191, 1055-1057.

Tanguay, P.E., Taub, J.M., Doubleday, C. and Clarkson, D. An inter-
    hemispheric comparison of auditory evoked responses to conso-
    nent-vowel stimuli. Neuropsychologia, 1977, 15, 123-131.

Vaughan, H.G. and Ritter, W. The sources of auditory evoked res-
    ponses recorded from the human scalp. Electroenceph. Clin.
    Neurophysiol., 1970, 28, 360-367.

Wolpaw, J.R. and Penry, J.K. A temporal component of the auditory
    evoked response. Electroenceph. Clin. Neurophysiol., 1975,
    39, 609-620.

Wolpaw, J.R. and Penry, J.K. Hemispheric differences in the audi-
    tory evoked reponse. Electroenceph. Clin. Neurophysiol., 1977,
    43, 99-102.

DIFFERENT VARIANTS OF ENDOGENOUS NEGATIVE BRAIN POTENTIALS IN

PERFORMANCE SITUATIONS:   A REVIEW AND CLASSIFICATION

R. Naatanen and P.T. Michie

University of Helsinki

Helsinki, Finland

INTRODUCTION

After the discovery of the CNV (Walter et al., 1964), the existence of many other, mainly endogenous negative shifts have been claimed in different situations.   The common feature of these ERPs is their unclear relationship to the original CNV and, of course, to each other.   The present paper attempts to list these negative shifts and shed some dim light on the question of their mutual relationships.


ENDOGENOUS NEGATIVE POTENTIALS AS SEPARATED
MAINLY ON THE BASIS OF SITUATION OR PERFORMANCE

CNV, readiness potential, Sl-related slow negativity.   In 1965 the existence of a long-duration premotion negative shift called Bereitschaftspotential (readiness potential, RP), quite closely resembling the CNV, was reported (Kornhuber and Deecke, 1965). Thereafter these two negativities have lived in peaceful coexistence and mutual respect, often being studied without the necessary methodological and theoretical integration.   Every now and then the question of their mutual relationship was, however, raised mainly because of their conspicuous similarities.   Both are negative shifts of quite long duration.   Both have a central focus approximately at the vertex.   RPs show a clear asymmetry, with a larger amplitude contralateral to the responding limb (this difference being maximal over the respective motor area); this asymmetry starts during the long negative ramp several hundreds of milliseconds before the EMG onset (Deecke and Kornhuber, 1977).   Many CNV studies have also shown such an asymmetry, but less clearly (for a review,

see Donchin et al., 1978). RPs only exist during preparation for a
movement, whereas the latter condition has proven ideal for eliciting a CNV. In fact, there has been some dispute as to whether a
CNV can ever be completely nonmotor (see Donchin et al. , 1978).
Many of the factors affecting the amplitude of the CNV also affect
the amplitude of RPs, such as motivation (for a review emphasizing
these similarities, see McAdam, 1973).

Besides (1) the eliciting paradigm (and the often larger amplitude of the CNV), there have been at least the following two important differences between the two shifts: (2) A morphological difference: whereas RPs show a ramp-like rise, the CNV often develops
abruptly; (3) A topographical difference: contrary to RPs, the CNV
usually has a high frontal amplitude especially when measured at an
early phase. It appears to be mainly due to these three differences
that the two shifts have been kept that separated. However, quite
recently data were obtained that suggested the existence of an S1-
related fronto-central slow wave, with a sharp onset, which often
overlaps the S2-related slow wave ("true CNV") in the CNV paradigm
(e.g., Loveless and Sanford, 1974; Gaillard, 1976). Consequently,
as the latter two differences (2-3) were, in fact, attributed to
another wave, usually called the "orienting component of the CNV",
some workers suggested that the residual S2-related slow potential
is, in fact, an RP (e.g., Gaillard, 1976; Rohrbaugh et al., 1976).
Hence the original CNV would be composed of an orienting component
and RP. Such thinking was supported by data indicating artificial-
ity of paradigm differences, e.g., it has been shown that a CNV can
exist with no S1 and S2 and that an RP can exist during the S1-S2
interval.

There is, however, one weak loop in this reasoning. The evidence that the S1-related fronto-central slow wave is separable
from the S2-related slow wave is strong - though calling it an
orienting component appears to be premature. On the other hand,
the role in RPs of a "true CNV"-type widespread, central, nonspecific, negative shift (Syndulko and Lindsley, 1977) associated with
motivation, preparation, expectancy, etc., i.e., with increased
activity, appears likely. It is possible that the RP is a hybrid
wave consisting of (1) the CNV and (2) some slow negative potential
specific to response initiation (Hillyard, 1973). The first possibility (1) is supported by data showing that the RP is affected by
similar variables as the CNV (McAdam, 1973). Interestingly, even
the scalp distribution of the RP shifts anteriorly (and hence becomes more CNV-like) under the influence of such variables (Mc
Callum, 1978). Moreover, usually the Cz amplitude is larger than
that above the contralateral hand area (in manual tasks), and the
amplitude above the ipsilateral hand area is substantial (e.g.,
Syndulko and Lindsley, 1977). It might well be that even in a most
boring RP situation with frequent repetitions of a movement there

still is some CNV-inducing element left - a movement is some activity, something to do and concentrate on, after a period of intertrial silence and rest.

As to the second possibility (2), the aforementioned contralateral hemispheric asymmetry is well established. This asymmetry starting well before the onset of the movement speaks in favor of the existence of some negative shift specific to response initiation. This shift, as such, may be of a relatively low amplitude. Hence, the negative shift known as RP is suggested to be composed of a low amplitude motor-specific slow negativity and of a CNV of varying amplitude.

What, then, is the traditional CNV? Besides the "true CNV" defined above, it appears to be composed of an S1-related slow negative wave and, when a motor task is involved, a slow negativity specific to response initiation. The latter component is lent credence by hemispheric asymmetries contralateral to the responding limb found also in the CNV paradigm (Donchin et al., 1978). The S1-related component (appearing mainly with an auditory S1) might reflect the arousing and facilitatory properties of a stimulus (Loveless and Sanford, 1974; Gaillard, 1976; Gailllard and Naatanen, 1976), probably activation of some reticular and thalamic activation systems. The S2-related negative shift ("true CNV") is somewhat more posterior and, presumably, is also related to the activation of such nonspecific systems (Naatanen, 1967). [Skinner's (1971) cryogenic lesion studies have identified frontal and central negative shifts having separate relations with the thalamus.] This activation is presumably associated with sustained activity required between S1 and S2 (e.g., preparation for a task performance). Additionally, there may exist during the S1-S2 interval some modality-specific slow potentials (Gaillard and Naatanen, 1976; Syndulko and Lindsley, 1977) and some other function-specific potentials such as those associated with word and pattern processing (Rebert et al., this conference).

Speech-related negativity. A number of studies have reported an RP preceding speech production. For example, McAdam and Whitaker (1971) observed that it shows a small hemispheric asymmetry with the potential being maximal over Broca's area in the left hemisphere, an area known to play a major role in articulation. This negativity appeared up to 1 sec before articulation. However, there has been continuing controversy as to the cerebral versus extracerebral origin of this negativity. Szirtes and Vaughan (1977) conclude that the scalp recorded speech-related potentials either represent volume conducted activity from muscles involved in speech production or are heavily contaminated by such activity. In view of the continuing controversy over the validity of the speech-related negativity, this potential is not considered further in this review.

Sustained negativity. So far we have dealt with "slow" potentials elicited in paradigms with stimuli of a short duration. If
the stimulus duration is prolonged, say, to 1 sec, a negative shift,
called the sustained potential (SP), lasting for the whole duration
of the stimulus, has been observed in addition to the onset and offset EPs (Keidel, 1971; Hillyard et al., 1978). SPs have been observed for stimuli in the auditory (Keidel, 1971; Jarvilehto and
Fruhstorfer, 1973; Picton and Woods, 1975; Hillyard et al., 1978),
visual (Keidel, 1971; Jarvilehto et al., in press) and somatosensory (Hillyard et al., 1978) modalities. The auditory SP was
reported to have a maximum at the vertex and frontal locations, the
focus being slightly more anterior than that of either the N1 or
P2 components of the auditory EP and showing no reversal of polarity over the Sylvian fissure (Picton and Woods, 1975). The topography of the visual and somatosensory SPs has not been investigated in detail although Keidel (1971) found that the visual SP is
larger over the occipital area than over the vertex and frontal
sites.

The auditory SP exhibits an intensity function similar to that
of the auditory N1-P2 component at the vertex. On the other hand,
the auditory SP is much more resistant to decreasing ISI than the
auditory N1 (Picton and Woods, 1975; Hillyard et al., 1978), and
furthermore the recovery cycle of the SP shows little or no pitch
specificity compared with the N1-P2 onset potentials (Hillyard et
al., 1978).

It was suggested by Keidel (1971) that SP is an objective correlate of perception. This interpretation was regarded as having
been contradicted by Jarvilehto and Fruhstorfer (1973) who showed
that a break of 1 sec in a continuous tone elicits a negative shift
very similar to the SP. It appears likely, however, that the shift
observed by the authors was a CNV of a much larger amplitude than
the SP caused by the continuous tone, and hence this result would
not invalidate Keidel's interpretation. In fact, presently there
is clear evidence that the SP is composed of two coincident negative
potentials: (1) "true SP" (specific shift caused by the stimulus);
(2) CNV. "True SP" (1) is supported by the findings that the SP
occurrence is not dependent on the subject being given any particular task involving the stimuli (Jarvilehto and Fruhstorfer, 1973;
Jarvilehto et al., in press) and that the auditory SP has been
recorded during sleep (Picton and Woods, 1975). Moreover, the
findings suggesting modality-specific topography reviewed in the
aforegoing lend credence to (1). CNV (2) is suggested by Picton
and Wood's (1975) result that instructing subjects to detect an
occasional tone of longer duration results in an increase in the SP
amplitude. It is possible that this attentional enhancement of the
SP is due to the superimposition of a CNV on the SP. However, the
clearest evidence for separability of these two components comes

from Jarvilehto et al. (in press) in which the effect of repetition
of the stimulus on SPs was studied.  Auditory and visual stimuli of
1 sec duration were presented in trains of six stimuli with an ISI
of 1 sec.  Repetition rate was 1 train/min.  The EEG was recorded
from Cz, Pz and Oz.  Both auditory and visual stimuli elicited SPs
which during the first stimuli of the trains were maximal in amplitude at the vertex.  Repetition of the stimulus in the stimulus
train resulted in almost complete disappearance of the SPs.  For
auditory stimulation, a small negative shift remained only at Cz,
whereas for visual stimulation a small SP was seen only at Pz and
Oz.  The authors suggested that the large component susceptible to
habituation is associated with neural processes underlying orienting
behavior, whereas the resistant component might reflect stimulus
processing in the specific projection area.

     Processing negativity.  For some time it was generally accept-
ed that (provided stimulus delivery rate is sufficiently fast)
directing attention to one source of stimuli while ignoring other
sources results in an increase in the amplitude of the N1 component
of the EPs to stimuli from the attended source (Hillyard et al.,
1973).  This is the so-called N1 selective-attention effect.  More
recent evidence, however, indicates that the N1 effect is not the
result of the enhancement of a true N1 component of the EP to
attended stimuli but rather is due to a negative component of endogenous origin superimposed on the attended EP, a component which
may only partly overlap the N1 component (Naatanen et al., 1978a,b).
They observed a long-duration negative displacement of the EP to
the attended ear stimuli in comparison to that to the unattended
ear stimuli (randomized stimuli delivered at a regular ISI of 800
msec).  The negative shift called 'processing negativity' began
quite late at about 150 msec on the falling phase of the N1 component and continued for a further 500 msec.  With a shorter ISI
(250 msec) this shift began before the N1 peak (Naatanen et al.,
1978c).  Corroborating data were provided by Desmedt and Robertson
(1977) who used a selective attention task to somatosensory stimuli
randomly delivered to either hand at a mean ISI of 410 msec.  EPs
to attended stimuli exhibited a small negative shift with a mean
onset latency of 78 msec, approximately 60 msec before the mean
peak latency of the N1 component, which persisted in many cases
beyond 200 msec poststimulus.

     In their recent review, Naatanen and Michie (1978) have drawn
attention to the fact that many of the early Hillyard findings
should also be interpreted as due to the superimposition of a
negative wave on the attended EP since the attention effects were
often not entirely coincident in time with the N1 component.  For
example, in Schwent et al. (1976) the attended EP to central stimuli in their two single-cue conditions exhibits no clear N1 effect
but does exhibit a negative displacement with an onset latency on

the falling phase of N1 giving the appearance of a filled P2.

Most experiments designed to study the effects of selective attention on EPs involve the presentation in random order of a number of different stimuli of brief duration, the stimuli differing on one or more cue dimensions. One of the stimuli is usually designated as a target on a given run, and the direction of attention is controlled by instructing the subject to count the number of occurrences of the target during the run or to make some response on detecting a target. One of the nontargets is usually more similar to the target than other nontargets because it shares a common cue characteristic with the target; for example, it may arise from the same spatial location as the target [the same ear as in Hillyard et al. (1973), or the same hand as in Desmedt and Robertson (1977)] or have the same pitch [as in the pitch-alone condition of Schwent et al.(1976)]. It is usually assumed that subjects adopt the strategy of paying attention to the most target-like nontargets (stimuli in the attended source or channel) in order to be able to detect the (infrequently occurring) targets.

The earliest observed onset of the processing negativity is 60-70 msec (Hillyard et al., 1973; Desmedt and Robertson, 1977). Naatanen (1975) and Naatanen and Michie (1978) have argued that 60-70 msec is sufficient time for an easy discrimination between stimuli from different sources to be completed, and therefore the processing negativity is related to operations carried out after the decision relating to stimulus source has been made. What, then, determines the actual onset latency and duration of the processing negativity since an easy discrimination does not necessarily result in an early onset latency of the processing negativity? Naatanen and Michie have proposed that its onset latency and duration are determined by the difficulty of discriminating stimuli from the attended and unattended sources and the time pressure of the task which, in turn, is determined by the ISI structure and task requirements such as the difficulty of distinguishing targets from nontargets on the attended source. When an easy between-source discrimination is combined with a fast delivery rate, the processing negativity is early and of short duration and under these circumstances (Hillyard et al., 1973) can give rise to an apparent N1 facilitation. On the other hand, an easy discrimination combined with a slow delivery rate results in a prolonged-duration negativity with a considerably later onset as observed by Naatanen et al. (1978a,b). Thus it appears that while the onset of the negativity can begin early when the between-source discrimination is easy, it will only do so when the time pressure of the task requires that whatever processing associated with the negativity be completed early. On the other hand, when the discrimination between attended and unattended sources is more difficult, the onset latency of the processing negativity must of necessity be later as was observed for the central channel of the two single-cue conditions of the Schwent et al.

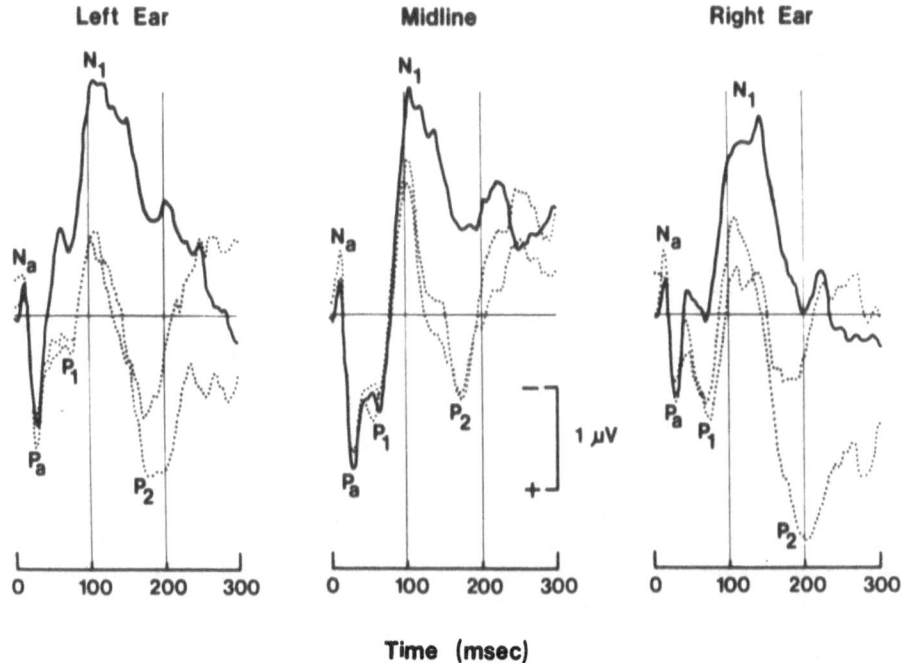

Fig. 1.   Vertex EPs to left ear, midline (binaural) and right ear
stimuli when attended (solid line) and when unattended (dotted lines).
(From Van Voorhis et al., unpublished data.)

(1976) experiment.   [See also the onset latency in Fig. 1 from an
unpublished experiment conducted by Van Voorhis et al. (1976)].

     Available evidence suggests that the processing negativity
associated with attention to stimuli in the auditory modality has
a frontal maximum (Naatanen et al., 1978c).   A small amplitude negative displacement is also evident at T3 and T4 when referred to
linked mastoids (Naatanen et al., 1978a,b).   The processing negativity in the somatosensory modality is larger over contralateral
parietal areas than the ipsilateral areas and smaller at central
and frontal midline and lateral sites (Desmedt and Robertson, 1977).
The topography of the processing negativity elicited by attention
to stimuli in the visual modality has not been investigated in any
detail although Van Voorhis and Hillyard (1977) have evidence that
in some subjects an effect of selective attention at the N1 latency
can be produced at an occipital site (O2) when the stimulated visual
field is contralateral to the scalp location but not when the stimulated visual field is ipsilateral.   Much more investigation of the

scalp topography of the processing negativity is obviously required, but the available evidence is suggestive of a modality-specific topography.

Mismatch negativity. There is solid evidence for the existence of an endogenous negative component with a peak latency of approximately 200 msec (in the auditory modality) in response to a deviating stimulus (e.g., a click of a slightly stronger or weaker intensity than the other clicks) in a repetitive stimulus background (Squires et al., 1975; Snyder and Hillyard, 1976; Ford et al., 1976; Simson et al., 1977; Naatanen et al., 1978a,b,c). Stimulus deviation appears essential as infrequently presented single clicks did not evoke this component (Snyder and Hillyard, 1976). This component, called N2 or N200, or mismatch negativity, as Naatanen et al. call it, was elicited by a stimulus deviation whether attention was directed to the stimuli or not. Unlike the N1 and P2 components of the EP, it was very resistant to increased frequency of the background stimuli (Snyder and Hillyard, 1976). N2, or mismatch negativity, often had a short, EP component-like waveform which could be easily observed as the "N2 component" in the EP to the deviating stimuli. On the other hand, Simson et al. (1977) and Naatanen et al. (1978a,b) revealed the mismatch negativity by subtracting the EP to background stimuli from that to the deviating stimuli. The latter authors observed it to last for at least 200 msec. In many studies (e.g., Squires et al., 1975; Synder and Hillyard, 1976), the mismatch negativity was followed by P3a, a frontally dominated late positivity (with somewhat shorter latency than the parietal P3), and they were often regarded as intimately linked ("N2-P3a complex"). It was, however, demonstrated by Naatanen et al. (1978b) that under dichotic listening conditions the mismatch negativity with no later positivity is elicited by a deviating input among repetitive background stimuli to the unattended ear (while in the attended ear this positivity was observed).

A fronto-central topography of the (auditory) mismatch negativity was generally observed in these studies. Naatanen et al. (1978b) found that there was another focus near the specific sensory areas of audition, as the amplitudes from the T3 and T4 sites were even larger than those from the vertex. Clear data lending credence to the modality-specific distribution of the auditory mismatch negativity were presented by Simson et al. (1977) who also showed a similar effect within the visual modality. In contrast to the auditory modality, frontal activity did not contribute appreciably to the visual mismatch negativity.

Detection negativity. In Cooper et al.'s (1977) study on vigilance of operators watching a visual display for a long time, a videotape recording was made by televising a model landscape across which correctly scaled vehicles moved singly at infrequent, unpredictable times. Vehicles entered along any of the four roads

from the left or right or from behind clumps of trees in the middle
of the picture.  The observer was instructed to press a switch
whenever a vehicle appeared in the display.  The mean detection time
was 4.3 sec.  About 1 sec before the switch was pressed to indicate
detection, the gaze transferred to the region of the vehicle, and
detailed scanning of this part of the display began.  During this
scanning a large centro-parietal positive shift was reported to
occur.  (This potential was not directly related in time to the eye
movements or to the switch press.)  Interestingly, this positivity
was often preceded by a slow centro-parietal negative shift which
could start while the eyes were scanning other parts of the display.
According to the authors, it presumably starts when something seen
in peripheral vision directs the eye scan towards the area of the
display containing the vehicle.  This negativity was reported to
be similar in form to the CNV and was suggested to indicate preparation for action.  (It is uncertain to what extent this negativity
is an RP preceding the fixation of the gaze to the target).

Missing-stimulus negativity.  It has now been well established
that the nondelivery of an expected stimulus gives rise to an
"emitted" potential, the missing-stimulus potential, which consists
of a long latency positive component which is preceded by a negative component (Klinke et al., 1968; Ford et al., 1976; Simson et
al., 1976).  The late positive component of the missing-stimulus
potential appears to be identical to the P300 component elicited
by stimuli which deliver task-relevant information as shown by their
similar scalp distributions (Simson et al., 1977) and by the fact
that they respond similarly to changes in event probability (Ruchkin et al., 1975).  The negative component of the missing-stimulus
potential, henceforth called the 'missing-stimulus negativity'
(MSN), has been most successfully elicited by paradigms in which a
stimulus omission occurs in a regular train of stimuli.  Under
these circumstances the MSN appears to begin at the point in time
at which the missing stimulus would have occurred (Simson et al.,
1976; Ford et al., 1976).

The MSN has been observed for omission of stimuli in the visual
(Simson et al., 1976), auditory (Simson et al., 1976; Ford et al.,
1976) and somatosensory modalities (Klinke et al., 1968).  Simson
et al. (1976) have shown that the scalp topography of the MSN is
modality-specific in the visual and auditory modalities.  The visual
MSN shows a pre-occipital maximum and, in many cases, a secondary
focus at the vertex.  The topography of the visual MSN is, in fact,
quite similar to the scalp topography of the P2 (and to a lesser
extent N1) component of the visual EP, suggesting that they arise
from similar cortical regions, probably visual areas 18-19 for the
posterior focus and the frontal premotor cortex for the central
focus.  The auditory MSN, on the other hand, has a posterior frontal
maximum which appears to extend laterally toward the posterior
superior temporal region.  Simson et al. (1976) have suggested that

the auditory MSN arises from activity in the cortex of the supra-
temporal plane which is projected to the surface of the central
region and a field overlying the auditory association cortex on
the lateral surface of the superior temporal gyrus.  The scalp
topography of the somatosensory MSN has not yet been investigated.

Further modality differences in the MSN are evident from modality effects on the MSN peak latency.  In the paradigm used by
Simson et al. (1976) (involving the omission of a stimulus in a
train of stimuli occurring regularly at a rate of 1/sec) the visual
MSN peaked at a mean latency of 275 msec while the auditory MSN
peaked at 230 msec.  The peak latency of the MSN also appears to be
affected by ISI as Picton et al. (1974) found that progressive increases in the ISI of the train of stimuli produced MSNs of longer
latency and smaller amplitude.  The smaller amplitude of the averaged MSN with increasing ISI could well be in part due to greater
variability of the MSN latency over single trials.  Both effects
presumably reflect the longer, more variable and flatter time
course of expectancy observed when the ISI is prolonged (Naatanen
adn Merisalo, 1977).

The occurrence of the missing-stimulus potentials is not dependent on the subject being given any particular task relating to
the missing stimuli since the negative-positive complex can be recorded when the subject is instructed to "keep as alert as possible
and to direct attention to the stimuli" (Klinke et al., 1968) or
when the subject is instructed to ignore the stimuli and read a
book (Ford et al., 1976).  Instructions to attend to the missing
stimuli and to push a button as quickly as possible on detecting
a stimulus omission does not affect the amplitude of the MSN recorded at the vertex but does increase its latency (Ford et al.,
1976).  Possible changes in the scalp topography of the MSN with
attention have not been investigated.


CONCLUSION

The above review appears to suggest that the negative shifts
classified on the basis of eliciting situation or performance are
composed of one or several of the following components:

1) Frontal nonspecific negative shift.  This is a fronto-central negative shift reaching its peak some 500-700 msec from the
stimulus onset observed most clearly when an auditory stimulus is
used.  In an S1-S2 paradigm, it can exist even without S2.  Its
amplitude reflects the intensity and significance of the stimulus,
and its time course appears to be independent of ISI.  There is much
evidence for its being associated with some subcortical nonspecific
activation processes.  This negative shift is often associated with
a slow positive shift maximal over the parietal area.

2) <u>Central</u>, <u>nonspecific</u> <u>widely</u> <u>distributed</u> <u>negative</u> <u>shift</u>.
Called the "true CNV" in the aforegoing, this is S2-related in
S1-S2 paradigms and is very sensitive to ISI and task demands but
can also exist outside or independently of the S1-S2 paradigm.  It
was suggested to reflect the degree of activation of the subcortical nonspecific activation mechanisms mainly reflecting the nature
of the task and task demands in performance situations.  This view
appears to clarify two persistent issues in the field:

(a) The generally low correlations between the amplitude of CNV
and performance: if CNV mainly reflects the degree of increased
activity in some nonspecific activation centers rather than some
more specific factors in performance and preparation for it (e.g.,
expectancy or attention), the low correlations between various
"activation measures" (varying within the relatively narrow limits
of the test situation) and performance (see Naatanen, 1973);

(b)  Reaction time and other motor tasks as optimal conditions for
CNV elicitation: there is plenty of evidence for large physiological changes regarded as indicating "activation" increase during the
S1-S2 interval of the reaction time paradigm.  On the other hand,
for example a sensory discrimination task is performed by the or-
ganism with much less extensive mechanisms which would explain why
no large ERPs are generated.  Moreover, in sensory tasks there is
emphasis on accuracy (rather than speed of performance) for which a
calm, relaxed attitude might be ideal.

3) <u>Modality-specific</u> <u>negativity</u>.  The reviewed evidence
points to the conclusion that various performances with a sensory
aspect are associated with a modality-specific negative shift.
There seem to exist three types of such shifts.  The first is
associated with template mismatch (missing stimulus negativity
appears to be a mismatch negativity too) underlying automatic pas-
sive-attention and may play a role in the initiation of the orienting response.  The second type is processing negativity, that associated with voluntary attention to and further processing of certain
stimuli selected in preliminary processing.  (Many other types of
tasks probably induce such shifts as well.)  Detection negativity
probably is one form of processing negativity; it is associated
with intensive processing on detection of a preliminary cue for a
target.  As to the differences between the mismatch and processing
negativities, the former appears to be of relatively larger size
over the sensory-specific areas and has a ramp-like, short waveform
while the latter often is a steady, long-duration shift.  (Both
have a quite strong nonspecific component.  This might be intimately interlinked with the specific process to the degree that they
cannot be disassociated.  In such a case it would be appropriate
to deal with the mismatch negativity and the processing negativity
as if each were composed of one component.  Generally the division
into different components is based on the idea that the latter are

experimentally separable in that they show different relations to
some experimental manipulations.  (For an elegant example, see the
Jarvilehto et al. experiment reviewed above.)  The third type is
suggested to be the specific component of the sustained potential.

4)  Motor-specific negativity.  Topographical data showing
hemispheric asymmetries contralateral to the responding limb suggest
that in tasks with a motor performance there also exists a motor-
specific slow negative shift.

5)  Some other forms of function-specific negativities.  Examples include those associated with word and pattern processing.

The traditional CNV was suggested to be composed of several of
these components.  Perhaps they all are present when an auditory S1
(producing the frontal negativity) is used in a reaction time task
with word stimulus.  The RP was regarded as being composed of motor-
specific negativity and the central type of nonspecific negativity.
(There is evidence for a lack of frontal negativity, even for frontal positivity, during the RP).  On the other hand, the S1-related
slow negativity known as the orienting component of the CNV appears
the same as component 1), but it is possible that there are modality-specific aspects in its topography too.  The remaining five
negativity shifts classified on the basis of situation or performance
(speech-related negativity is omitted here), sustained negativity,
processing negativity, mismatch negativity, detection negativity
and missing-stimulus negativity, all appear to be composed of a
nonspecific (either frontal or central type) and a modality-specific component.

Of these five, mismatch and missing-stimulus negativities
appear to be closely related as stated above, and their topography
is similar.  They both seem to represent an automatic type of detection of, or response to, an environmental change.  Sustained
negativity (its sensory-specific component) also appears to be a
relatively inflexible, automatic type of negativity, depending to
a great extent on physical stimulus characteristics.  The nonspecific central negativity, motor-specific slow negativity, processing
negativity and detection negativity, on the other hand, appear to
be of voluntary or flexible character, reflecting to a great degree
higher cognitive functions.  For example, processing negativity
seems to be elicited by the stimulus the subject is instructed to
pay attention to.  As discussed above, detection negativity might
be one form of processing negativity.  The suggested components of
negative shifts as classified into two main categories are presented in Table I.  In light of the available evidence the nonspecific
frontal component appears as a borderline case between the negative
shifts associated with "first-order" and "higher-order" processes.

Table 1.  Suggested components of negative shifts.

| | |
|---|---|
| -NONCOGNITIVE | -COGNITIVE |
| -INFLEXIBLE | -FLEXIBLE |
| (not much effect of variables such as learning, stimulus significance, attention, task, etc.) | (effect of variables such as learning, stimulus significance, attention, task, etc.) |
| -DETERMINED BY PHYSICAL STIMULUS FEATURES | -NOT DETERMINED BY PHYSICAL STIMULUS FEATURES |
| -"FIRST ORDER" | -"HIGHER ORDER" |

| | |
|---|---|
| SUSTAINED POTENTIAL (specific) | NONSPECIFIC CENTRAL ("true CNV") |
| MISMATCH NEGATIVITY | RP (specific) |
| | PROCESSING NEGATIVITY |

| |
|---|
| NONSPECIFIC FRONTAL |

## SUMMARY

As research in the neurophysiology of higher cerebral functions progresses, more and more different types of brain potentials in performance situations are discovered.  The recent years have especially brought up candidates for new variants of endogenous negative potentials.  It appears that besides the CNV we have at least the following negative shifts:  Bereitschaftspotential; "orienting component" of the CNV; speech-related negativity; sustained negativity; processing negativity; mismatch negativity; detection negativity; missing-stimulus negativity.  The present paper attempts to systematize these more or less overlapping negative shifts which have mainly been named on the basis of situation or performance eliciting them.  Especially the lack of detailed knowledge of the scalp topography of most of these negative shifts in different situations makes it difficult at the present stage of research to determine their mutual relationships.

## REFERENCES

Cooper, R., McCallum, W.C., Newton, P., Papakostopoulos, D., Popcock, P.V. and Warren, W.J.  Cortical potentials associated with the detection of visual events.  Science, 1977, 196, 74-77.

Deecke, L. and Kornhuber, H.H.  Cerebral potentials and the initiation of voluntary movement.  In J.E. Desmedt (Ed.), Attention, Contraction and Event Related Cerebral Potentials, Progress in Clinical Neurophysiology, Vol. I, Basel: Karger, 1977.

Desmedt, J.E. and Robertson, D.  Differential enhancement of early and late components of the cerebral somatosensory evoked potentials during forced-paced cognitive tasks in man.  J. Physiol., 1977, 271, 761-782.

Desmedt, J.E., Robertson, D., Brunko, E. and Debecker, J.  Somatosensory decision tasks in man:  Early and late components of the cerebral potentials evoked by stimulation of different fingers in random sequences.  Electroenceph. Clin. Neurophysiol., 1977, 43, 404-415.

Donchin, E., Ritter, W. and McCallum, W.C.  Cognitive psychophysiology: The endogenous components of the ERP.  In E. Callaway, S. Koslow and P. Tueting (Eds.), Event Related Brain Potentials in Man, Academic Press: New York, in press.

Ford, J.M., Roth, W.T. and Kopell, B.S.  Attention effects on auditory evoked potentials to infrequent events.  Biol. Psychol., 1977, 4, 65-77.

Gaillard, A.W.K.  Effects of warning signal modality on the contingent negative variation (CNV).  Biol. Psychol., 1976, 4, 139-154.

Gaillard, A.W.K. and Naatanen, R.  Modality effects on the contingent negative variation in a simple reaction time task.  In W.C. McCallum and J.R. Knott (Eds.), The Responsive Brain, J. Wright: Bristol, 1976.

Hillyard, S.A.  The CNV and human Behavior.  A review.  In W.C. McCallum and J.R. Knott (Eds.), Event Related Slow Potentials of the Brain: Their Relations to Behavior, Electroenceph. Clin. Neurophysiol. Suppl. 33, 1973, 161-171.

Hillyard, S.A., Picton, T.W. and Regan, D.M.  Sensation, perception and attention: Analysis using ERPs.  In E. Callaway, S. Koslow and P. Tueting (Eds.), Event Related Brain Potentials in Man, Academic Press: New York, in press.

Hink, R.F., Hillyard, S.A. and Benson, P.J.  Event related brain potentials and selective attention to acoustic and phonetic cues.  Biol. Psychol, 1978, 6, 1-16.

Jarvilehto, T. and Fruhstorfer, H.   Is the sound evoked DC poten-
    tial a contingent negative variation?  In W.C. McCallum and
    J.R. Knott (Eds.), Event Related Slow Potentials of the Brain:
    Their Relations to Behavior., Electroenceph. Clin. Neurophys-
    iol. Suppl. 33, 1973, 105-108.

Jarvilehto, T., Hari, R. and Sams, M.   Effect of stimulus repetition
    on negative sustained potentials elicited by short auditory and
    visual stimuli in the human EEG.  Biol. Psychol., in press.

Keidel, W.D.   DC potentials in the auditory evoked response in man.
    Acta Otolaryng., in press, 71, 242-248.

Klinke, R., Fruhstorfer, H. and Finkenzeller, P.   Evoked responses
    as a function of external and stored information.  Electroen-
    ceph. Clin. Neurophysiol., 1968, 25, 119-122.

Kornhuber, H.H. and Deecke, L.   Hirnpotentialanderungen bei Will-
    kurbewegungen und passiven Bewegungen des Menschen.  Bereit-
    schaftspotential und reafferente Potentiale.  Pflugers Arch.
    ges. Physiol., 1965, 284, 1-17.

Loveless, N.E. and Sanford, A.J.   Slow potential correlates of
    preparatory set.  Biol. Psychol., 1974, 1, 303-314.

McAdam, D.W.   Physiological mechanisms.  A review.  In W.C. Mc-
    Callum and J.R. Knott (Eds.), Event Related Slow Potentials
    of the Brain:  Their Relations to Behavior.  Electroenceph.
    Clin. Neurophysiol. Suppl. 33, 1973, 79-86.

McAdam, D.W. and Whitaker, H.A.   Language production: Electroen-
    cephalographic localization in the normal human brain. Science,
    1971, 172, 499-502.

McCallum, W.C.   Relationships between the Bereitschaftspotential
    and the CNV.  In D. Otto (Ed.), New Perspectives in Event
    Related Potential (ERP) Research, Washington, D.C.: U.S.
    Government Printing Office, in press.

Naatanen, R.   Selective attention and evoked potentials.  Ann. Acad.
    Scient. Fenn., B, 1967, 151, 1-226.

Naatanen, R   The inverted-U relationship between activation and
    performance: A critical view.  In S. Kornblum (Ed.), Attention
    and Performance IV, Academic Press: New York, 1973.

Naatanen, R.   Selective attention and evoked potentials in humans:
    A critical review.  Biol. Psychol., 1975, 2, 237-307.

Naatanen, R. and Merisalo, A.  Expectancy and preparation in simple
    reaction time.  In S. Dornic (Ed.), Attention and Performance
    VI., Erlbaum: New Jersey, 1977.

Naatanen, R. and Michie, P.T.  Early selective attention effects on
    the evoked potential: A critical review and reinterpretation.
    Submitted for publication.

Naatanen, R., Gaillard, A.W.K. and Mantysalo. S.  The N1 effect of
    selective attention reinterpreted.  Acta Psychol., 1978a, 42,
    313-329.

Naatanen, R., Gaillard, A.W.K. and Mantysalo, S.  N1 component of
    the evoked potential does not reflect selective attention.
    Unpiblished manuscript, 1978b.

Naatanen, R., Gaillard, A.W.K. and Varey, C.  The N1 component of
    the evoked potential as reflecting selective attention and
    voluntary orienting.  Unpublished data, 1978c.

Picton, T.W. and Woods, D.L.  Human auditory evoked sustained po-
    tentials.  Electroenceph Clin. Neurophysiol., 1975, 38, 543.

Picton, T.W., Hillyard, S.A. and Galambos, R.  Cortical evoked res-
    ponses to omitted stimuli.  In M.W. Livanov (Ed.), Major
    Problems in Brain Electrophysiology, Academy of Sciences: Mos-
    cow, 1974.

Rebert, C.S., Lowe, R.C. and Hatchel, J.M.  Electrocortical mani-
    festations of complementary hemispheric specialization in an
    expectancy task.  This symposium.

Rohrbaugh, J.W., Syndulko, K. and Lindsley, D.B.  Brain wave compo-
    nents of the contingent negative variation in humans.  Science,
    1976, 191, 1055-1957.

Ruchkin, D.S., Sutton, S. and Tueting, P.  Emitted and evoked P300
    potentials and variation in stimulus probability.  Psychophys-
    iol., 1975, 12, 591-595.

Schwent, V.L., Snyder, E. and Hillyard, S.A.  Auditory evoked po-
    tentials during multichannel selective listening: Role of pitch
    and localization cues.  J. Exp. Psychol.: Human Perception and
    Performance, 1976, 2, 313-325.

Simson, R., Vaughan, H.G. and Ritter, W.  The scalp topography of
    potentials associated with missing visual or auditory stimuli.
    Electroenceph. Clin. Neurophysiol., 1976, 40, 33-42.

Simson, R., Vaughan, H.G. and Ritter, W.   The scalp topography of
    potentials in auditory and visual discrimination tasks.   Elec-
    troenceph. Clin. Neurophysiol., 1977, 42, 528-535.

Skinner, J.E.   Abolition of a conditioned, surface-negative, corti-
    cal potential during cryogenic blockade of the nonspecific
    thalamocortical system.   Electroenceph. Clin. Neurophysiol.,
    1971, 31, 197-209.

Snyder, E. and Hillyard, S.A.   Long latency evoked potentials to
    irrelevant deviant stimuli.   Beh. Biol., 1976, 16, 319-331.

Squires, N.K., Squires, K.C. and Hillyard, S.A.   Two varieties of
    long latency positive waves evoked by unpredictable auditory
    stimulus.   Electroenceph. Clin. Neurophysiol., 1975, 38, 387-
    401.

Szirtes, J. and Vaughan, H.G.   Characteristics of cranial and facial
    potentials associated with speech production.   Electroenceph.
    Clin. Neurophysiol., 1977, 43, 386-396.

Syndulko, K. and Lindsley, D.B.   Motor and sensory determinants of
    cortical slow potential shifts in man.   In J.E. Desmedt (Ed.),
    Attention, Voluntary Contraction and Event Related Cerebral
    Potentials, Progress in Clinical Neurophysiology, Vol. 1,
    Basel: Karger, 1977.

Van Voorhis, S. and Hillyard, S.A.   Visaul evoked potentials and
    selective attention to points in space.   Perc. Psychophys.,
    1977, 22, 54-62.

Van Voorhis, S., Hillyard, S.A. and Naatanen, R.   Unpublished data,
    1976.

Walter, W.G., Cooper, R., Aldridge, V.J., McCallum, W.C. and Winter,
    A.   Contingent negative variation: An electric sign of sensori-
    motor association and expectancy in the human brain.   Nature,
    1964, 203, 380-384.

EVENT RELATED POTENTIALS IN LANGUAGE AND NON-LANGUAGE TASKS IN

PATIENTS WITH ALEXIA WITHOUT AGRAPHIA

H. J. Neville, E. Snyder, R. Knight and R. Galambos

The Salk Institute and University of California,

San Diego, La Jolla, California

The concurrent study of behavior and event related potentials (ERPs) from different scalp locations can provide converging evidence for the brain structures and functions which underlie normal human cognitive processes.  The study of behavior and ERPs in patients with localized brain damage that has resulted in specific behavioral deficits can, in theory, complement studies of normal subjects by: (1) describing changes in particular aspects of ERPs associated with disturbances in particular cognitive functions, and (2) permitting correlations between the absence or distortion of particular ERP components and damage to particular areas of the brain.  Results from studies like these may provide information as to those aspects of cognitive functions that are reflected in particular ERP components and may also provide information as to the neural origins of different ERP components.

We and others have looked for evidence of cerebral specialization of function in ERPs recorded from the two hemispheres of normal adults.  Cerebral specialization of function refers to the fact that the left and right cerebral hemispheres of man do not contribute equally to certain specific cognitive abilities.  In most normal adults the integrity of the left cerebral hemisphere is more important for language functioning, and the integrity of the right hemisphere is more important for the performance of certain non-language perceptual tasks.  Evidence for this differential functional specialization comes from studies showing greater deficits in language functioning following damage to the left hemisphere than damage to the right hemisphere, but greater deficits in perceptual functioning such as the recognition of faces and orientation in space after damage to the right than to the left

cerebral hemisphere (Luria and Karasseva, 1968; Teuber, 1974).
Studies of normal adults, showing better perception and recall of
language material presented to the right ear and right visual field
(which project more directly to the left hemisphere) and better
perception and recall of certain non-language material presented to
the left ear and left visual field (which project more directly to
the right hemisphere), reveal similar differential specializations
of the two hemispheres in the intact brain (Kimura, 1967; Klein
et al., 1976; Knox and Kimura, 1968). Over the last decade a
number of studies have reported left/right differences in the ERP
which are thought to reflect functional hemispheric asymmetries
(Wood et al., 1971; Brown et al., 1976). Many would agree, however, that the asymmetries reported have been elusive and, when
obtained, less prominent than one might expect from the neuropsychological studies of cerebral specialization. Many of these
studies have methodological shortcomings which make interpretation
of the results difficult (see the reviews of this literature by
Friedman et al., 1975; Galambos et al., 1975; Donchin et al., 1977).
Perhaps the primary shortcomings of many of these studies are the
lack of real language stimuli (for example, many investigators
employ meaningless syllables such as /ba/, /da/) and the failure
to engage the subject in a demanding task which requires language
processing.

We investigated the possibility that stronger ERP asymmetries
indicative of cerebral specialization might be obtained if we recorded ERPs in tasks which produce marked behavioral asymmetries
(Neville et al., 1977). This type of design, in addition to
engaging the subject in a demanding task, also has the advantage
of providing converging behavioral evidence for a functional
interpretation of any ERP asymmetries obtained. We found that
ERPs (N1) to auditory and visual language stimuli were significantly
larger from the left than the right hemisphere when subjects performed tasks which resulted in a lateral behavioral asymmetry. The
most difficult task, the simultaneous presentation of two different
words to the two visual fields, produced the most marked behavioral
and ERP asymmetries: in every subject who correctly reported more
words from the right than the left visual field, the N1 from the
left hemisphere was larger than that of the right hemisphere. Thus,
the functional specialization of the left hemisphere for language
processing is reflected in ERPs recorded from subjects engaged in
demanding tasks which result in behavioral asymmetries.

In the present investigation we employed paradigms similar to
those described above in the study of three patients with the
syndrome known as alexia without agraphia (Ajax et al., 1977;
Vincent et al., 1977). This disorder is of considerable interest
to the neuropsychologist because it is a striking example of how a
discrete structural lesion can selectively dissociate one particular

aspect of language (reading) from language functioning as a whole.
In these patients the ability to read is severely disrupted.  This
occurs without impairment of the ability to write.  These patients
can write normally, spontaneously or to dictation, but later cannot read what they have just written.  The patients may be able to
read individual numbers and letters and some simple words, although
slowly and laboriously.  Speech and the comprehension of speech are
normal in these patients as is the ability to name visually presented objects.

This rare syndrome was described by Wernicke (1885), who
proposed that it might be due to a lesion which spared the angular
gyrus (the 'storehouse for visual words'), thereby preserving the
ability to write, but destroyed the pathways whereby visual
information reaches this center and is decoded.  Dejerine's (1892)
description of the brain of such a patient who came to autopsy
confirmed Wernicke's hypothesis exactly.  Dejerine's patient had
suffered an infarct of the left occipital lobe (thereby rendering
him blind in the right visual field) and the splenium of the corpus
callosum (thereby preventing the transfer of visual information
from the left visual field and intact right occipital cortex to the
left angular gyrus).  The preserved left angular gyrus presumably
enabled the patient to write.

This 'disconnection' model of the functions of the brain
underlying the ability to read continues to receive support
(Geshwind, 1965).  While this theory can often predict the site of
a lesion on the basis of initial behavioral deficits, there is
little understanding of the possible mechanisms involved in the
improvement of function which some patients show.  Often in this
syndrome the reading deficit is not absolute immediately after
the injury and patients may show some improvement in the ability
to read months and years after the initial trauma.  Several explanations for this improvement are possible.  Conceivably, for
example, some recovery of function might occur if the right angular
gyrus somehow is able to assume certain functions that the left
angular gyrus normally performs.  Alternatively, perhaps over time
visual language information presented to the left visual field
could cross over to the left angular gyrus by portions of the
corpus callosum anterior to the splenium.  In the present investigation we recorded ERPs to visually presented language and non-
language stimuli from left and right, central, parietal and occipital electrode sites to determine whether the distribution and/or
form of the ERP might differ in these patients in a systematic way
from normal.

METHODS

Subjects

Our subjects were three men with the syndrome of alexia without agraphia and three normal controls matched for sex, visual acuity, age and handedness.

Patient 1. PW was a 28 year old, right-handed male.  Eight years prior to testing he suffered a penetrating head trauma which destroyed the left occipital cortex and splenium of the corpus callosum [as seen on computerized axial tomography (CAT) scan].  Immediately following his injury PW had a dense right hemianopsia and was severely impaired in his ability to read single numbers, letters or words.  He was never impaired in his ability to write, to name visually presented objects, to speak or to understand speech. This patient has shown considerable recovery in the 8 years since the injury and can now read single numbers, letters and some three- and four-letter words.

Patient 2. CP was a 60 year old, right-handed male who, 9 months prior to testing, suffered an occlusion of the left posterior cerebral artery (as seen by cerebral angiography) which compromised the left occipital lobe and splenium of the corpus callosum.  Immediately following the occlusion he had a dense right hemianopsia and made many errors in reading single letters and words.  He experienced no difficulty in writing, speaking or understanding speech.

Patient 3. BR was a 60 year old, left-handed male who, 1.5 months prior to testing, underwent surgery for the removal of a tumor involving the left occipital lobe and splenium of the corpus callosum (CAT scan).  Following surgery he had a dense right hemianopsia, had some difficulty reading single numbers and letters and had a severe deficit in reading words.  His abilities to write, to speak and to understand speech were not impaired.

At the time of testing the patients were out of the hospital and were functioning quite normally.  The major obstacle each patient had to adjust to was his right hemianopsia and the difficulty reading.  All patients have shown some recovery in the ability to read since their initial insult.  In fact, the youngest patient (PW) now reads at a third grade level.

Stimuli

We recorded visual ERPs to full field white and colored flashes and to unilateral squares of white light, numbers, letters, three-

and four-letter words and line drawings of common objects.  Here we
report only the methods and results for full field white flashes,
four-letter words and line drawings.

All visual stimuli consisted of slides back-projected onto a
translucent screen.  The edges of all slides coincided precisely
with the edges of the screen to yield a rectangular field 13° wide
and 8.5° high.  Subjects saw 1.25 meters from the screen and fix-
ated a red spot which was always at the center of the field.  Stimuli were tachistoscopically presented for 100 milliseconds (msec).
Except for the full field flashes, all stimuli were white patterns
(words and line drawings) on a black background.  They were presented so that their nearest edge began 2° to the left or right of
the fixation point.  All stimuli were presented at irregular
interstimulus intervals ranging from one to four seconds.

1.  Flashes of white light.  These covered the full field and were
690 candelas/meter$^2$ (cd/m$^2$).  Subjects simply viewed the screen
with no assigned task.

2.  Four-letter words.  Eighty-five different four-letter words
were randomly presented once to the left and once to the right visual field.  Each word was 2.5° in length.  The brightness of these
stimuli was 200 cd/m$^2$.  The subject's task was to verbally report
the word after each trial.

3.  Line drawings.  Thirty different line drawings of common objects (e.g., shoe, train) were presented randomly to the left and
right visual fields.  These stimuli were 2.5° in length and 2° high.
There were on average 170 cd/m$^2$.  After each trial subjects reported
the name of the object presented in the slide.


Procedure

During all stimulus presentations the EEG was recorded from
electrodes placed at O1 and O2, P3 and P4, C3 and C4 (International
10-20 system) and from beneath the right eye, all referred to the
linked mastoids.  Electrode impedances were all below 3000 ohms.
Signals were amplified with Grass 7P5 amplifiers (TC = .45 seconds)
and were recorded on an FM tape recorder (Vetter model A) for off-
line computer analysis.

Each control subject was tested on all stimuli in one four-hour
session.  Each patient was tested twice on all stimuli in two different four-hour sessions.  Stimuli were presented in blocks according to stimulus type.  During all tasks an experimenter sat next to
the subject and pointed to the fixation spot prior to each trial,
monitored the subject's eye movements to ensure central fixation,

indicated (about 1 sec after stimulus presentation) when the subject could respond and recorded his verbal response.  All subjects
wore earphones through which white noise was presented to mask
sounds produced in conjunction with stimulus delivery.


## Data Analysis

The EEG was digitized and averaged on a PDP 11/45 computer
employing programs which automatically rejected trials on which
excessive muscle artifact and eye movements occurred.  ERPs were
averaged separately according to stimulus type and according to
whether the subject responded correctly or incorrectly.  We
measured the peak amplitude of ERP components N1 and P3 relative to
an average prestimulus baseline of 100 msec.  We also measured the
area of the positivity between 200 and 300 msec relative to the
baseline.


## RESULTS


## Behavioral Data

On average, the controls accurately reported 67% of the four-
letter words.  All patients responded "nothing" to all right visual
field presentations of words (confirming their right hemianopsia).
Patient PW correctly reported 60% of left visual presentations of
four-letter words.  Patient CP accurately reported 24% of left
visual field presentations of four-letter words, and patient BR
accurately reported 30% of four-letter words.  All subjects
performed virtually perfectly in reporting the line drawings except
that the patients reported "nothing" to all right visual field
presentations.


## ERP Data

In general, the morphology of the ERP waveform in control subjects showed a prominent negativity around 180 msec post-stimulus
presentation (N1) and (except in the passive flash run) a positivity
maximal around 350 msec post-stimulus presentation (P3).

1.  Flashes of white light.  In control subjects these (full field)
stimuli evoked an N1 around 150 msec after stimulus presentation.
These responses were present at both left and right hemisphere leads.
In the patients (for whom this was a unilateral, left visual field
stimulus due to their right hemianopsia) the flash did not evoke an
N1 at the left hemisphere electrode sites but evoked an N1 of com-

MEAN ERP   3 CONTROLS
FOUR LETTER WORDS
CORRECT RESPONSES

LEFT VISUAL FIELD                          RIGHT VISUAL FIELD

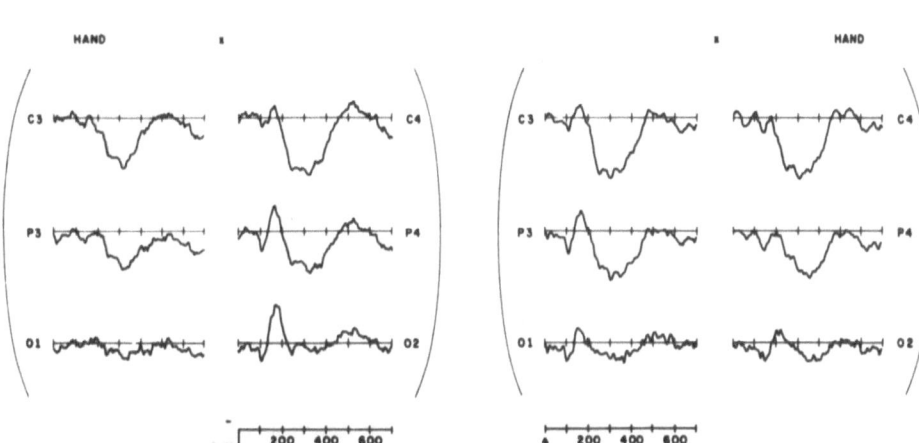

Fig. 1.   ERPs averaged over control subjects to correctly reported
presentations of four-letter words to the left and right visual
fields.

parable amplitude to the controls at the right hemisphere electrode
sites.   In this (no task) situation, no P3 was elicited.

2.   <u>Four-letter words</u>.  Figure 1 shows ERPs averaged over the three
control subjects to presentations of four-letter words (correctly
reported) to the left and right visual fields.

Left visual field presentations produced an N1 (170 msec)
over the right hemisphere at O2 (5.8 µV), P4 (3.9 µV) and C4
2.3 µV); at the left hemisphere sites N1, if present, was very
small.  In contrast, right visual field presentations produced a
large N1 at left hemisphere electrode sites (O1 3.6 µV; P3 3.7 µV;
C3 3.7 µV) and a small N1 at right hemisphere electrode sites
(O2 2.1 µV; P4 0.4 µV; C4 1.3 µV).  The ERPs to left and right
visual field presentations of words also contained a P3 (maximal
about 325 msec after word onset) at central (on average, 10.5 µV)
and at parietal leads (8.6 µV), but not at the occipital leads.
This P3, in contrast to the asymmetrical N1, was of equal amplitude
at the left and right hemispheres, and its amplitude was not altered
as a function of left or right field presentation.  A comparison
of the ERPs to four-letter words reported correctly and incorrectly
revealed no striking differences in morphology or left/right distribution.

MEAN ERP   3 PATIENTS
FOUR LETTER WORDS

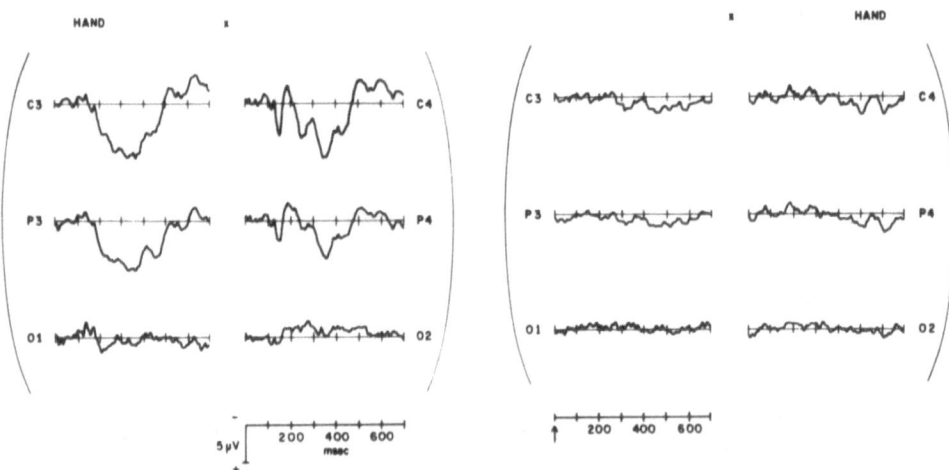

Fig. 2.   ERPs averaged over the three patients to correctly reported
presentations of four-letter words to the left visual field and ERPs
to right visual field presentations of the same stimuli.


    Figure 2 shows ERPs averaged over the three patients to cor-
rectly reported presentations of four-letter words to the left
visual field, and ERPs to right visual field presentations of the
same stimuli.  Presentations of these stimuli to the right (hemianopic) visual field produced no discernible ERP components.  Correctly reported four-letter words presented to the (preserved) left
visual field did not produce an N1 over the lesion (O1), and also
failed to evoke an N1 over the intact right occipital cortex (O2).
More anteriorly, the N1 was present at right parietal (mean 2.5 µV)
and at right central (mean 2.2 µV) leads.  Left visual field presentations of four-letter words also produced a P3, maximal
around 350 msec post-stimulus presentation, at central (mean
9.0 µV) and parietal (mean 7.5 µV) leads.  In contrast to the
symmetrical positivity in control subjects, the amplitude of this
positivity was asymmetrical in patients, especially at the parietal
leads: it was broader and larger at left (mean area between 200 and
500 msec in arbitrary units = 70) than at right (mean area 200 -
500 msec = 30) hemisphere leads.  There were no consistent differences in morphology, amplitude or distribution between ERPs
to left visual field presentations of four-letter words reported
correctly and incorrectly by the patients.

Figure 3 presents the left visual field data of Figures 1 and
2 in a different way.  ERPs from the left and right hemispheres are
superimposed.  In controls the N1 is larger from the right hemisphere than the left hemisphere, while the P3 response is essentially symmetrical.  In patients, the N1 is absent at all left
hemisphere sites and over the right occipital lead, but has an
essentially normal appearance at right central and parietal leads.
Note also the asymmetrical (left greater than right) positivity
(shaded area) between 200 and 500 msec which is most pronounced at
the parietal leads.  This ERP asymmetry to correctly and incorrectly
reported words was consistently present in all three patients during both recording sessions.

3.  _Line drawings_.  In control subjects left visual field presentations of line drawings evoked an N1 at occipital and parietal
leads which closely resembled the responses to words (asymmetrical,
right hemisphere larger than left).  Similarly, left visual presentations of line drawings also elicited a P3 which was symmetrical
at left and right hemispheres.

In contrast to the results for words, the patients' responses
to left visual field presentations of the line drawings contained
an N1 at right occipital (mean 4.1 μV) and right parietal (mean
3.5 μV) leads.  As with words, ERPs from the left hemisphere did

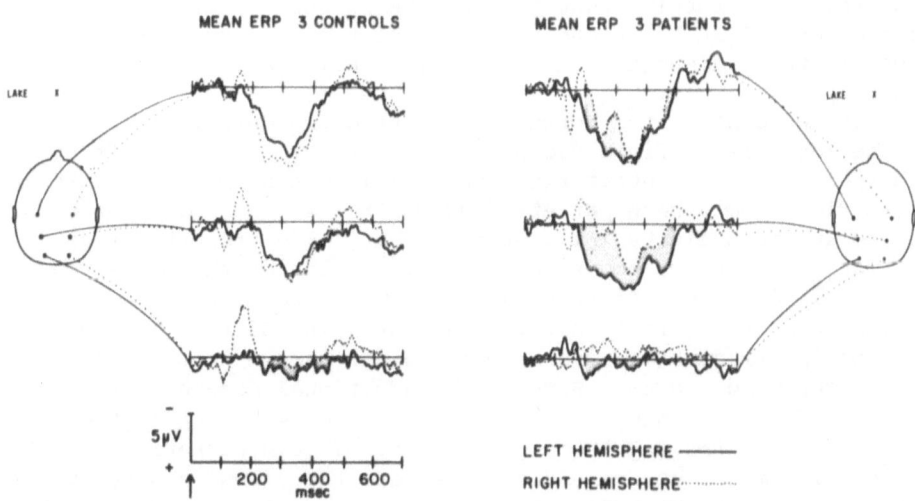

LEFT VISUAL FIELD
FOUR LETTER WORDS
CORRECT RESPONSES

MEAN ERP  3 CONTROLS                    MEAN ERP  3 PATIENTS

5μV

200   400   600
        msec

LEFT HEMISPHERE ———
RIGHT HEMISPHERE··········

Fig. 3.  Controls' and patients' ERPs from left and right hemispheres (superimposed) to correctly reported left visual field
presentations of four-letter words.

not contain an N1, and these stimuli elicited a P3 which was larger
from left than right parietal leads.


## DISCUSSION

In general, all left visual field and full field stimuli produced ERPs of similar morphology for control subjects and patients.
The waveform was characterized by an N1 (about 180 msec after
stimulus presentation) and, when subjects performed a task, a P3
(maximal around 350 msec after stimulus onset).  Differences between control subjects and patients were found in the anterior/
posterior and left/right amplitude distributions of these components.

In control subjects the lateralized presentation (to the
left or right visual field) of words and line drawings produced
ERPs in which the N1 was larger over the hemisphere contralateral
to the field of stimulation, and small or absent over the ipsilateral hemisphere.  This result is an agreement with what might
be expected on the basis of the anatomy of the visual pathways if
the N1 is generated in the hemisphere of the primary receiving
area.  Other investigators (Nakamura and Biersdorf, 1971; Shagass
et al., 1976) have reported similar results.  Here the N1 asymmetry,
seen over occipital cortex, extended to parietal and central leads
as well.

In patients, stimuli presented to the right visual field were
not perceived, and they did not evoke any discernible ERP components.  This result suggests that the N1 and later components
were generated at or beyond the level of the primary receiving
areas in the hemisphere contralateral to stimulation.

In these patients, correctly reported presentations of words
to the left visual field did not produce an N1 over the left hemisphere or over the intact right occipital cortex, but did evoke an
N1 at right hemisphere parietal and central sites.  Other studies
of hemianopic patients (Wildberger et al., 1976) report normal
ERPs over the intact hemisphere to stimulation of the preserved
visual field.  The different results found here might be a
consequence of the fact that our patients, in addition to having
left occipital damage, have also sustained damage to the splenium
of the corpus callosum.  Perhaps the additional damage to the
callosal fibers joining the two occipital lobes disrupted the
functioning of the right occipital lobe.  This hypothetical right
occipital damage, however, did not affect the visual acuity of the
patients, nor did it affect the N1 at right parietal and central
electrode sites.  Moreover, the suggestion that secondary right
occipital damage disrupted the occipital N1 is complicated by the
fact that left visual field presentations of line drawings did
produce an N1 over right occipital cortex in the patients.  The

different results for words and line drawings suggest that the
nature of the evoking stimuli may determine the distribution of
the N1 in patients such as these.  The anterior distribution of
the N1 over the right hemisphere for words, but not for line
drawings, may indicate that visual language information is relayed
to those areas of the right hemisphere where transfer across intact
portions of the corpus callosum is possible.

This interpretation of the N1 results is weakened by the
dissimilarities in the physical characteristics of the words and
the line drawings.  Although their average spatial luminance was
comparable (words 200 cd/m$^2$; line drawings 170 cd/m$^2$), other
optical parameters such as contour density and complexity are
virtually impossible to equate across these two categories of
stimuli.

Further tests of these and other patients may aid in the
interpretation of the results found for N1.  For example, if the
absence of the splenium is the important factor in the anterior N1
distribution for words, patients with an infarct of the splenium
(but intact left occiput) should show the same results as these
patients.  Patients with left occipital lesions which have spared
the splenium should show a normal N1 distribution to left visual
field presentations.

All subjects verbally reported the laterally presented words
and line drawings, and when they did so their ERPs contained a P3
at parietal and central leads.  In controls this P3 was symmetrical
over the two hemispheres independent of field of presentation.  This
dissociation between the distribution and symmetry of N1 and P3 supports current opinion which views these two ERP components as distinct, both in terms of their functional significance and in terms
of their neural origins (Hillyard and Picton, in press).  This symmetry of the P3 to unilateral stimulation might be attributed to
complete transfer across interhemispheric commissures of a response
generated in one hemisphere or to generation of the P3 by a midline
subcortical structure(s).

Whereas the P3 amplitude in control subjects was symmetrical
over the left and right hemispheres, it was asymmetrical in all
three patients.  The P3 at parietal leads was consistently broader
and larger from the left than from the right hemisphere.  Although
the precise nature of the psychological variables which determine
the amplitude of the P3 are poorly understood, it has been interpreted as a sign of the later stages of information processing
including response set selection, decision making and the reduction
of uncertainty (e.g. Hillyard and Picton, in press; Sutton et al.,
1967).  The parietal leads from which we recorded roughly underlie
the left and right angular gyri.  One might have expected, if
patients were able to use the right but not the left angular gyrus
in reading words presented to the left visual field, that a P3

would be elicited which was larger over right than left parietal areas. No evidence in support of this notion was found in the present investigation. Moreover, the asymmetry was found in ERPs to all task relevant stimuli. This suggests that perhaps the structural damage to the adjacent left occipital lobe was responsible for the larger P3 amplitude over the left parietal area; perhaps the larger P3 resulted from increased excitability at left parietal cortex resulting from loss of inhibition from the adjacent damaged occipital cortex. Similar tests of patients with left occipital lobe damage which has spared the splenium (and who have no reading deficit) may aid in the interpretation of this result.

To summarize, the major findings reported here are the absence, in patients with alexia without agraphia, of an N1 over intact right occipital cortex to correctly reported words presented to the left visual field and the asymmetrical (left larger than right) amplitude of the P3 in these patients. These results, although clear and consistent, are difficult to interpret from the point of view of the proposed mechanisms underlying the syndrome of alexia without agraphia and also from the point of view of current knowledge of the functional and structural correlates of the N1 and P3. Additional studies on these and similar patient populations may aid in the clarification of the neural bases of cognitive processes and ERPs.

## SUMMARY

We have simultaneously studied ERPs and performance on language and non-language tasks in normal control subjects and in three patients with the disconnection syndrome known as alexia without agraphia. This syndrome, in which every aspect of language functioning was intact except the ability to read, was produced by a lesion which compromised left occipital cortex and the splenium of the corpus callosum (as seen on CAT scan). We recorded ERPs from left and right central, parietal and occipital leads and from the eyes, all referred to linked mastoids. The stimuli were numbers, letters, three- and four-letter words and line drawings of common objects presented to the left and right visual fields. ERPs from left and right hemispheres were averaged separately according to stimulus type, visual field and whether or not subjects accurately perceived the stimuli.

Both the left/right and the anterior/posterior distributions of the patients' ERPs differed from those of control subjects. Most remarkable was the absence, in all three patients, of the N1 response over the intact right occipital lobe, even when patients accurately read words presented to the (good) left visual field. The N1 was present more anteriorly over right parietal and central sites, however. The other major result was a large asymmetry (left parietal greater than right parietal) in the P3

response of all three patients (but not in controls).  These
results are tentatively discussed in terms of possible functional
and structural changes in alexia without agraphia.

## ACKNOWLEDGMENTS

Supported in part by the National Institutes of Health,
USPHS Grants NS14365-01 and AG00712 and the Alfred P. Sloan
Foundation.  We are grateful to Wendy Borst for typing and for
valuable assistance in preparing stimuli and figures.

## REFERENCES

Ajax, E.T., Schenkenberg, T. and Kosteljanetz, M.  Alexia
    without agraphia and the inferior splenium.  Neurol.,
    1977, 27, 685-688.

Brown, W.S., Marsh, J.T. and Smith, J.C.  Evoked potential
    waveform differences produced by the perception of dif-
    ferent meanings of an ambiguous phrase.  Electroenceph.
    Clin. Neurophysiol., 1976, 41, 113-123.

Dejerine, M.J.  Contribution a l'etude anatomopathologique et
    clinique des differentes varietes de cecite verbale.
    Societe de Biologie - Comptes rendus et memoire, 1892,
    4, 61-90.

Donchin, E., McCarthy, G. and Kutas, M.  Electroencephalographic
    investigations of hemispheric specialization.  In J.E.
    Desmedt (Ed.) Progress in Clinical Neurophysiology.
    Language and Hemispheric Specialization in Man: Event
    Related Potentials.  Basel: Karger, 1977, Vol. 3.

Friedman, D., Simson, R., Ritter, W. and Rapin, I.  Cortical
    evoked potentials elicited by real speech words and human
    sounds.  Electroenceph. Clin. Neurophysiol., 1975, 38,
    13-19.

Galambos, R., Benson, P., Smith, T.S., Schulman-Galambos, C. and
    Osier, H.  On hemispheric differences in evoked potentials
    to speech stimuli.  Electroenceph. Clin. Neurophysiol.,
    1975, 39, 279-283.

Geshwind, N.  Disconnection syndromes in animals and man.  Brain,
    1965, 88, 237-294.

Hillyard, S.A. and Picton, T.W.  Event related brain potentials

and selective information processing in man.  In J. Desmedt
(Ed.) Cerebral Evoked Potentials in Man,  Basel: Karger,
in press.

Kimura, D.  Functional asymmetry of the brain in dichotic
listening.  Cortex, 1967, 3, 163-178.

Klein, D., Moscovitch, M. and Vigna, R.  Attentional mechanisms
and asymmetries in tachistoscopic recognition of words
and faces.  Neuropsychologia, 1976, 14, 55-66.

Knox, C. and Kimura, D.  Cerebral processing of nonverbal sounds
in boys and girls.  Neuropsychologia, 1968, 6, 1-11.

Luria, A.R. and Karasseva, T.A.  Disturbances of auditory-speech
memory in focal lesions of the deep regions of the left
lobe.  Neurosychologia, 1968, 6, 97-104.

Nakamura, Z. and Biersdorf, W.R.  Localization of the human
visual evoked response: Early components specific to visual
stimulation.  Amer. J. Ophthal. 1971, 72, 988-997.

Neville, H.J., Schulman, C. and Galambos, R.  Evoked potential
and behavioral correlates of functional hemispheric specialization.  Presented at the Fifth Annual Meeting of the International Neuropsychology Society, Sante Fe, 1977.

Shagass, C., Amadeo, M. and Roemer, R.A.  Spatial distribution
of potentials evoked by half field pattern reversal and
pattern onset stimuli.  Electroenceph. Clin. Neurophysiol.,
1976, 41, 609-622.

Sutton, S., Braren, M., Zubin, J. and John, E.R.  Information
delivery and the sensory evoked potential.  Science,
1967, 155, 1436-1439.

Teuber, H.-L.  Why two brains?  In F.O. Schmitt and F.G. Worden
(Eds.) The Neurosciences Third Study Program.  Cambridge,
Mass: Massachusetts Institute of Technology Press, 1974.

Vincent, F.M., Sadowsky, C.H., Saunders, R.L. and Reeves, A.G.
Alexia without agraphia, hemianopia or color naming
defect: A disconnection syndrome.  Neurol., 1977, 27,
689-691.

Wernicke, C.  Die neuren arbeiten über aphasie.  Fortschritt
der Medecin, 1885.

Wildberger, H.G.H., Van Lith, G.H.M., Wijngaarde, R. and Mak,
    G.T.M.  Visually evoked cortical potentials in the evaluation
    of homonymous and bitemporal visual field defects.  Brit.
    J. Ophthal., 1976, 60, 273-278.

Wood., G Goff, W.R. and Day, R.S.  Auditory evoked potentials
    during speech perception.  Science, 1971, 173, 1248-1251.

SPATIAL AND TEMPORAL DISTRIBUTION OF OLFACTORY EVOKED POTENTIALS

AND TECHNIQUES INVOLVED IN THEIR MEASUREMENT

K.-H. Plattig and G. Kobal

Institute of Physiology and Biocybernetics

Universitatsstr. 17, D-8520 Erlangen

Finkenzeller (1966) and Allison and Goff (1967), in studying the olfactory system, succeeded in finding olfactory evoked potentials (OEPs) on the intact skull of awake humans. Partly due to the technical difficulties associated with olfactory stimulation, however, there has been little subsequent progress in this area.

In order to properly record and analyze OEPs from awake humans and relate them to the underlying olfactory processes it is necessary to:

1. Use an olfactory stimulus with precisely determined intensive and temporal characteristics (including an instantaneous onset and offset time);

2. Eliminate (or minimize) the artifactual components that distort or mask the OEPs; and

3. Present many repetitions of the stimulus in order to improve the signal-to-noise ratio of the recorded potentials.

In regards to the first requirement, several serious technical problems have made it quite difficult in the past to produce an exactly reproducible olfactory stimulus. The first part of this paper includes the description of a new stimulating device that enables us to produce, as often as desirable, a stimulus with constant characteristics.

Satisfying the second requirement cited above has proven to be equally difficult. Several sources of artifactual intrusions have been described previously. Some of them include (listed according

285

to increasing difficulty): thermoreceptive disturbances, auditory responses, synchronization of the potentials with respiration, somatosensory (tactile) responses, eye blinking and somatosensory responses by chemical stimulation of free trigeminal nerve endings by the odorous substances.

The latter two sources of artifactual disturbances have been particularly bothersome. Eye-blinking is a disturbance well known to investigators of EEG phenomena in other sensory modalities. Chemical stimuli, however, are even more prone to elicit eye-blinking responses since cornea and conjunctiva are particularly sensitive to such stimulation. Uncontamined OEPs can be expected only when no chemical stimulation occurs at the eye. Moreover, eye-blinking is also elicited by chemical and mechanical stimulation of the nasal mucosa.

Smith et al. (1971) suggested that there were no olfactory EEG responses and that all OEPs, including those reported by Finken-zeller and by Allison and Goff, were produced by chemical irritation of the intranasal free trigeminal nerve endings. To support their suggestion, Smith and his group reported on results obtained on patients who had lost trigeminal sensitivity on one side of their nose. In those cases they were not able to find EEG responses to odorous substances. It is our opinion, however, that odorous substances produce both olfactory and somatosensory evoked potentials in man and animals. In the second part of this paper we will present suggestions that olfactory and somatosensory responses are separate phenomena that might be differentiated both in terms of their topographical distribution on the skull and in terms of the time course of the adaptation of each.

In regard to the third requirement cited above the repetitious presentation of an olfactory stimulus to improve signal-to-noise ratio causes serious difficulties when studying olfaction due to the rapid and significant adaptation and habituation that occurs. As a result, in most experiments that have been reported, no more than thirty consecutive stimulus presentations have been used. Knowledge of the time course of adaptation and habituation for the different components of the OEP is considered to be particularly important in these considerations.

STIMULUS DEVICE AND CONTROL OF ARTIFACTS

The "pulse method" of presenting odorous substances has been one of the more common techniques of olfactory research on animals. The method involves typically the presentation of an air-puff that is blown towards the olfactory mucosa. The air-puff can be varied in its duration, and the concentration of odorous substances contained within it can be controlled (e.g., see Giesen and Mrowinski, 1970; Herberhold, 1973). The major advantage of the pulse method is that the stimulus onset time is very rapid. The maximum concentration of odorous substance can be reached in approximately 20 msec (Plattig and Kobal, 1977; Kobal and Plattig, 1978).

The major disadvantage of the pulse method is that, inherently in its use, it elicits strong, artifactual nonodorous responses which are synchronized to the presentation of the odorant. The only method of stimulus presentation, in our opinion, that completely avoids this artifact is the "flow method" of stimulation. In the flow method a constant gaseous flow continuously flows over the nasal mucosa. At the time of stimulus presentation an odorous substance is substituted for the neutral gas without altering the rate or volume of air flow. The major difficulty of the flow method, of course, is to develop an ability to substitute the odorant substance for the neutral gas in such a manner that the maximum concentration is reached rapidly and yet no flow turbulences are generated.

The olfactometer developed in our laboratory is illustrated in Fig. 1. When using the flow method compressed air is cleaned and dried with charcoal and $CaCl_2$ and then delivered to three air cylinders. Prior to the observation interval when an odorous stimulus is presented, clean air is delivered via Tube C (Control) to Flask I which contains distilled water. The air is then delivered from the air cylinder to the most important part of the olfactometer - the 3-Y shaped nasal exit - where it is presented to the human observer. During this period in which neutral air is being delivered to the nasal exit all other (odorous) air is exhausted via Tube $E_1$. In order to present an odorous stimulus with a controlled concentration, clean and dried air is delivered via Tube O (odorant) to Flask II containing the odorous substance. If maximum saturation of this odorant is required, the air is delivered to the nasal exit in an undiluted form. During the presentation of the odorant, the neutral air that had been delivered to the nasal exit is exhausted from the nasal exit via Tube $E_2$. The switching of the exhaust tubes from $E_1$ to $E_2$ is accomplished with a magnetic valve (M) also developed in our laboratory. If an odorous substance with a lower-than-maximum saturation is required, the odorous air from Flask II can be diluted by replacing part of the air with neutral air from Flask III. To do so, a volume of odorant air equal to that being added from Flask III is exhausted from the output of Flask II via Tube $E_0$. In this manner any saturation of odorant from 0% to 100% may be delivered at the nasal exit.

All tubing in the olfactometer is constructed of teflon or glass. A thermostabilized water cover keeps the temperature of all tubing at a constant 37°C. At the beginning of the observation

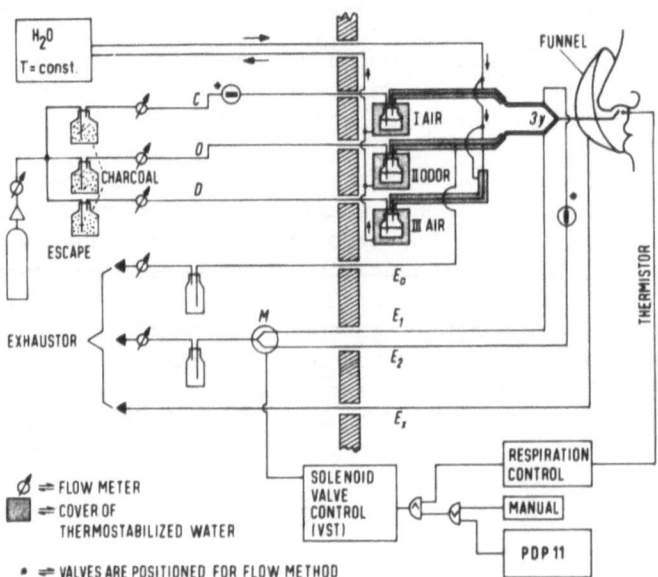

Fig. 1.   Olfactometer for both the flow method and the pulse method.
To use the pulse method the two valves designated by asterisks have
to be closed, but to use the flow method they have to be open so
that the path C-Flask I-$E_2$ can be opened by the magnetic valve M
while $E_2$ is closed.  Flask I and Flask II contain distilled water
and Flask II the odorant

interval, when the odorant air is substituted for the neutral air,
the air exhausted from the nasal exit via $E_2$ is equivalent in flow
and temperature to that being delivered at the nasal exit from Flask
II (and III).  The odorant air reaches the nasal cavity 2 msec
after the neutral air is replaced by the odorant air at the input
to the nasal exit.  Because of the effectiveness of the air flow
system and the magnetic valve, it is possible to select a stimulus
onset time as fast as 40 msec when using the flow method.  Even at
the maximal flow rate of 500 ml/sec no flow turbulences are observed
when a 40 msec rise-fall time is employed.

     In our research the nasal exit terminates in a funnel located
directly, but loosely, in front of the observer's nose and is
connected to an exhauster.  When using a prenasal application,
however, it is necessary to initiate each stimulus presentation at
the same moment in the inhalation process.  For this purpose a
thermistor located directly in front of the nose and a suitable
electronic circuit are used to synchronize the respiration cycle
and stimulus presentation.  The disadvantage to this synchrony, of

course, is the confounding that occurs due to the recording of
extra- or intracranial potentials associated with respiratory
activity.  These confounding effects can be minimized (Kobal and
Plattig, 1978).

The olfactometer may also be used in the pulse method of
stimulation.  By switching the valves on Tubes C and $E_2$ (designated with asterisks in Fig. 1) the continuous flow of neutral air
prior to and following the presentation of the odorant are eliminated.  In addition, the rise-fall time of the stimulus may be
reduced to approximately 20 msec when using this method.

During stimulation the clicking noise of the valves and, when
using the pulse method, the hissing sound generated by the air flow
may be masked by white noise presented via headphones.

Typical results obtained while using the olfactometer in
both the flow method and the pulse method are shown in Fig. 2.
Trace 1 (the upper trace) shows the resulting waveform that occurred
when nonodorous air was presented to the observer via the flow
method.  As can be noted, no meaningful potentials occurred.  Trace
2 shows the results obtained when eucalyptol was presented to
observers using the flow method.  Definite positive and negative
deviations with readily measurable latencies occurred.  Trace 3
shows the results obtained in response to nonodorous air when using
the pulse method of stimulation.  The potentials seen are the result
of tactile somatosensory stimulation.  Trace 4 indicates the results
in response to eucalyptol when using the pulse method.  The potentials were somewhat different than those elicited by the same
odorant when using the flow method.  The magnitude of N1 was notice-
ably smaller, and the latency was approximately 20 msec shorter.
These differences resulted presumably from the interaction of the
positive component of the somatosensory potential and the negative
deviation of the olfactory response.  Further, since the influence
of the tactile somatosensory potential is not always phase-coherent
to the olfactory response, the shape of the resulting potentials
varies considerably.  This variance eliminates the possibility of a
meaningful evaluation of amplitudes or areas of the potentials when
using the pulse method.

Table I summarizes the latencies for the various positive and
negative potentials that occurred in response to the eucalyptol in
the flow method conditions.

Another source of artifact cited earlier was the central and
peripheral potentials associated with eye-blinking.  The presentation of high concentrations of an odorant often elicits eye-
blinking responses, particularly in the early minutes of a data
gathering session.  The associated electrical activity (e.g.,

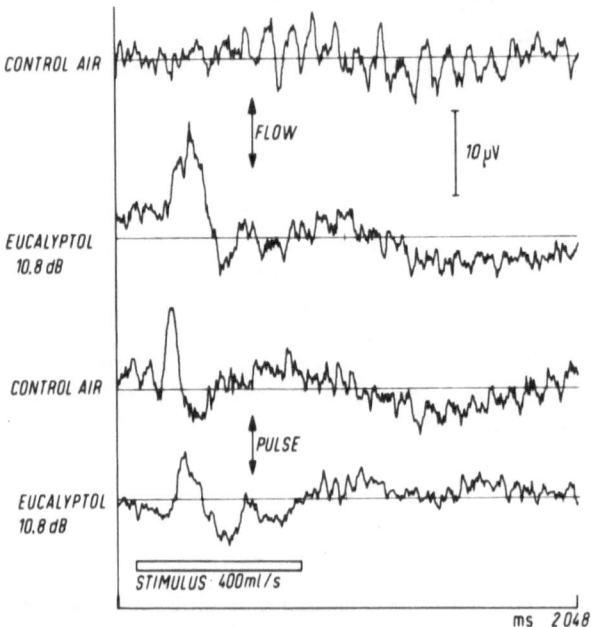

Fig. 2.  Comparison of OEPs obtained by the flow method (trace 1+2) and by the pulse method (trace 3+4).  Lead Cz/Al.  Negativity up. N=16.  Likewise in all following records.

the electonystogram record, ENG) usually results in a positive potential (approximately 200 uV) when the record is obtained at the vertex (EEG position Cz/Al).  The interaction of the ENG and the OEPs may result in a variety of distortions depending upon the

Table I.  Average latencies for OEPs from Cz/Al of twelve subjects. The mean latency and the standard deviation ($\pm$s) in msec for twelve subjects are indicated.  Each individual subject's waveform represented the averaged result of sixteen stimulus presentations.  The latency values shown include the physiological time for excitation and conduction as well as the stimulus transportation time from the prenasal thermistor to the olfactory epithelium.  Although results for only one stimulus intensity (12.04 dB re threshold) are shown, other results indicated that the latency of the OEP was dependent upon stimulus intensity.

| P1 | N1 | P2 | N2 | P3 |
|---|---|---|---|---|
| $222.2\pm 46.0$ | $317.2\pm31.9$ | $455.7\pm43.2$ | $572.7\pm47.3$ | $695.0\pm64.4$ |

phase relations of the two potentials. Frequently an increase in
the magnitude of P2 is seen, and occasionally the complete masking
of N1 occurs. As a result we have adopted a procedure (OFFLAB)
developed by Spreng (1976) to eliminate or minimize the contribution of artifacts to the evoked potential record (Kobal and Plattig,
1976).

An added benefit of the application of the OFFLAB program to
eliminate contamination from eye-blink is that contamination from
other sources may also be eliminated. Gaardner (1964), for example,
has described the visual evoked potentials associated with eye
movements. We consider, then, the method of averaging only uncon-
taminated OEPs to be the most reliable procedure currently available.

CHEMICAL STIMULATION OF THE TRIGEMINAL NERVE

Many substances that evoke an electro-olfactogram (EOG) in
experiments on animals excite the trigeminal nerve by stimulating
its free nerve endings. Beidler (1965) demonstrated this by
recording the activity of small branches of the trigeminal nerve
while stimulating the nasal epithelium. Dawson (1962) was able to
record electrical activity in the trigeminal nerve while chemically
stimulating the cornea of the rabbit. In unpublished experiments
in our laboratory we have recorded local potentials from the cornea
of the frog while stimulating the cornea and conjunctiva with
linalool and eucalyptol. The local potentials resemble closely the
EOG potentials in shape but have a positive deviation rather than
the negative potential of the EOG. The amplitude of the potential
is dependent upon stimulus intensity and has an initial latency of
about 2 sec (slightly longer than the corresponding peak of the
EOG).

This direct stimulation of the trigeminal nerve by odorants
has long been a difficulty for scientists studying the olfactory
system. Tucker (1971) suggested: "The dream of finding an odorant
that is purely olfactory in its stimulating capabilities is still
unrealized." Smith (1971), as discussed earlier, argued that
"olfactory" potentials are elicited solely by the excitation of the
somatosensory modality. In our opinion this discussion of olfactory
and somatosensory interaction will continue until a patient whose
trigeminal sensitivity is completely lost can be examined. Unfortunately no such opportunity has as yet arisen for us. We have,
however, examined patients whose filia olfactoria were torn off
following aneurismarrhaphy. In these patients we found a distinct
decrease in the amplitude of evoked potentials recorded in response
to odorants on the affected side. We presume, in these patients,
that both the olfactory and somatosensory modalities were responsible for the recorded activity.

To examine this problem further we have performed the following experiment.  A thin teflon tube, 2 mm in diameter and connected
to the olfactometer exit, was inserted into the nose approximately
2-3 cm.  The air flow was directed either through the lower nasal
duct (Condition A) or towards the olfactory cleft parallel to the
dorsum of the nose (Condition B).  This procedure was repeated on
both the left and right sides.  Amyl butyrate and eucalyptol were
used as odorous stimuli.  The evoked potentials based on sixteen
stimulus presentations in each condition are shown in Fig. 3.  In
each case the potentials recorded in Condition B were greater in
amplitude.  Further, and particularly when amyl butyrate was presented, an additional potential component appeared approximately
300-400 msec after the onset of the stimulus (either another peak
was discernible or the existing peak broadened in shape).  The
subjective responses reported in the two conditions were notice-
ably different.  In Condition A the cooling effect of eucalyptol
was felt in the "lower" part of the nose.  In response to the amyl
butyrate the subjects reported the odor of raspberry but were
unable to localize the sensation.  In Condition B the sensation of
the two substances was more "upward" in the nasal cavity.  Further,
the subjects reported that the perceptions that occurred in
Condition B suggested the stimulus had a much sharper ("steeper")
rise time than the perceptions elicited in Condition A.

Also shown in Fig. 3 are results obtained in Condition A in
response to eucalyptol following the application of a local anesthesia to the lower and middle nasal duct.  The resulting evoked
potentials were considerably smaller in amplitude except for an
unusual characteristic.  Following a substantial delay, a late
positive potential appeared.  The potential occurred according to
a perception reported by the subjects that was localized in the
pharynx.

Two possible explanations for the data reported in the experiment described above are noteworthy.  First, it was our intent to
vary the manner in which the odorant reached the olfactory mucosa.
In Condition A we imagined the odorant would infiltrate upwards
relatively slowly through the nasal cavity.  In Condition B, however,
we were assuming the odorant would reach the olfactory mucosa more
directly and more rapidly.  The perceptual results of the experiment
as reported by the subjects apparently confirm our intentions.
Further the electrophysiological results suggest that the rise-time
of the stimulus may be of critical importance in determining the
magnitude of the OEP.

Another explanation of the potentials shown in Fig. 3 is that
stimulation in Condition B may have elicited responses in trigeminal
receptors that are different from and more sensitive than those
receptors stimulated in Condition A.  Finally the results reported

in this experiment may also help account for the negative results reported by Smith, et al. (1971). Using the flow method of stimulation the design of their olfactometer required a large volume of gas resting in the odorous cylinder to be accelerated and then transported a considerable distance to the subject. As a result the onset time of the stimulus may have been too slow to elicit the OEP.

## DISTRIBUTION OF AMPLITUDES AND LATENCIES ON THE HUMAN SKULL

As suggested in the introductory remarks, an examination of the topographical distribution of evoked responses on the human skull may provide information helpful in the separation of ol-

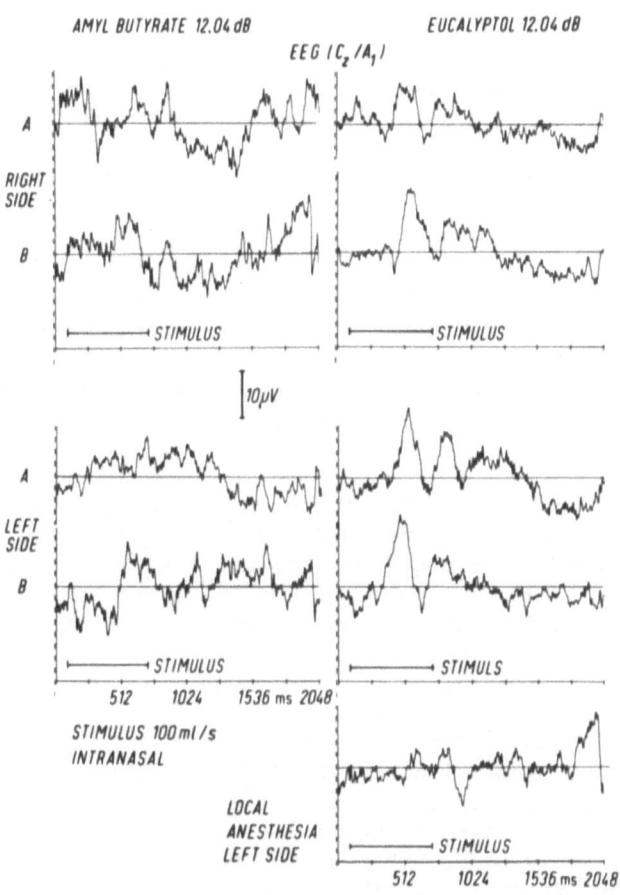

Fig. 3. AEPs after stimulation of the lower (A) and of the upper (B) parts of the nasal cavity by amyl butyrate and by eucalyptol.

factory and somatosensory responses. Additionally information
provided by such an analysis can be used to determine the optimal
number of recording sites that should be employed in the measurement of OEPs.

To conduct such an examination EEG records were obtained at
nineteen positions (on the 10/20 classification) on the skull in
response to eucalyptol presented at the right nostril via the flow
method. The recordings were made in two separate sessions. In
the first session ten positions in the frontal part of the skull
were used. Eight positions in the rear of the skull were examined
in a second session. In addition, position Cz (vertex) was included
in both sessions for comparison purposes. Position Al (the left
mastoid) was the reference point for all positions. All EEG records
were recorded on a 12-channel Siemens-mingograph as well as stored
on magnetic tape (Sangamo Sabre VI: PCM by Johne and Reilhofer
3K12).

Ten subjects were initially employed in the experiment. Three
of the ten subjects had to be eliminated due to heavy eye-blinking.
Of the remaining seven subjects, five were examined in all conditions on two separate sessions (i.e., the recordings on both the
frontal and rear positions of the skull were repeated). The
remaining two subjects were examined entirely on one occasion. An
overload of artifactual components required the omission of some
of the sessions. As a result final data analysis was computed on
eight sessions recorded at the frontal sites and eleven sessions
recorded at the rear positions. A further complication resulted
when some of the recording sites yielded no measurable potentials
(or a minimal number of non-zero values). As a consequence no
analysis of variances could be employed.

Some of the results of the experiment are shown in Fig. 4. At
the upper left position of the figure a typical evoked response is
illustrated. Additionally the N1/P2 amplitude (a), the P2/N2
amplitude (b), the area under N1 (F1) and the area under N2 (F2)
are illustrated. At the lower left of the figure are the evoked
potentials obtained on one subject at both the frontal sites
(lower) and the rear sites (upper) on the skull. On the right side
of Fig. 4 are the results of the amplitudes and area measurements.
Under "a" are the N1/P2 measurements summarized on a 9-point scale
from black (maximum amplitude) to white (minimum amplitude). The
results under "b" summarize the P2/N2 amplitude measurements, etc.
The illustration of each skull is divided into a 5 X 5 matrix which
corresponds to the international 10/20 classification. The illustration immediately under "a" and "b" (row 1) summarizes the results
obtained at the frontal positions, and the illustrations just below
(row 2) summarize the results at the rear positions. The combined
results are shown in row 3. The results of the area measurements

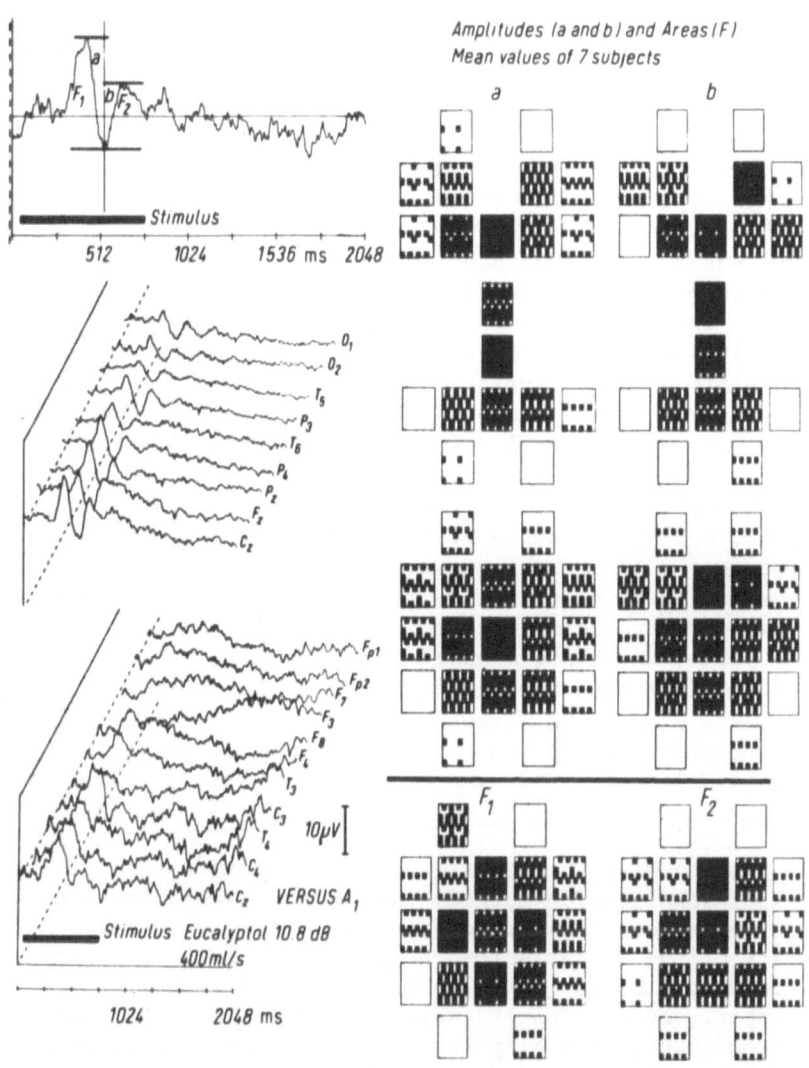

Fig. 4.   Distribution of amplitudes and areas of OEPs (maximum black).

have been combined into the row four illustration (even though they are collected in two separate sessions).   The results shown in Fig. 4 are the mean values for seven subjects.

In general the late unspecific potentials reached their greatest amplitude at recording sites near the vertex.   The maximum Nl/P2 amplitude occurred directly at the vertex, and the second highest amplitude occurred at C3 (the position adjacent to the ver-

tex and contralateral to the stimulated nostril). The maximum P2/N2
amplitude occurred at Fz and F4. The results of the measurements
of the area under N1 and under N2 were distributed similarly to the
amplitude results.

The upper half of Fig. 5 summarizes the results of amplitude
measurements of each of the five identifiable peaks (P1, N1, P2,
N2, P3) when the measurements were made from the "baseline of the
EEG". The baseline, illustrated as a straight horizontal line in
the evoked response shown in Fig. 4, is the linear average of each
EEG record. The results shown in Fig. 5, like those in Fig. 4, are
the mean values obtained from seven subjects. The results indicating the distribution of amplitudes on the skull for N1 are similar
to the distribution measured on N1/P2. Further, the topographical
distribution of N2 was similar to that for N2/P2.

Results concerning the averaged latencies for the five peaks
(P1, N1, P2, N2, P3) relative to the onset of the stimulus are
summarized in the lower half of Fig. 5. Again a 9-point scale from
black (maximum latency) to white (minimum latency) was employed.
An examination of these results points out that, at least for the
N1 and N2 peaks, the topographical distribution of the minimum
latencies is similar to the distribution of the maximum amplitudes
(and, conversely, maximum latencies are similar to minimum amplitudes). The relationship between the topographic distribution of
amplitudes and latencies for the other peaks (P1, P2, P3) is more
complex.

The results displayed in Fig. 4 were submitted to a factor
analysis (diagonalization method, varimax rotation), omitting those
positions which sometimes yielded no measurable potentials. Although
the results of the analysis for the amplitude and latency measures
of each component of the potentials are too numerous to summarize
in this paper, several results were noteworthy. In the examination
of the topography of the N1 potential (amplitude), three factors
with loads greater than 0.7 ($p < 0,05$) were noted. Factor I pointed
towards the central positions (loads: -0.96 for Cz, -0.95 for C3);
Factor II to the precentral positions (loads: 0.82 for T4 and 0.86
for F3); Factor III to the contralateral positions (loads: 0.89
for F7 and 0.90 for T3). Similar results and loads were obtained
when the latency of N1 was analyzed. In our opinion these results
suggest the presence of three underlying variables. The first
relates to the central positions (vertex), the second to the precentral positions and the third to the left-right displacement.

When the amplitude of N2 was examined similarly, three factors
were again extracted. They also exhibited loads of similar magnitude (Factor I: 0.92 for Cz, 0.84 for C4 and 0.79 for C3; Factor
II: 0.89 for T3; Factor III: 0.71 for T4). The results of the

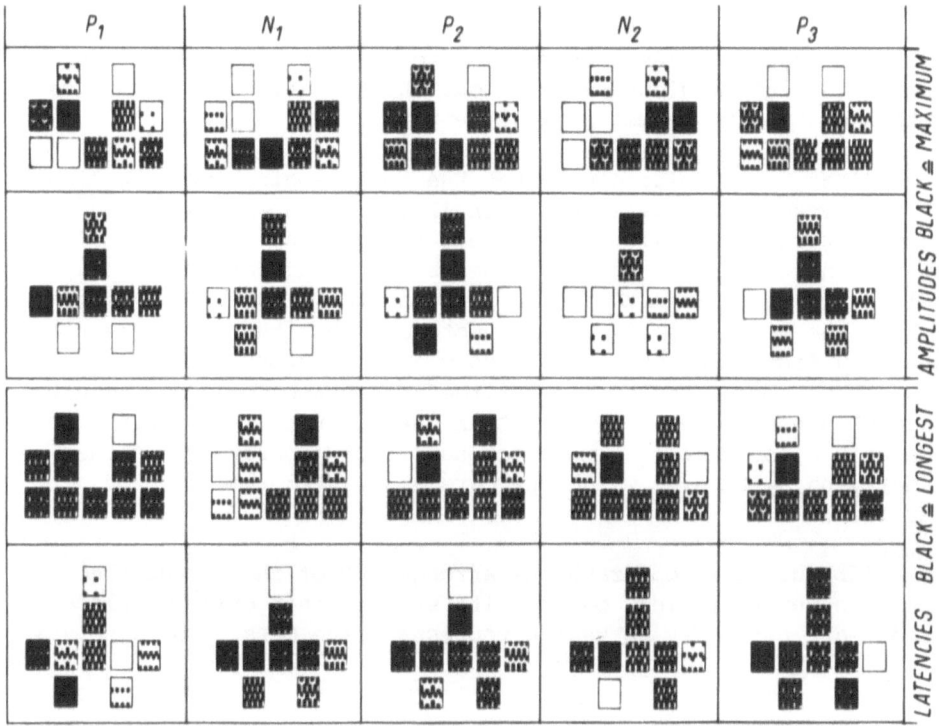

Fig. 5.  Distribution of amplitudes and latencies of OEPs (maximum black).

analysis of the latency of N2 were similar.  Again we interpret these results as suggesting the presence of three underlying variables which relate to the central positions, to the left side and to the right side.

The analysis of the potentials (amplitude and latency) on the occipital parts of the skull brought up only one factor.  The factor corresponded quite nicely with the distribution of the OEPs which become smaller as the electrode is moved in an occipital direction (see Fig. 4).

CONCLUSION

Although much research remains to be completed and we are
only at an intermediate point in our investigations; the results
obtained thus far permit several tentative conclusions.

First it is quite clear that the topographical distribution
of the evoked potentials on the skull are a nonrandom arrangement that reach a maximum at or near the vertex.  The amplitude
and latency of the various components of the potentials displayed
relatively specific patterns in response to stimulation by eucalyptol at the right nostril.  Our hypothesis that the OEP reflects
activity from both the somatosensory and olfactory systems, however,
has not yet been completely confirmed.  Nevertheless, our results
suggest there is probably more than one generator responsible for
the evoked potentials.  The exact number of generators and the
underlying systems to which they are associated remain to be
verified.

Although the topographical arrangement of the OEP on the
skull is quite complex, our results suggest that only two electrodes are necessary to record representative OEPs.  To do so, one

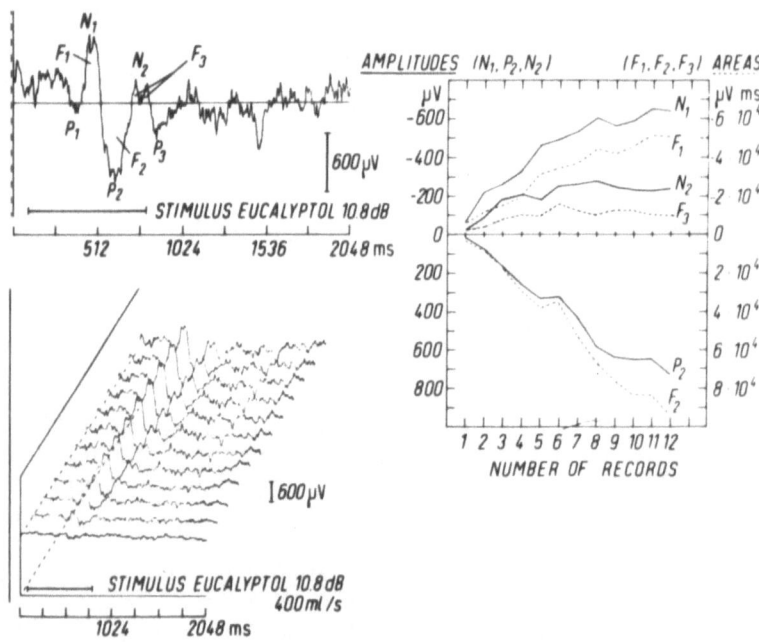

Fig. 6.    Time course of single components of OEPs during averaging
Cz/Al.

electrode should be located at Cz and the other at a precentral
position (e.g., F4). Of course, for omitting eye-blinking artifacts
as discussed earlier it is also necessary to record the ENG
potentials.

Finally, we feel that further confirmation of our hypothesis
concerning the generators of the OEP may be gained by examining
the time course of adaptation of the various components of the OEP.
The details of an experiment we are conducting currently and some
early results are shown in Fig. 6. Briefly, we are examining the
changes in amplitude that occur in N1, P2 and N2 (designated on the
upper left of Fig. 6) as well as the changes in the magnitude of
the areas of N1 ("F1" in Fig. 6), P2 ("F2") and N2 ("F3") as an
odorant is presented twelve times in succession. The odorant we
are examining is eucalyptol at an intensity of 10.8 dB re threshold. The interstimulus interval in the succession of twelve
presentations is 50-60 sec.

A cumulative record of the EEG recordings made on one subject
during a single session are shown in the lower left portion of Fig.
6. The lower record was elicited in response to the first presentation of the stimulus; the second record is the cumulative EEG
response to the first two stimulus presentations, etc. The twelfth
record, then, is the cumulative EEG of all twelve stimulus presentations. On the right-hand side of the figure some of our results
are summarized. Each function displays the cumulative result
that occurred during the twelve presentations of the odorant. The
amplitude values are displayed on the left ordinate (for N1, N2
and P2) and the area values for N1 (F1), P2 (F2) and N2 (F3) on
the right-hand ordinate. (A cumulative function that increased
linearly throughout the twelve presentations would indicate that
the component being measured remained constant in response to each
stimulus presentation. A horizontal cumulative function would
indicate the component had disappeared.)

Several interesting findings can be noted. For example, the
amplitude of the N1 wave remained relatively constant throughout
the first five presentations of the stimulus, was somewhat reduced
in magnitude through the eighth presentation and had completely
adapted and disappeared during the latter presentations. The
amplitude of the P2 wave, on the other hand, remained relatively
constant throughout the twelve stimulus presentations. The magnitude of the N2 wave, in contrast, seemed to oscillate somewhat
during the session. The results of the area measurements indicated
a pattern of adaptation similar to that exhibited by the amplitude
measures.

At the present time we are making similar analyses on data
collected on many subjects in several experimental conditions. We
continue to believe that the time course of adaptation of the

various components will be useful in distinguishing those aspects
of the OEP attributable to the somatosensory system and those parts
resulting from olfactory processes.


SUMMARY

An improved device is described for olfactory stimulation via:
(a) the "pulse method", and (b) the "flow method".  Only the flow
method (with stimulus onset and offset times of 40 msec each)
guarantees reproducible records of olfactory sensory activity by
avoiding mechanoreceptive artifacts; additional control of thermo-
ceptive, auditory and eye-blinking artifacts is necessary.  Human
olfactory evoked responses from nineteen different sites of the
skull are demonstrated.  The components N1, N2 and P2 with different rates of adaptation are more clearly recognizable than P1 and
P3.  N1 (which is possibly of somatosensory origin) occurs 270–350
msec, N2 (possibly of olfactory origin) 520–620 msec and P2 occurs
410–500 msec following the stimulus onset.  The maximum amplitude
of N1 is recorded in the central, contralateral (to the stimulated
nostril) area of the skull and the maximum of N2 is found at the
precentral ipsilateral area.


ACKNOWLEDGEMENTS

We would like to acknowledge and express our appreciation to
the "Umweltbundesamt (Federal Office of Environmental Protection)
Berlin" for supporting this research.  Further we thank the Haar-
mann and Reimer GmbH, Holzminden, for supplying us with odorous
substances and Prof. Dr. W. Schiefer, Head of the Department of
Neurosurgery, University of Erlangen-Nurnberg, for the loan of the
12-channel "Mingograph".  We also wish to express our appreciation
to U. Brandl for writing our "OFFLAB" program and Prof. Dr. T.
Dolan, on leave from the National Science Foundation, Washington,
D.C. for his assistance in writing this manuscript.  Finally, we
wish to dedicate this chapter to the pioneer physiologist in olfaction, Prof. Dr. Yngve Zotterman, Stockholm, on the occasion of
his eightieth birthday.


REFERENCES

Allison, T. and Goff, W.R.  Human cerebral evoked responses to
    odorous stimuli.  Electroenceph. Clin. Neurophysiol., 1967,
    23, 558-560.

Beidler, L.M.  Comparison of gustatory receptors, olfactory
    receptors and free nerve endings.  Cold Spring Harb. Symp.
    Quant. Biol., 1965, 30, 191-200.

Dawson, W.W.   Chemical stimulation of the peripheral trigeminal
    nerve.   Nature, 1962, 196, 341-345.

Finkenzeller, P.   Gemittelte EEG-Potentiale bei olfaktorischer
    Reizung.   Pflugers Arch. ges. Physiol., 1966, 292, 76-80.

Gaardner, K., Krauskopf, J., Graf, B., Kropfl, W. and Armington,
    J.C.   Averaged brain activity following saccadic eye movements.
    Science, 1964, 146, 1841-1843.

Giesen, M., Mrowinski, D.   Klinische Untersuchungen mit einem
    Impuls-Olfaktometer.   Arch. Ohr. Nas. - Kehlk. Heilk., 1970,
    196, 377-380.

Herberhold, C.   Nachweis und Reizbedingungen olfaktorisch und
    rhinosensibel evozierter Hirnrindensummenpotentiale sowie
    Konzept einer klinischen Computer-Olfaktometrie.   Opladen:
    Westduetscher Verlag, 1973, 126.

Kobal, G., Plattig, K.-H.   Methodische Anmerkungen zur Gewinnung
    olfaktroischer EEG-Antworten des wachen Menschen.   EEG-EMG,
    1978, 9, 135-145.

Plattig, K.-H., Kobal, G.   Olfactory and gustatory responses in
    the human electroencephalogram (EEG).   In Y. Katsuki, M. Sato,
    S.F. Takagi and Y. Oomura (Eds.), Food Intake and Chemical
    Senses, Tokyo: Tokyo Univ. Press, 1977.

Smith, D.B., Allison, T., Goff, W.R., and Princitato, J.J.   Human
    odorant evoked responses:  Effects of trigeminal or olfactory
    deficit.   Electroenceph. Clin. Neurophysiol., 1971, 30, 313-
    317.

Spreng, M.   Zusatzmethoden zur Verbesserung der Aussagekraft
    gemittelter evozierter Potentiale.   EEG-EMG, 1972, 3, 49-56.

Tucker, D.   Nonolfactory responses from the nasal cavity:  Jacob-
    son's organ and the trigeminal system.   In L.M. Beidler (Ed.)
    Handbook of Sensory Physiology, Vol. IV/1, Berlin/Heidelberg/
    New York: Springer, 1971.

EVENT RELATED SCALP POTENTIALS DURING A BIMANUAL CHOICE R.T. TASK:

TOPOGRAPHY AND INTERHEMISPHERIC RELATIONS

R. Ragot and A. Remond

Electrophysiology and Applied Neurophysiology Laboratory

Salpetriere Hospital, 75634 Paris Cedex 13 (France)

## INTRODUCTION

The general purpose of this experiment is to evaluate the specificity of electrophysiological correlates of decision making in the brain; in particular, its main goal is to investigate possible relationships between right and left hemisphere scalp recorded electrical activity during a choice reaction time task and either the stimulated or the responding side of the body.

Much work has recently been devoted to the study of electrical correlates of prepatory mechanisms before movement. In man, tools for investigation range from purely behavioral (RT and performance) to scalp recorded EEG activities (readiness potentials, premotor and motor potentials, contingent negative variation, the P300 wave of the evoked potential, etc.) through electromyography and other indexes.

The readiness potential (RP), a large negative shift, appears on the scalp prior to a voluntary movement (Kornhuber et al., 1965; Gilden et al., 1977; Vaughan et al., 1968; Deecke et al., 1968; Gerbrandt et al., 1973). It is well established now that the final phase of this component and the motor potential (MP)(also negative) that occur during the movement tend to peak precentrally on the scalp contralaterally to the part of the body involved in the movement (Kutas and Donchin, 1977). This negative phase is followed by an abrupt positive postmovement deflection called the "reafferent potential".

If the preparatory stimulus warns the subject that he will have to make a movement with the right hand on the arrival of the imperative stimulus, the negative shift appears larger in the left hemisphere and vice versa (Syndulko and Lindsley, 1977).

The P300 (latency 250-500 msec), a late component of the sensory evoked potential, appears, or is greatly enhanced, if the stimulus is task relevant (Sutton et al., 1967), or uncertain (Sutton et al., 1965), rare (Cooper et al., 1977; Squires, 1977), if it is expected but does not occur (Weinberg et al., 1970; Simson et al., 1976; Renault and Lesevre, in press; Klinke et al., 1968; Renault et al., in press) or if the occurring stimulus is different from the expected stimulus (Demaire and Coquery, 1977; Courchesne et al., 1975). If visual stimuli are delivered in random order either in the right or left peripheral visual field, and if the subject is required to respond only to one of these stimuli, the components of the VEP, and the P300 in particular, appear enhanced after the presentation of this stimulus (Van Voorhis and Hillyard, 1977).

The above mentioned studies demonstrate that the topography and amplitude of both the CNV in preparation for a motor act and the P300 following the reception of an expected stimulus depend on afferent (sensory) and efferent (motor) information. The present study investigated whether any of the electrical events occurring between the stimulus and the response during a bimanual choice RT task were correlated, either with the responding hand or with the stimulated side of the body. Because the stimuli are task relevant, this experimental paradigm was expected to induce P300 components.

This situation was, however, preceded by a simple, self-paced movement task in order to compare the electrical pattern due to a complex stimulus-response paradigm to that produced by the movement alone.

EXPERIMENTAL PROCEDURE

General Setup

Four male and three female volunteers, aged 21-32, all right-handed, served as subjects for the experiment. Handedness was determined using a playing card dealing test (Zazzo, 1960); all subjects used the right hand spontaneously to perform the test, and dealing duration was more than twice as long when they were asked to employ the left hand instead of the right hand.

Subjects were seated in a comfortable chair in a dark, sound attenuated room; they were asked to relax all muscles as much as possible, contracting only those involved in the motor act. The movement consisted in a right or left index finger press on a micro-switch. Pressure required for contact closing was 300 ± 20 g, and

displacement of the index finger was 3 mm.  Switches were fixed on
a light cardboard cylinder grasped with both hands by the subject
and resting on his knees.  In order to avoid any auditory feedback
from the switch operation, earplugs were worn by the subjects.  Similarly a small luminous cross was used as a gaze fixation point to
prevent eye movements during stimulation.

Scalp potentials were recorded with seven collodion-affixed
Beckman electrodes placed along a transverse line running between
two points situated 1 cm in front of the auditory canal via the vertex.  This electrode placement was chosen in order to detect both
motor potential components and P300s, and especially to evaluate
their lateral topography.  Interelectrode distance was 3.5 cm, and
the mean of the two earlobe potentials was taken as a reference.
Simultaneous vertical and horizontal electro-oculograms were also
recorded; this permitted the elimination from the average of all
self-paced movements or responses which were affected by eye
movements.

The time constant of the EEG channels was 1.5 sec; the time
constant of the oculogram, .3 sec.  Analog-to-digital conversion was
performed on-line; data were stored on digital tape and processed
later by computer (BGE M40).

## Self-Paced Movements

The task consisted of a self-paced, right and left index finger
pressing on the microswitch.  A regular pace of 2 sec was required
in order to compare the situation with the reaction time procedure,
and subjects succeeded in keeping this pace within reasonable limits
(1.8 to 2.5 sec).

## Choice Reaction Time Situation

The stimuli consisted of a brief flash (3 msec duration) from
light emitting diodes placed on a panel standing approximately 40
cm in front of the subject.  These stimuli appeared within a fixed
period (2 sec) and, at random, either $10°$ to the right or the left
of the fixation point; their color also varied randomly, either red
or green.  The subject was required to press with the right index
(R) if the light flashed green and with the left index (L) if it
flashed red, irrespective of the location of the stimulus [on the
right (r) or on the left (l) of the fixation point].

Consequently the four possible situations that appear randomly
can be labeled lR, rL (when the response must be given contralaterally to the stimulus), rR and lL (if the response is to be given on
the same side as the stimulus).  Prior to event related potential

recordings, subjects were given practice runs.  Error-free performance was achieved after an average of twenty to thirty trials.

## DATA ANALYSIS

### Computer Data Processing

After suitable filtering (elimination of 50 cycle interference), responses were averaged, and spatiotemporal (equipotential) maps were plotted (Remond, 1961).  Each map is the average of seventy to ninety responses, and the time reference (trigger) corresponds to contact closing of the index operated microswitches.

### Statistical Analysis

The data between subjects exhibit large standard deviation interindividual variabilities which are greater than those due to differences between situations; in this case, a good practice is to calculate differences between situations for each subject and then to test whether the mean of these differences is statistically different from zero or not.  The data obtained here exhibit Gaussian distributions, and samples are independent; it is, therefore, legitimate to use Student's "T" for comparisons.  Data were also analyzed with a nonparametric sign test.

## RESULTS

### Self-Paced Movements

In agreement with the literature, all subjects exhibited a large negativity before the movement and a positive wave after the movement.  However, interindividual differences between spatiotemporal characteristics were important and appeared largest when compared to intersituation (right or left index flexion) differences. Typical spatiotemporal maps of these results are shown in Fig. 1.

The premotion negativity (readiness potential or "RP") started at a mean latency of 200 msec before the motor act, slowly rising towards a peak culminating approximately 30 msec after the motor act.  This peak, called motor potential (MP), appeared significantly contralateral to the movement ($t = 3.45$, $p < .02$) with a Student's test, and $p < .05$ with a sign test; see Table I and Fig. 2).

For six subjects out of seven, the amplitude of the MP was larger during the left-hand movement; this result is not, however,

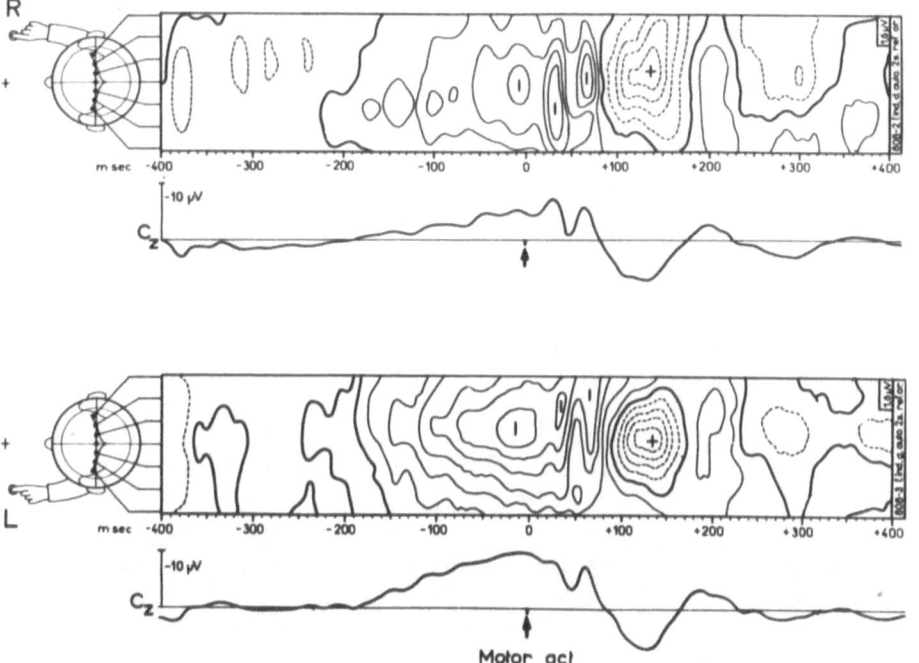

Fig. 1.   Spatiotemporal maps during a self-paced right (R) and left
(L) index flexion.   Underlying chronogram represents activity at
the vertex electrode.   Average responses of eighty movements, at a
rate of approximately 2 sec, triggered on the mechanogram.   1.6 µV
potential difference on all maps between two successive isopotential
lines; linked earlobe references; + and - signs indicate peaks or
dips of potential.

statistically very significant (t = 1.99, p < .10 with a Student's
test).

The MP was sometimes preceded by a relative positivity (subjects ER, BG, CR) occurring just during the motor act and called
premotion positivity (PMP).   However, this event was not reliable
enough to be taken into account in the present analysis.

The positive component that followed movement completion,
called the "reafferent potential", appeared bilaterally distributed,
except for subject RR for whom it peaked contralaterally to the
movement.   Its mean latency was 140 msec after the motor act with
very small variability.

Table I. Experimental data for right (R) and left (L) index self-paced flexions: Topography and amplitude of MPs for the seven subjects. Mean and SP values are plotted in Fig. 3, whereas mean differences are used for statistical analysis. Topography is referred to Cz counted positive towards the right hemisphere and negative towards the left.

|      | MP topography (cm) | | | MP Amplitude (µV) | | |
|------|------|------|------|------|------|------|
|      | R    | L    | R-L  | R    | L    | R-L  |
| ER   | -4   | +6   | -10  | -7.8 | -10.0 | +2.2 |
| BG   | -1.5 | +2   | -3.5 | -4.0 | -7.0 | +3.0 |
| GG   | -1   | 0    | -1   | -4.3 | -4.3 | 0    |
| CR   | -1   | +4.5 | -5.5 | -3.8 | -8.0 | +4.2 |
| AA   | -3   | +5.5 | -8.5 | -6.4 | -10.0 | +3.6 |
| RR   | -1   | +4   | -5   | -4.9 | -2.1 | -2.8 |
| JMA  | 0    | 0    | 0    | -1.8 | -4.5 | +2.7 |
| Mean | -1.6 | +3.1 | -4.78 | -4.7 | -6.6 | +1.84 |
| S.D. | 1.4  | 2.5  | 3.66 | 1.9  | 3.0  | 2.44 |

## Choice Reaction Time Task

During this task a few errors (response given with the wrong hand) occurred (one out of eighty responses, approximately). These were not taken into consideration and were deleted from the average.

In all possible situations, 1R, rL, rR, 1L, i.e., irrespective of the stimulus color and location, all subjects produced a large positive wave between the stimulus and the response with a mean latency of approximately 370 msec (Fig. 3).

These P300 waves were sometimes followed by a small relative negativity. This event exhibited the same latency as the motor potential of the corresponding self-paced motor potential for a given subject.

When detectable, this negativity was followed by a further positive event that peaked on the vertex (subjects ER, BG) or appeared contralateral to the movement (subjects AA, RR) with a mean latency of about 140 msec after the motor act. The topography and latency of this component was similar to those of the reafferent potentials observed during the self-paced movement.

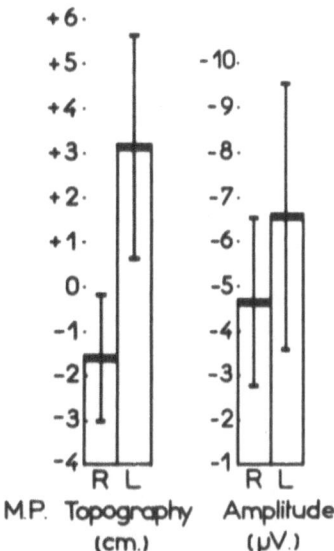

Fig. 2.   Average topography and amplitude of MPs for the seven
subjects.   Topography is counted positively towards the right hemisphere and negatively towards the left with respect to Cz.   MP
maxima are contralateral to the movement, and their absolute amplitude is larger for a left index flexion.   Standard deviation is
across the seven subjects.


The P300 waves reached their maximum amplitude later in the
contralateral than in the ipsilateral situation (Table II and Fig.
4).   This was observed in all subjects, the mean increase in latency
being equal to 34 msec.   This difference is statistically significant
(p < .05 with sign test; t = 5.44, p < .005 with Student's test).
Conversely, there was no marked difference in the latency of P300
with respect to the responding hand.

This difference in the latency of the P300 wave was accompanied
by a similar difference (28 msec) in the reaction time between the
contralateral and ipsilateral situations which was also observed in
all seven subjects (p < .05 with sign test; T = 5.27  p < .005 with
Student's test).   These results are in agreement with purely behavioral experiments (Craft and Simon, 1970).   The responding hand
had no effect on the RT either.

Together with this effect on RT and latency of the P300 waves,
the amplitude of the P300s was also modified; they appeared larger
(mean amplitude equal to 10.9 μV with respect to the baseline) in
the contralateral situation than in the ipsilateral situation (mean

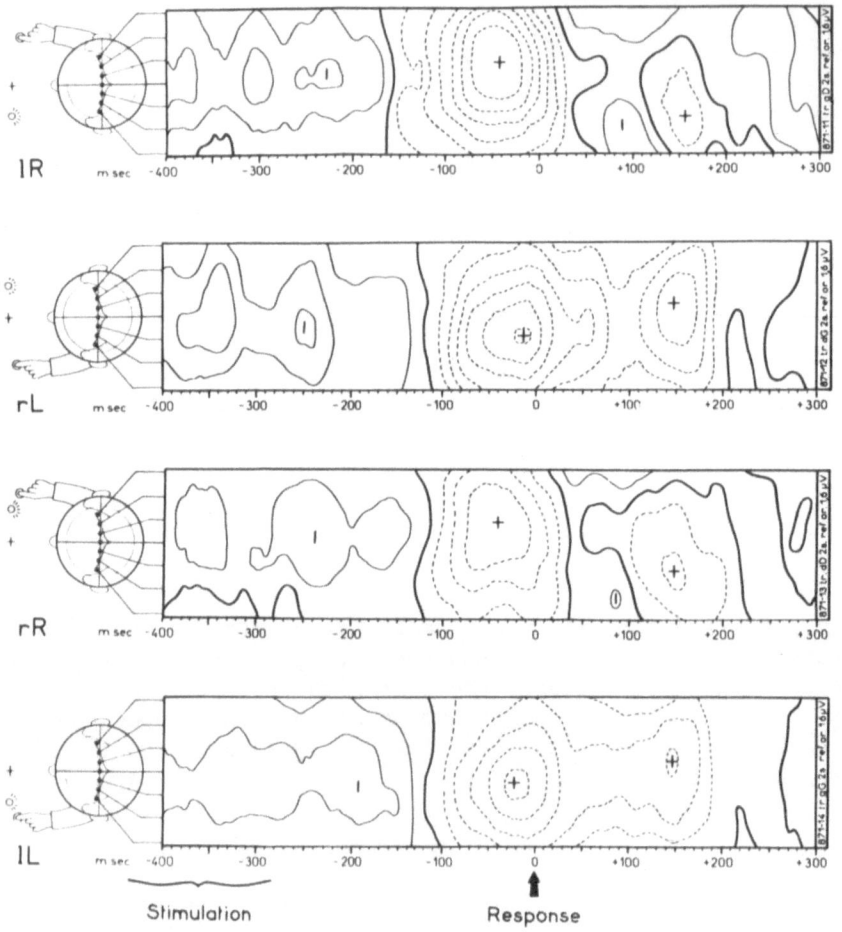

Fig. 3.   Spatiotemporal maps during bilateral choice RT task.
Stimulus appearing regularly every 2 sec, either in the right (r)
or in the left (l) visual half-field, randomly and requiring either
a right (R) or left (L) index flexion.  Average responses to eighty
movements triggered on the mechanogram; linked earlobe reference.

amplitude = 8.5 µV).  This difference was also observed in all seven
subjects (p < .05 with sign test; t = 8.77, p < .001 with Student's
test).

The responding hand had no marked effect on the absolute amplitude of the P300, but it modified the topographical distribution of
the P300 wave which culminated slightly on the right (1.7 cm) of the
vertex for a right hand movement and on the left (1.8 cm) for a left
hand movement.  These differences are significant (p < .05 with sign
test; t = 4.54, p < .005 with Student's test).

Table II: RT, and latency, topography and amplitude of P300 peaks for the seven subjects in the four possible situations during the choice reaction time task.

| | Reaction Time (msec.) | | | | | P300 Latency (msec.) | | | | | P300 Topography (cm.) | | | | | P300 Amplitude (µV) | | | | |
|---|---|---|---|---|---|---|---|---|---|---|---|---|---|---|---|---|---|---|---|---|
| | 1R | rL | rR | 1L | (1R+rL)/2 -(rR+1L)/2 Contra-Ipsi | 1R | rL | rR | 1L | (1R+rL)/2 -(rR+1L)/2 Contra-Ipsi | 1R | rL | rR | 1L | (1R+rR)/2 -(rL+1L)/2 Right-Left | 1R | rL | rR | 1L | (1R+rL)/2 -(rR+1L)/2 Contra-Ipsi |
| ER | 468 | 488 | 426 | 447 | +41.6 | 406 | 390 | 370 | 349 | +19.3 | 1 | -1 | 0 | 0 | +1 | 9 | 9.2 | 6.2 | 6 | +3 |
| BG | 405 | 432 | 384 | 400 | +26.5 | 311 | 362 | 294 | 330 | +12.2 | 2 | -1 | 2 | 0 | +2.5 | 10 | 12.5 | 6.5 | 10.5 | +3 |
| GG | 381 | 394 | 363 | 366 | +23.1 | 369 | 386 | 351 | 354 | +12.0 | 0 | -1 | 0 | -1 | +1 | 18 | 15.6 | 13.2 | 14 | +3.2 |
| CR | 414 | 374 | 398 | 360 | +14.7 | 346 | 394 | 314 | 300 | +31.3 | 5 | 0 | 5.5 | -1 | +5.7 | 12.4 | 14.8 | 10.4 | 12.4 | +2.2 |
| AA | 422 | 391 | 400 | 396 | +8.3 | 378 | 379 | 356 | 372 | +7.1 | 3 | -3 | 3.5 | -2 | +5.7 | 10.8 | 9.8 | 5.8 | 8.4 | +3.2 |
| RR | 535 | 500 | 479 | 488 | +33.7 | 485 | 446 | 419 | 440 | +13.3 | 1 | -4 | 1 | -3 | +4.5 | 6.6 | 6 | 6.6 | 3.7 | +1.6 |
| JMA | 453 | 455 | 407 | 408 | +47.0 | 405 | 399 | 343 | 364 | +24.5 | 0 | -4 | 1.5 | -5 | +5.2 | 10 | 8 | 7.6 | 8.6 | +1.4 |
| Mean | 440 | 433 | 408 | 409 | +27.8 | 386 | 394 | 350 | 358 | +17.2 | 1,57 | -1,86 | 1,93 | -1,71 | +3.68 | 10,97 | 10,84 | 8,04 | 9,08 | +2.52 |
| S.D. | 51 | 49 | 37 | 45 | +14.0 | 55 | 26 | 40 | 43 | +8.3 | 1,90 | 1,77 | 1,99 | 1,80 | +2.14 | 3,57 | 3,57 | 2,74 | 3,57 | +0.76 |

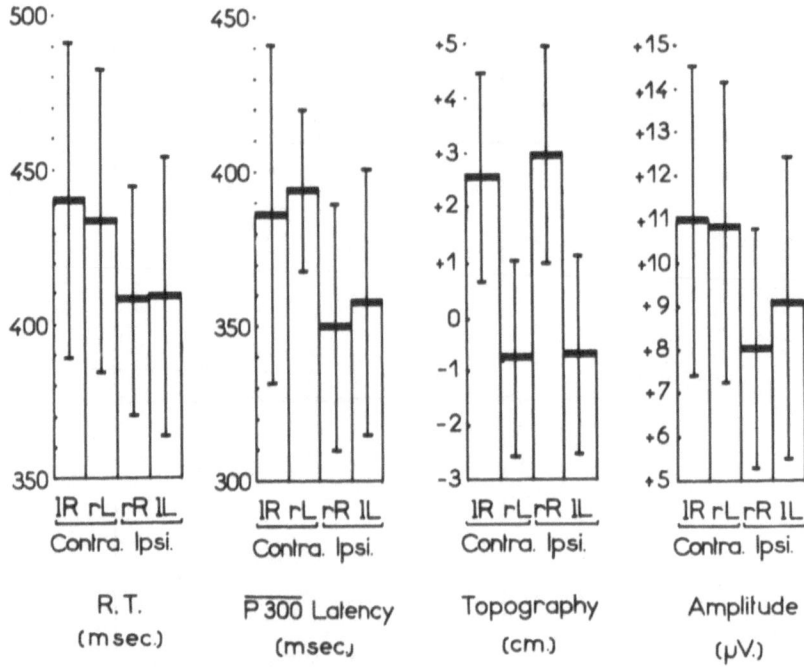

Fig. 4. Average RT, and latency, topography and amplitude of P300
peaks for the seven subjects. The topography of the P300s is ipsilateral to the responding hand. RT is longer in contralateral
situations, together with the latency of P300 peaks. In the contralateral situations P300 amplitudes are larger.


DISCUSSION

    In the RT situation subjects have to act in response to the
color of the stimulus; here the movement programming is subsequent
to a decision which requires a certain amount of information processing.

    The electrical patterns observed on the scalp in this situation
differ from the self-paced task mainly in that they all exhibit
a large positive wave (P300) before the response. This P300 component seems to appear superimposed on the emerging negative readiness potential. In a few cases a slight negativity can be observed
following the P300, and at the same latency, that of the self-paced
motor potential. This could explain why the P300 topography appears
to be dependent on the responding hand. Indeed, if the MP (negative)
or the last part of the RP (also negative) does superimpose on the
P300, partial cancellation would occur on the potentials recorded on

the hemisphere contralateral to the responding hand, thus making
the P300 predominate on the ipsilateral hemisphere.

The P300s are much smaller, or even absent, with stimulus alone
when no task is required (this well known fact has been verified in
the present experiment for two subjects).  Nor are these waves
present during the self-paced task.  Consequently they appear to
reflect a decision-making process; if the P300 is accepted as being
such an index of relevant response evaluation, then the results
obtained in the present experiment can be explained as follows: in
the contralateral situation longer RTs, accompanied with a longer
P300 latency indicate (a) that the response takes more time for the
subject to evaluate and (b) that the response is dependent on the
P300.

Moreover, the fact that P300 amplitude is larger in the contralateral than the ipsilateral situation is an additional argument in
favor of the above mentioned significance of the P300 index.

The logical relationship from cause to effect of this succession
of events could be traced in this way:  contralateral stimulus-
response evaluation takes a longer time, this leads to a longer
latency for the P300 and this,  in turn, increases the RT. Why
evaluation itself takes a longer time remains to be explained, but
two hypotheses can be formulated:

(1) Afferent information takes a longer time to reach the contralateral hemisphere (approximately 10 msec), but this fact alone
cannot be responsible for the long difference observed concerning
the P300 increase in latency (34 msec) as well as the RT increase
(28 msec).

(2) Innate and learned body responses are better organized to be
carried out by the limbs ipsilateral to the stimulation (Simon,
1969); this would seem to be a logical process as a defense reflex
or as a simple energy saving process.


CONCLUSION

A negative shift occurred prior to the self-paced movement
becoming contralateral towards the end, and a positive shift followed
the movement.

During the bilateral choice RT task the P300 culminated on the
hemisphere ipsilateral to the stimulation; this could be the result
of partial cancellation of the P300 and the negative MP on the
hemisphere contralateral to the movement.

The contralateral situation appeared to have two significant

effects on the P300s: their latency was increased, as was the mean
RT; their amplitude was also increased compared to that obtained
in the ipsilateral situation.  This can be explained by assuming
that the P300 is an index of decision-making.  A contralateral
stimulus-response task, which is more difficult to evaluate (having
larger P300s), takes more time for the decision to be accomplished
(having delayed P300s) which, in turn, leads to a longer RT.

SUMMARY

This study was undertaken in order to investigate the specificity of the electrical events observed on the scalp during a choice
reaction time task, particularly when the response is contralateral
or ipsilateral to the stimulation.

Seven right-handed subjects were requested to press a switch
as fast as possible with their right index finger in response to
a green light and with their left index finger in response to a
red light.  These stimuli appeared at random, within 2 sec intervals
and at a $10^{\circ}$ angle, either on the right or the left of a fixation
point.

For the seven subjects in these four situations, a large positive potential (P300) appeared, peaking approximately 50 msec before
the response.  This peak was shifted towards the right hemisphere
before a right hand response and vice-versa.  This result could be
related to the fact that the ends of the readiness potential and
the motor potential were contralateral to the movement, thus partially cancelling the P300 contralaterally to the response.

The latency of this P300 was longer in the contralateral situation, as was the RT; also the amplitude of the P300 was larger in
this case with respect to the ipsilateral situation.  Consequently
the P300 latency and amplitude appear as electrophysiological
indexes of the difference in information processing required when
the response is or is not to be given on the same side as the stimulus.

REFERENCES

Cooper, R., McCallum, W.C., Newton, P., Papakostopoulos, D., Pocock,
    P.V. and Warren, W.J.  Cortical potential associated with the
    detection of visual events.  Science, 1977, 196, 74-77.

Courchesne, E., Hillyard, S.A. and Galambos, R.  Stimulus novelty,
    task relevance and the visual evoked potential in man.
    Electroenceph. Clin. Neurophysiol., 1975, 39, 131-144.

Craft, J.L. and Simon, J.R.  Processing symbolic information from a visual display: Interference from an irrelevant directional cue.  J, Exp. Psychol., 1970, 83, 415-420.

Deecke, L., Scheid, P. and Kornhuber, H.H.  Distribution of readiness potential, premotion positivity and motor potential of the human cerebral cortex preceding voluntary finger movements.  Exp. Brain Res., 1969, 7, 158-168.

Demaire, C. and Coquery, J.M.  Effects of selective attention on the late components of evoked potentials in man.  Electroenceph. Clin. Neurophysiol., 1977, 42, 702-704.

Gerbrandt, L.K., Goff, W.R. and Smith D.B.D.  Distribution of the human average movement potential.  Electroenceph. Clin. Neurophysiol., 1973, 34, 461-474.

Gilden, L., Vaughan, H.G. and Costa, L.D.  Summated human electroencephalographic potentials associated with voluntary movements.  Electroenceph. Clin. Neurophysiol., 1966, 20, 433-438.

Klinke, R., Fruhstorfer, H. and Finkenzeller, R.  Evoked responses as a function of external and stored information.  Electroenceph. Clin. Neurophysiol., 1968, 29, 119-122.

Kornhuber, H.H. and Deecke, L.  Hirnpotentialanderungen bei Willkurbewegungen und passiven Bewegungen des Menschen: Bereitschaftpotential und reafferente Potentiale.  Pflugers Arch. Ges. Physiol., 1965, 284, 1-17.

Kutas, M. and Donchin, E.  The effects of handedness, or responding hand and of response force on the contralateral dominance of the readiness potential.  In J. Desmedt (Ed.), Attention, Voluntary Contraction and Event Related Cerebral Potentials, Karger: Basel, 1977.

Remond, A.  Integrated and topographical analysis of the EEG.  Electroenceph. Clin. Neurophysiol., Suppl. 20, Computer techniques in EEG analysis., 1961b, 64-67.

Renault, B. and Lesevre, N.  Topographical study of the emitted potential obtained after the omission of an expected visual stimulus.  In D.A. Otto (Ed.), Multidisciplinary Perspectives in Event Related Brain Potential Research, U.S. Government Printing Office, in press.

Renault, B., Ragot, R., Furet, J. and Lesevre, N.  Etude des relations entre le potentiel emis et les mecanismes de preparation perceptivo-motrice.  In J. Requin (Ed.), Anticipation et Processus Psychologiques, CNRS, in press.

Simon, J.R.   Reactions toward the source of stimulation., J, Exp.
    Psychol., 1969, 81, 174-176.

Simson, R., Vaughan, H.G. and Ritter, W.   The scalp topography of
    potentials associated with missing visual or auditory stimuli.
    Electroenceph. Clin. Neurophysiol., 1976, 40, 33-42.

Squires, K.C., Donchin, E., Herning, R.I. and McCarthy, G.   The
    influence of task relevance and stimulus probability on event
    related potential components.   Electroenceph. Clin. Neuro-
    physiol., 1977, 42, 1-14.

Sutton, S., Braren, M. and Zubin, J.   Evoked potential correlates
    of stimulus uncertainty.   Science, 1965, 150, 1187-1188.

Sutton, S., Tueting, P., Zubin, J. and John, E.R.   Information
    delivery and the sensory evoked potential.   Science, 1967,
    155, 1436-1439.

Syndulko, K. and Lindsley, D.B.   Motor and sensory determinants of
    cortical slow potential shifts in man.   In J. Desmedt (Ed.),
    Attention, Voluntary Contraction and Event Related Cerebral
    Potentials, Karger: Basel, 1977.

Van Voorhis, S. and Hillyard, S.A.   Visual evoked potentials and
    selective attention to points in space.   Perception and Psycho-
    physics, 1977, 22, 54-62.

Vaughan, H.G., Costa, L.D. and Ritter, W.   Topography of the human
    motor potential.   Electroenceph. Clin. Neurophysiol., 1968,
    25, 1-10.

Weinberg, H., Walter, H.G. and Crow, H.J.   Intracerebral events in
    humans related to real and imaginery stimuli.   Electroenceph.
    Clin. Neurophysiol., 1970, 29, 1-9.

Zazzo, R.   Manuel pour l'examen psychologique de l'enfant.   Dela-
    chaux et Niestle, 1960.

A TRIAL BY TRIAL STUDY OF THE VISUAL OMISSION RESPONSE IN REACTION

TIME SITUATIONS

B. Renault and N. Lesevre

Electrophysiology and Applied Neurophysiology Laboratory

Hopital de La Salpetriere - 75634 Paris Cedex 13

## INTRODUCTION

The present work was undertaken in order to study the mechanisms underlying the various stages of perceptive and perceptivo-motor processes by analyzing the characteristics (latency, amplitude and topographical distribution) of its electrophysiological correlates.

The brain response to a relevant stimulus which delivers information the subject has to process in order to perform a task (in particular, a motor task) is quite a complex response made up of stimulus and motor related components (occurring usually during the first 200 msec), followed by slow components which are considered to be chiefly related to cognitive processes. These slow components include, in particular, the so-called P300 wave which is often preceded by a negative component, N200. N200 is difficult to analyze since it occurs (at least in the case of visual stimuli) at the same time as the P200 visual component. Indeed, this P200 component usually has so large an amplitude and so wide a topographical distribution on the scalp that not only does it hide N200 but since the scalp acts as a spatial averager, it sometimes also mingles with P300.

For the above reasons we have used in this study the "missing stimulus" paradigm requiring a motor response from the subject whenever the stimulus is omitted. This experimental situation is particularly suitable for studying the preparatory stage of perception; moreover, with such a paradigm the electrical correlates of perceptivo-motor processes are not distorted by the stimulus-related potentials.

317

In a previous work dealing with the same missing stimulus paradigm in which either a motor task or a counting task was required of the subject in response to each missing stimulus (Renault et al., in press), two types of responses to omission were differentiated on the basis of spatio-temporal criteria: a "vertex type", in which both components (the negative and the positive) peaked at the vertex, and a parietal one. These topographical characteristics were related to the nature of the task required from the subject. The parietal type of omission response was significantly more frequent, and the parietal activity was of higher amplitude during the counting task. The vertex type was more frequently observed during the motor task. On the other hand, during the motor tasks, contrary to the positive waves which often appeared during or just after the motor act, the negative component always occurred before the motor act. The latency of the negative component was strongly correlated with the reaction time (RT). This last result suggested that the negative components could reflect a preparatory stage of decision depending upon sensorimotor processing, whereas the positive waves might be related more to the execution of the task. These assumptions were based on the high correlation observed between the latency of each component of the omission response and the reaction time (RT). In fact, such a high correlation between these two phenomena (omitted response and reaction time) is not necessarily the sign of causal relationships since they could both depend upon a third internal event, e.g., the subject's estimation of the moment the omission should have occurred.

Therefore, after having designed an experiment enabling evaluation of the accuracy of this "time estimation" of the subject, the present work was undertaken in order to shed some light on the nature of the internal events which determine response. This was achieved by analyzing the relationships between the "time estimation of the omission" and the various characteristics of the scalp recorded omission response, as well as those of the performance of the required task.

METHODOLOGY

Experimental Design

Seven normal adults (six right-handed and one left-handed) served as subjects for this study. The responses to omitted stimuli were obtained in situations during which 450 visual stimuli (appearance, in the center of a screen, of a $20^\circ$ checkerboard for 22 msec) were delivered at a rate of one per second. Ten percent of the stimuli were randomly omitted. In order to minimize eye movements, subjects were asked to fixate the center of the screen.

Two different omission situations were tested. In the first situation subjects were asked to beat the rhythm (with the second finger of their preferred hand) at the same frequency as that of the visual stimuli; whenever the visual stimulus was missing they were required to give, as quickly as possible, an additional motor response (RT) with the same finger. The "beaten rhythm" was considered as an index of the subject's time estimation of the moment the stimulus should have occurred; its latency with respect to this moment was taken as a measure of the subject's accuracy of time estimation (ATE). In order to estimate the modifications introduced by the "beaten rhythm", a second situation was used in which subjects were only asked to give, as quickly as possible, a motor response after each omission. Both movements (beaten rhythm and RT movements) consisted of a finger displacement towards a photoelectric cell and thus required very little strength. This kind of movement was chosen in order to minimize scalp recorded potentials related to the motor act (Kutas and Donchin, 1977).

In addition, in order to study motor related potentials in absence of all other event related potentials, a third situation was recorded during which the subject was asked to perform self-paced finger displacements at approximately the same rate of one per second with any visual stimuli occurring.


Electrophysiological Recordings

Recordings were made with a montage of eight equally spaced electrodes (10% of the nasion-inion distance apart) extending from inion to Fz and thus including Oz, Pz and Ca. Electrodes were referred to linked ears. The time constant was 1.5 sec with an upper bandpass limit of 220 Hz. Horizontal and vertical electro-oculograms were recorded and every response occurring during or after an eye movement was suppressed from the analyzed data.

On-line analog-to-digital conversion was performed at a 500/ sec sampling rate. The data were displayed off-line by computer (BGE Gamma M40) in form of chronograms and spatio-temporal maps (Remond, 1961). Spatio-temporal maps were obtained for each subject from single trial data following each missing stimulus as well as from averaged data. In this case for each subject the averaging process was triggered successively by the moment of occurrence, by that of the "beaten rhythm" and that of the motor response (RT) to the missing stimulus. Besides, all the single trial omission responses (45 per subject in each situation) were averaged across subjects, the time trigger for this averaging process being one of the peaks of the response.

Recognition Procedure in the Trial by Trial Study

For each subject, the missing stimulus response obtained from average spatio-temporal maps was utilized as a template in order to visually identify each component of each single trial response to omission. The single trial peaks were visually identified on each map prior to knowing the time of occurrence of each motor act (beaten rhythm and reaction time response). This visual analysis was performed within a time window extending from one second before an omission to one second after. The only responses taken into account were those for which the signal-to-noise ratio made it possible to measure the values of latency, amplitude and topography for each component.

RESULTS

Organization of the Single Trial Omission Responses

As seen on the average single trial maps obtained across subjects, in both situations (with and without the presence of a "beaten rhythm") the response to the missing stimulus was made up of a negative component beginning in the parieto-occipital region (Na) which peaked later towards the vertex (Nb) followed by two positive components, the first one peaking at the vertex (Pa) and the second one (Pb) peaking in the parieto-occipital region (Fig. 1). It must be noted that during both situations (with and without the beaten rhythm) the parieto-occipital activity began around the moment of the omission and lasted for 600 msec, whereas the central activity (Nb and Pa) began approximately 200 msec after the omission and stayed on for 250 msec (this vertex activity disappeared about 450 msec after the omission). A slow late negative wave was also seen peaking posterior to the central area. It followed in time the vertex positivity and ended approximately at the onset of the next visual stimulus.

In fact, such an organization of the omission response, including Na, Nb, Pa and Pb, was found in 76% of all single trial responses. The remaining 24% of responses could be distributed into three groups: the first one was composed of only one negative wave followed by one positive wave, both peaking at the vertex (13% of the cases); the second one was made up of two components both peaking in the parieto-occipital region (6%); the remaining 5% were made up of omission responses in which the peaks of the two negative waves (Na and Nb) were clearly differentiated, the first one peaking in the parieto-occipital region, the second one on the vertex, both of them followed by a positive wave peaking in the same region.

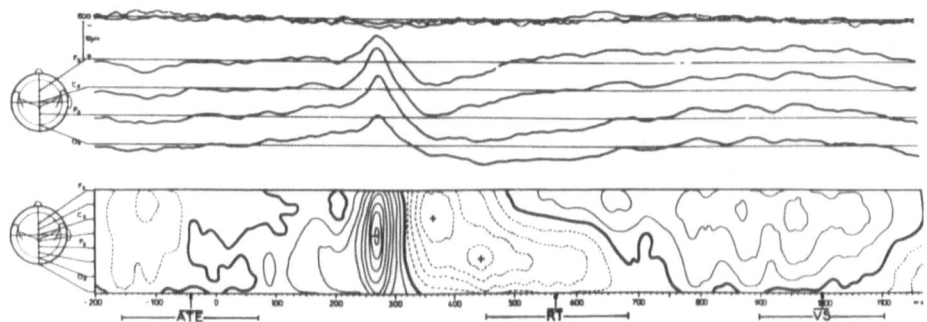

Fig. 1.   Average of 165 single trial omission responses (across
subjects) triggered by the negative vertex peak.   Above, the data
obtained from four derivations of the montage are represented in
the form of chronograms.   Average horizontal (broken line) and
vertical (plain line) eye movements are superimposed in the upper
traces.   Below, the spatiotemporal map obtained from the whole
montage.   Amplitude is plotted in the form of isopotential lines as
a function of time (in abscissa) and space (electrode location in
ordinate); the values between two successive electrodes are obtained by interpolation.   From one isopotential line to the next the
difference of potential is equal to 1.6 µV.   Plain thick lines
indicate potential 0; plain thin lines indicate negative potentials,
broken lines positive potentials.   The omission response extends
from 50 to 650 msec; the exact location of the peaks is indicated
by the sign - or + according to their polarity.   The mean and standard deviation values of RTs, ATEs and moments of occurrence of the
next visual stimuli (VS) are indicated in the abscissa.

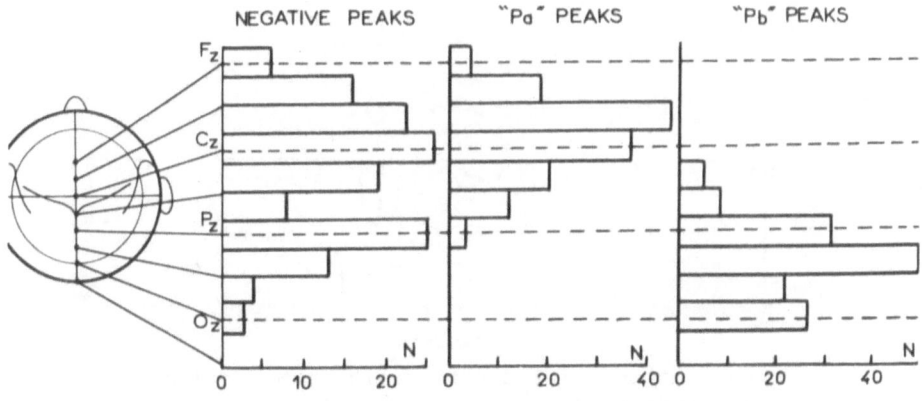

Fig. 2.   Histograms of the peaks' locations obtained from the most
typical type of omission response (76% of the cases, see text).

This spatio-temporal organization - in particular that illustrated by the single trial responses made up of four well differentiated peaks - suggests that two cortical regions play a role in
the genesis of both the negative and positive components of the
omission response: the parieto-occipital area for the negative Na
and positive Pb waves, and the central area for the negative Nb and
positive Pa waves.  This assumption is supported by the topographical analysis of the most typical response to omission which has been
described above (76% of the single trial responses, Fig. 1).  Indeed
as shown by the peak location histograms of their components (Fig. 2),
the distribution of the positive components Pa and Pb differed quite
significantly (t = 30, p < .0001); moreover the peak location histogram of the negative component appeared as bimodal, thus corroborating the existence of two active regions - a parietal and a central
one - which might show the maximum of their activity either simultaneously or successively.


### Average Scalp Potentials Related to the Motor Act

The spatiotemporal organization of the average potentials
related to self-paced movement (third situation) was quite different from that of the omission response (Fig. 3).  It mainly consisted of two successive waves, a negative one appearing before the
movement (readiness potential) followed by a postmotor wave.  Both
these motor related components peaked more anteriorly than did the
omission response in the fronto-central region.  As it could be
expected on account of the nature of the required movements, their
amplitudes were quite small (less than 3 μV) compared to the amplitudes of the components of the omission response which all had a
mean value of approximately 20 μV (Table I).

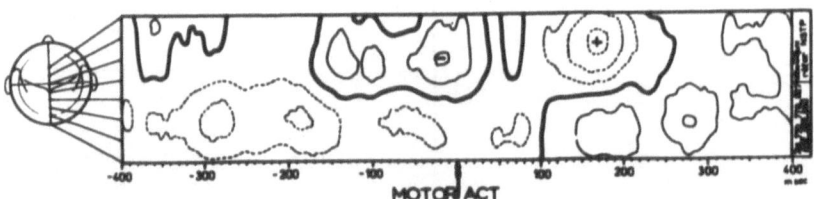

MOTOR ACT

Fig. 3.  Averaged motor related potentials obtained during the self-
paced movement situation (seven subjects, eighty motor acts per subject).  On the time scale, 0 indicates the occurrence of the acto-
gram which triggered the average process.  Between two successive
isopotential lines the difference of potential is equal to .8 μV.

Table 1.  Characteristics of the peaks of the omission response
(average of each trial across subjects).  ATE and latencies (L) are
measured in msec with respect to the instant of the omission; topographies (T) are measured in % of the nasion-inion distance with
respect to the inion; amplitudes (A) are measured in μV with respect
to the baseline.

| | | Negative Peak | | | Pa "Vertex" | | | Pb "Parietal" | | | RT | ATE | N |
|---|---|---|---|---|---|---|---|---|---|---|---|---|---|---|
| | | Lmsec | AμV | T% | Lmsec | AμV | T% | Lmsec | AμV | T% | msec | msec | |
| Situation 1 | x̄ | 265 | 19,5 | 42 | 383 | 22 | 55 | 508 | 20 | 22 | 568 | -42 | 165 |
| | s.d. | 101 | 8,4 | 14 | 104 | 9,6 | 10 | 114 | 9,7 | 8,3 | 113 | 110 | |
| Situation 2 | x̄ | 274 | 21 | 39 | 386 | 21 | 52 | 507 | 18 | 23 | 503 | / | 140 |
| | s.d. | 115 | 10 | 11 | 107 | 8,6 | 8,4 | 106 | 7,3 | 10 | 127 | | |

## Time Relations Between Omission Responses, "Beaten Rhythms" and RTs

For each situation (with and without beaten rhythm) Table I
depicts the mean characteristics (obtained across subjects) of the
single trial omission responses, RTs and ATEs.  It must be noted
that the latencies of the components of the omission response did
not significantly vary across the two situations (with and without
beaten rhythm), whereas RTs were significantly longer in the beaten
rhythm situation (t = 4.54, p < .001).  As the duration of the
movement is approximately 60 msec, this RT lengthening must be due
to a mechanical inertia phenomenon since the beaten rhythm and the
motor act are performed by the same finger.

As seen in Table II, all components of the omission response
always occurred after the beaten rhythm.  Concerning the RT response, the negative components always occurred before the motor
reaction time response, whereas Pa could peak just after the motor
act in some cases (10%), and Pb either just before or a long time
after this motor act.  The large range of variation of the RTs with
respect to the latency of the peaks of the omission response must
be noticed (Table II).

However, in both missing stimuli situations the latencies of
the different waves of the omission response were strongly and
positively correlated with the RTs, whereas their correlations with
ATEs were much lower (Fig. 4).  Moreover, ATEs and RTs were weakly
correlated (r = .35).  Thus the variability of ATEs cannot explain
either the variability of the latencies of the omission response
or that of the RTs, and consequently those two latter variables
(RTs and ATEs) do not depend on each other.

This absence of correlation between ATE and RT prompted us

Table II.  Time relations between peaks of the omission response, RTs and ATEs.

| | | SITUATION 1 | | | SITUATION 2 | | |
|---|---|---|---|---|---|---|---|
| | | Negative Peak | Pa "Vertex" | Pb "Parietal" | Negative Peak | Pa "Vertex" | Pb "Parietal |
| Time occurrence | min. max | -592 ; -152 | -468 ; 20 | -320 ; 124 | -580 ; -102 | -440 ; 56 | -318 ; 172 |
| / RT | $\bar{x}$ | -304 | -186 | -60 | -229 | -116 | 4 |
| (msec) | s.d. | 98 | 96 | 99 | 81 | 79 | 87 |
| Time occurrence | min. max | 68 ; 714 | 168 ; 838 | 260 ; 968 | | | |
| / ATE | $\bar{x}$ | 307 | 425 | 550 | | | |
| (msec) | s.d. | 130 | 133 | 143 | | | |
| Peak latency and RT correlation | | .62 | .61 | .56 | .66 | .64 | .59 |
| Peak latency and ATE correlation | | .23 | .19 | .14 | | | |

minus (-) indicates that the peak occurs before the RT.

to process our data in the following way in order to better understand the time relationships between these various events:  Across
subjects all single trial reaction times were divided into quartiles
as a function of their duration, and the corresponding single trial
omission responses were then averaged together as a function of
the RT quartiles (Fig. 5).  A significant relation was then found
between the duration of RTs and that of the negative parietal wave.
The longer the RT, the longer this wave lasted.  The onset of this
parietal wave was not correlated to the RT, nor was the duration
of the other components.  In addition, the increase in duration of
the parietal negative component of these average omission responses
was less important than that of the corresponding RT quartile
(Fig. 5).

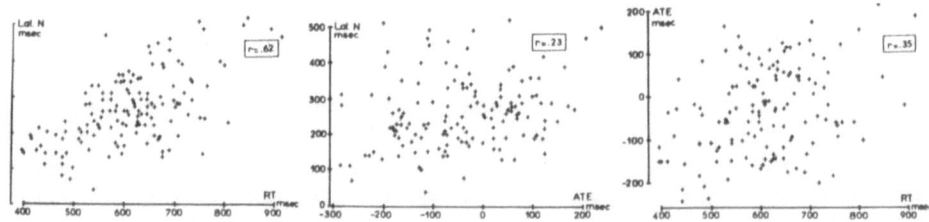

Fig. 4.  Latencies of the negative peak of the omission response
plotted against RTs (on the left) and against ATEs (in the middle);
ATEs against RTs are plotted on the right.  The corresponding
coefficients of correlation are noted in a cartridge.

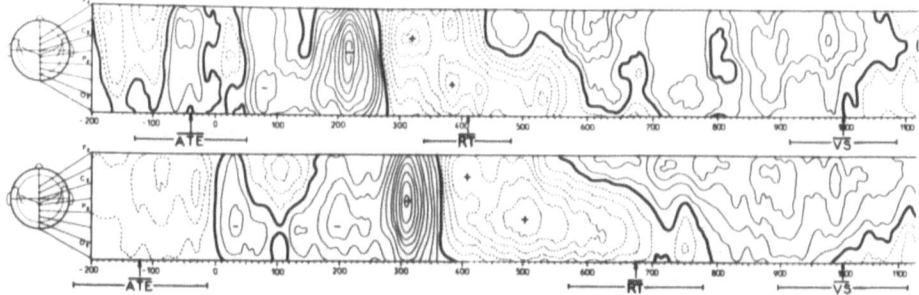

Fig. 5.  Averaged spatio-temporal maps (across subjects) triggered
by the negative peak of the omission response for the first RT
quartile (above) and the fourth RT quartile (below).  Between two
successive isopotential lines the difference of potential is equal
to 1.6 μV.


DISCUSSION


Hypothetical Underlying Generators

The spatiotemporal organization of the omission response
analyzed in the present study confirms the existence of two active
cortical regions playing a role in the genesis of this potential:
the parieto-occipital area and the central one, the former being
active for a longer time than the latter.  Since the scalp acts as
a spatial averager, the activities from both generators (the
parietal and the central one) most of the time add up, yielding
a complex response which exhibits an apparent flowing of activity
going from the parietal towards the central area for the negative
components and from the central to the parieto-occipital region
for the positive components.

These results confirm our previous findings concerning this
omission response (Renault and Lesevre, in press; Renault et al.,
in press) as well as the existence of the two types of P300 (a
central Pa and a parietal Pb) first reported by Squires et al.
(1975).  Moreover, they confirm the existence of negative waves
preceding each P300, a vertex one (reported by Courchesne et al.,
1976; Squires et al., 1977) and a long duration parietal one described by Simson et al.(1976).

This omission response was followed by a negative frontal
potential of long duration (Figs. 1 and 5) which spread all over
the scalp and lasted until the occurrence of the next visual
stimulus.  This late negative potential cannot be due to the

readiness potential related to the motor act (illustrated in Fig.
3) since its spatio-temporal organization is quite different and
its amplitude much higher, and also because it still goes on a long
time after the performance of the motor act.  Squires et al.(1975)
were the first to report the existence of a slow wave (S.W.) which
was described as being negative at Fz, near zero at Cz and positive
at Pz; our spatiotemporal data (Figs. 1 and 5) suggest that, in
fact, the negative Fz and positive Pz must probably represent two
distinct phenomena, one (positive) ending in the parieto-occipital
region when the other one (negative) is starting in the frontal
region.  The fact that this negative frontal activity lasts until
the onset of the next expected visual stimulus is in favor of its
probably being a CNV.


Omission Response and Timing of Perceptivo-Motor Processes

     Concerning the time relationships between the various electro-
physiological and behavioral events analyzed in the present study,
the following results have emerged:

     a)  The latency of each component of the omission response,
i.e., of the parietal as well as the vertex peaks, was positively
correlated with the RT but appeared to be independent of the subject's estimation of the moment the omission should occur, evaluated by the beaten rhythm.  These findings are consistent with
the assumption that all peaks of the omission response reflect
decision-making, but not with the hypothesis that the time estimation of the moment the stimulus should appear represented the
internal time trigger on which depends the spatiotemporal organization of the omission response.

     b)  The increase of the latencies of all peaks of the omission
response, which was observed when RTs increased, was, in fact, due
to an increase of the duration of the first parietal wave and not
to a delayed time estimation of the moment the stimulus should
have occurred.  This finding suggests that this parietal negative
wave could reflect some stimulus evaluation process.  The longer
this process would last, the later the decision to respond would
occur.  Besides, it must be noted that several previous findings
are consistent with the hypothesis that this negative component
is chiefly related to stimulus characteristics, in particular its
topography has been said to change according to sense modality
(Simson et al., 1976), or in the case of missing visual stimuli,
according to the position of the expected stimulus in the visual
field (Renault and Lesevre, in press).

     c)  Two other results of ours must be taken into account: on
the one hand, the fact that the increase in RTs was always more
important than that of the duration of the negative parietal wave,

and, on the other hand, that there were large variations of the time of occurrence of all peaks in respect to the occurrence of the motor act. These findings show the complexity of these time relationships and fit with the view developed by Kutas et al. (1977) regarding the existence of two concurrent processes initiated by task relevant stimuli, i.e., a stimulus evaluation process, which would be reflected in our data by the duration of the negative parietal wave, and a response selection process. In addition, our results suggest that the vertex peaks (Nb-Pa) could index the "coupling" between these two parallel processes. Indeed, this coupling would produce some sort of a surprise effect (vertex response) which, in turn, would permit quickly giving an overt response whenever the selection response process is already over (quick RT cases) or starting this selection response process (slow RTs).

In conclusion, our results support the assumption that the negative parietal activity (Na wave) could reflect the stimulus evaluation time, whereas the vertex Nb-Pa waves would index the instant when the two above-mentioned parallel processes (the motor and the sensory one) get coupled. Therefore, the parietal positive activity (Pb) would last as long as the sensorimotor processing. It should be noted that in such a speculative model the time occurrence of the Pb wave with respect to the motor act would be an electrophysiological correlate, depending upon the "strategy" the subject uses during such complex motor RT tasks. This strategy can, indeed, favor either speed or accuracy of reaction (Kutas et al., 1977) or, in other words, either the motor or the sensory aspect of the task evaluation (Renault et al., in press). When speed or motor evaluation is emphasized, the motor act occurs before the parietal positive wave, and on the contrary, when accuracy or stimulus evaluation are emphasized the motor act then occurs after this Pb wave.

## SUMMARY

This study was intended to explain the relations between event related potentials obtained in a missing stimulus paradigm and i) the estimation of the moment of occurrence of the missing stimulus; ii) the sensorimotor processes involved when the subject is asked to give a motor response after having detected the missing stimulus. These results support the assumption that two processes are initiated after the time estimation of the omission: a stimulus evaluation process reflected by the duration of the negative parietal wave and, concurrently, a response selection and execution process, indexed by the overt motor response. Moreover, it is assumed that the coupling between these two processes could be reflected by the vertex negative-positive potentials, whereas the relative timing of the RT with respect to the parietal positive activity would be related to the strategy used by the subject.

## ACKNOWLEDGEMENTS

We wish to express our gratitude to J. Martinerie for his important help concerning the statistical analysis of our data. We also want to thank A. Ripoche and R. Grob for their most helpful technical assistance.

## REFERENCES

Courchesne, E., Hillyard, S.A. and Galambos, R.  Stimulus novelty, task relevance and the visual evoked potential in man. Electroenceph. Clin. Neurophysiol., 1975, 39, 131-144.

Kutas, M., McCarthy, G. and Donchin, E.  Augmenting mental chronometry: The P300 as a measure of stimulus evaluation time. Science, 1977, 197, 792-795.

Kutas, M. and Donchin, E.  The effect of handedness, of responding hand and of response force on the contralateral dominance of the readiness potential.  In J.E. Desmedt (Ed.), Progress in Clinical Neurophysiology, I, Basel: Karger, 1977.

Remond, A.  Integrated and topographical analysis of the EEG. Electroenceph. Clin. Neurophysiol., 1961, Sup. 20, 64-67.

Renault, B. and Lesevre, N.  Topographical study of the emitted potential obtained after the omission of an expected visual stimulus.  In D.A. Otto (Ed.), Multidisciplinary Perspectives in Event Related Brain Potential Research, Washington, D.C.: U.S. Government Printing Office, in press.

Renault, B., Ragot, R., Furet, J. and Lesevre, N.  Etude des relations entre le potentiel emis et les mecanismes de preparation perceptivo-motrice.  In J. Requin (Ed.), Anticipation et Processus Psychologiques, CNRS, in press.

Roth, W.T., Ford, J.M. and Kopell, B.S.  Long latency evoked potentials and reaction time.  Psychophysiol., 1978, 15, 17-23.

Ruchkin, B.S. and Sutton, S.  Latency characteristics and trial by trial variation of emitted potentials.  In J.E. Desmedt (Ed.), Cognitive Components in Event Related Cerebral Potentials, Basel: Karger, 1978.

Simson, R., Vaughan, H.G. and Ritter. W.   The scalp topography of
    potentials associated with missing visual and auditory stimuli.
    Electroenceph. Clin. Neurophysiol., 1976, 40, 33-42.

Squires, N.K., Squires, K.C. and Hillyard, S.A.   Two varieties of
    long latency positive waves evoked by unpredictable auditory
    stimulus.  Electroenceph. Clin. Neurophysiol., 1975, 38, 387-
    401.

Squires, K.C., Donchin, E., Herning, R.I. and McCarthy, G.   On the
    influence of task relevance and stimulus probability on event
    related potential components.  Electroenceph. Clin. Neuro-
    physiol., 1977, 42, 1-14.

EVENT RELATED POTENTIAL RESEARCH IN PSYCHIATRY

Walton T. Roth, Judith M. Ford, Adolf Pfefferbaum, Thomas
B. Horvath, Carol M. Doyle and Bert S. Kopell

Stanford University School of Medicine
Stanford, California 94305

Over the last few years our laboratory has applied event related potential (ERP) techniques in three main research areas:
psychopathology, normal aging and drugs of abuse.  In this research
we have used a variety of paradigms eliciting a variety of ERP components.  It is a matter of efficiency to administer a battery of
paradigms to subjects from populations that are difficult to select
and recruit.  The paradigms in a battery are chosen to elicit ERP
components at various recording sites and latencies, and which reflect various stages and types of brain activity.

The sensory modality we have used has been primarily auditory.
Our subjects sit in a sound attenuated chamber and hear clicks,
noise bursts or shaped tone bursts.  Depending on the paradigm,
brain stem potentials, middle latency and auditory evoked potentials
(P1, N1, P2) or the sustained potential (SP) are elicited.  Under
the proper task conditions the potentials representing cognitive
processes more remote from sensation are elicited: P3, or the late
positive wave, the CNV and the slow wave.  The sensitivity of a
component to the clinical phenomena under study depends on the precise conditions under which the component is elicited.  Important
sensory parameters are intensity and interstimulus interval (ISI).
Cognitive parameters are as varied as the scope of the word cognition.  We have used target detection tasks, dichotic selective
attention tasks and memory retrieval tasks, as well as non-task
paradigms.

## SCHIZOPHRENIA

Our research in schizophrenia encompasses three studies.  The

331

first compared twenty-one schizophrenics at St. Elizabeths Hospital
with twenty-one age-matched controls (Roth and Cannon, 1972).  Subjects were exposed to non-task relevant sequences of tones and noise
bursts at about 70 dB sound pressure level (SPL).  The noise bursts
occurred randomly with a probability of 1/15 and elicited a positive
wave at about 220 msec which was prominent in control subjects for
the first twenty presentations of the noise bursts.  In retrospect
this wave is probably a composite of P2 and P3 components.  Schizophrenics generally showed no such wave.  Only seven of forty-two
subjects were misclassified when a criterion voltage of 3.2 $\mu$V was
set for P3 amplitude to the first ten stimuli.

     We explored this positive wave in a series of experiments
(Roth, 1973; Ford et al., 1973, 1976a, 1976b) and, after developing
a paradigm that we thought would elicit a reliable P3 in passive
subjects (Roth et al., 1976a), we did a second study comparing
schizophrenics and controls (Roth et al., 1978a).  Subjects were
twenty-five schizophrenics meeting the Research Diagnostic Criteria
(RDC) from a Veterans Administration Hospital and twenty age-matched
controls.  Over one-third of the patients were drug-free.  The stimulus eliciting P3 was an 80 dB SPL noise burst that occurred randomly in a sequence of background 65 dB SPL 800 c/sec tone pips.
Half of the noise bursts were immediately preceded by a 1200 c/sec
tone pip which served as warning.  The probability of the warning
tone and the unwarned noise burst were both 0.1, and both elicited
P3s.  Unfortunately this paradigm failed to show significant P3
differences between our schizophrenics and controls.  Although mean
values of P3 were more than 2.5 times larger in controls, there was
much overlap of P3 amplitude between the two populations.  The chief
problem appears to be that some controls produced negligible P3s,
while others produced large ones.

     In addition to the P3 paradigm, two other paradigms were in-
cluded in this test battery: a CNV paradigm and a tone-intervals
(recovery function) paradigm.  The CNV was elicited by a warning
tone (S1) followed 1 sec later by a series of light flashes (S2)
to which subjects pressed a button as quickly as possible.  The
intertrial intervals were 33-58 sec since we wanted to be sure that
CNV resolution was complete by the time a new trial was started.
The EEG amplifiers were set to have a time constant of 10 sec.
Electrodermal activity was eliminated by using pin electrodes.
Averages were computed from 5.5 sec epochs of EEG which had been
edited for various artifacts.  Eye blinks were compensated for by
a subtraction procedure.  Fig. 1 shows grand averages for 3.5 sec
of the epoch.  Although at Cz the CNV appears to remain more negative
after S2 for the schizophrenics than for controls, this difference
is not significant.  We considered this failure to replicate the
results of Timsit-Berthier et al. (1973) and the Montreal group
(Dobrovsky and Dongier, 1976) possibly to be due to differences in
the kinds of patients tested.  The Montreal group found the most

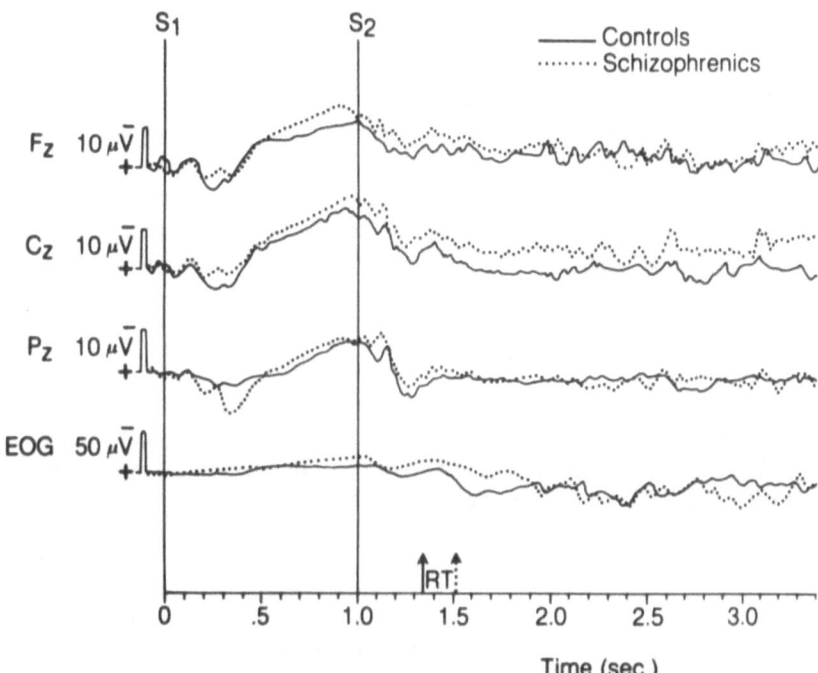

Fig. 1.  ERPs for controls and schizophrenics combined across all
subjects.  The averages are comprised of about eleven trials/subject
X 25 subjects.  Sl marks the warning tone and S2 the onset of the
imperative light flashes.  The arrows on the abscissa indicate mean
RTs.

striking prolongation in patients who had been ill for less than
six months, whereas almost all our patients had been ill for more
than a year.  In general our patients' illnesses, although chronic,
had not required continuous hospitalization.

The tone-intervals paradigm delivered 65 dB SPL 50-msec tone
pips at ISIs of 0.75, 1.5 and 3.0 sec in a random sequence.  The
amplitudes of N1 and P2 varied with ISI, as we knew they would (Roth
et al., 1976b), but there were no differences between schizophrenics
and controls.  Differences in temporal recovery had been shown previously for earlier peaks using somatosensory (e.g., Shagass, 1972)

and visual stimuli (Floris et al., 1968; Speck et al., 1966).

Our third and most recent study of fifteen schizophrenics and fifteen age-matched controls used a modified and expanded test battery of six paradigms, the first three of which were under the direction of Dr. Pfefferbaum. About half of the patients had been free of medication for at least two weeks prior to testing. In all except the last paradigm the subjects were given no task but asked to sit quietly. Briefly, the paradigms were as follows:

1. Click intensities: Clicks were delivered every 40 msec at 60, 70, 80 or 90 dB above an individual's sensation level (SL) threshold in random order. Averages of 2048 trials were computed for a 10 msec epoch. Fig. 2 illustrates sample waveforms for this paradigm. The amplitude and latency of wave V of the brain stem potential were measured.

2. Click intervals: 2048 90 dB SL clicks were delivered with an ISI of 20 msec, followed immediately by a series of identical stimuli delivered at an ISI increased to 80 msec. Wave V was measured as in the first paradigm.

3. Tone intensities: 500 c/sec tones 480 msec long were delivered with an ISI of 1.5 sec from tone onset to tone onset. Tone intensities were 50, 60, 70 or 80 dB SL presented in random order. Averages were computed for 64 trials of each intensity. Fig. 2 illustrates the N1, P2 and sustained potential (SP) components of a typical normal subject. The amplitudes and latencies of these components were measured.

4. Tone intervals: 1000 c/sec 50 msec tones were given at 85 dB sound pressur level (SPL). Tones occurred at ISIs of 0.75, 2.25 or 6.75 sec in random order. Averages were computed for forty trials of stimuli preceded by each ISI. Fig. 2 illustrates the N1 and P2 peaks elicited in this paradigm. The amplitudes and latencies of these components were measured. N1 and P2 were much smaller after ISIs of 0.75 sec than after ISIs of 6.75 sec.

5. Noise tone: Four types of stimuli, each 1 sec in duration with an ISI of 4 sec from stimulus onset to onset, were delivered in random order. Stimuli were either 1000 c/sec tones or white noise and were either 100 dB SPL or 70 dB SPL. Averages were computed for forty stimuli of each type. N1, P2, P3 and SP were elicited. All components were measured in all conditions. P3 was most prominent in the EP to the 100 dB noise bursts.

6. Reaction time: 85 dB SPL 50 msec tones were given with a 1 sec ISI. Tones were 800 or 1200 c/sec. The sequential probabilities were 0.85 for the 800 or 1200 c/sec tone and 0.15 for the 1200 c/sec tone. Hence the former tones are referred to as "fre-

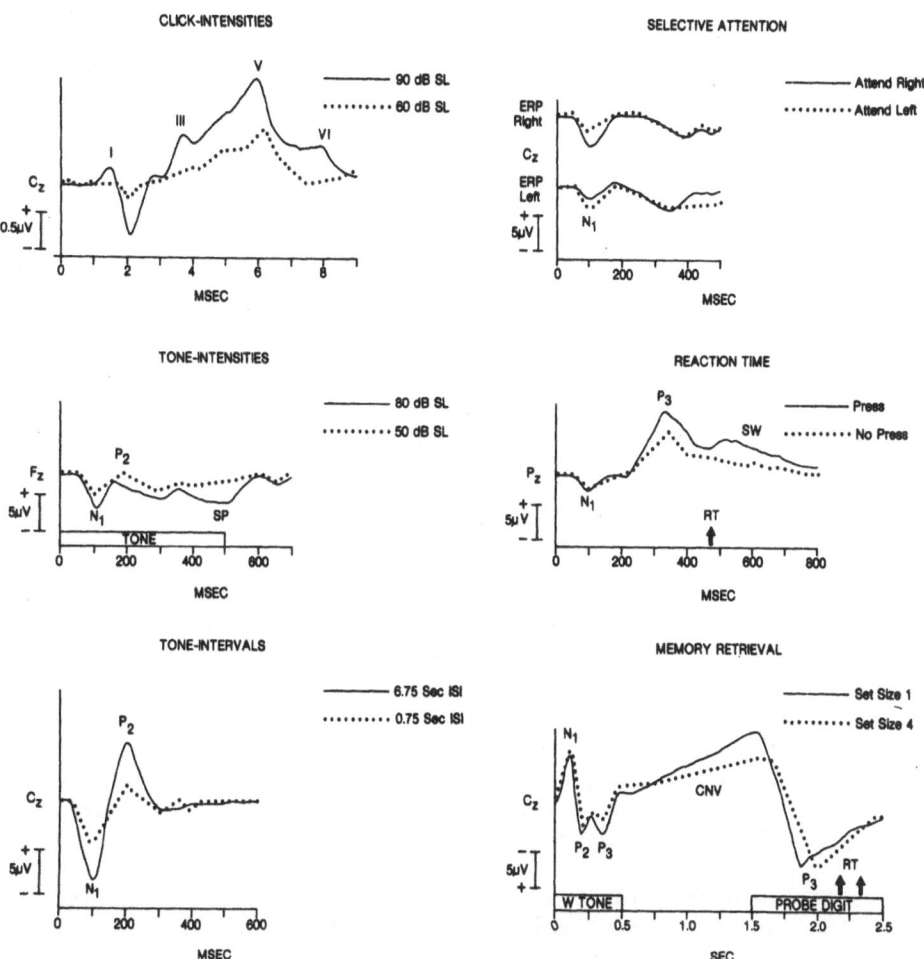

Fig. 2.    Sample ERPs from six paradigms described in the text.

quents" and the latter as "infrequents". Subjects were instructed
to press a button as quickly as possible upon hearing an infrequent
tone. Averages were computed for seventy-five infrequent tones and
430 frequent tones. The frequent tones elicit N1 and P2; the infrequent, N1, P2, P3 and a slow wave (SW) (illustrated in Fig. 2).
Amplitudes of all these peaks and latencies of all but the SW were
measured.

The click-intensities and click-intervals paradigms showed the
well known decrease in wave V latency as click intensity increased
or as ISI became longer, but there were no differences between
schizophrenics and controls. The tone-intensities paradigm showed
complex effects depending on lead and intensity. In general, P2
was smaller and later in controls, and SP was greater. Larger P2s
in schizophrenics were possibly due to a lack of the SP negativity

in their ERPs.  The tone-intervals paradigm gave smaller N1s for
schizophrenics than for controls at the 6.75 sec ISI but not at
shorter intervals.  Our hypothesis had been that endogenous auditory stimuli might be experienced by schizophrenics who, in general,
are liable to auditory hallucinations, and this would effectively
reduce the ISI.  If this is so, our data implies that such endogenous interference in the auditory system manifests itself most
clearly when the rate of exogenous stimulations is decreased.

The most striking differences between the groups were in the
noise-tone and reaction time paradigms.  N1, P2 and P3 amplitudes
were considerably smaller in the schizophrenics, the P2 and P3
differences being largest in the 100 dB noise condition.  Considerable startle blink reflex contaminated N1, but P2 and P3 were too
late to be affected.  The reaction time task was performed more
poorly by schizophrenics.  RTs were considered valid if they occurred between 100 and 600 msec after the targets.  Schizophrenics made
fewer responses within these limits (51 $\pm$ 22) than controls (68 $\pm$
10).  Schizophrenics were slower when they did respond (329 $\pm$ 51
vs. 283 $\pm$ 43 msec) and their RTs had larger standard deviations within an individual subject (70 $\pm$ 22 vs. 51 $\pm$ 13 msec).  The amplitudes
of P3 to the infrequents was considerably smaller in schizophrenics,
while N1, P2 and SW to the infrequents showed no such effects.  The
latency of P3 was the same for both groups (mean 320 msec at Cz).
The main difference between the groups in the evoked potentials to
frequent stimuli lay in P2 latency which had a mean of 18 msec for
schizophrenics and 217 msec for controls.

Stepwise discriminant analysis of the eight best variables as
determined by analysis of variance selected P2 latency to the fre-
quents as the best variable to discriminate schizophrenics from
controls.  It classified 13/14 controls correctly but only 7/12
schizophrenics.  The next variable entered was P3 amplitude to the
infrequents, but this did not improve the classification.  When the
P2 latency variable was excluded the first two variables picked
were P3 amplitude to infrequents and N1 amplitude after the 6.75
sec ISI.  These two variables correctly classified 11/14 controls
and 9/12 schizophrenics.  P3 and N1 amplitude to the 100 dB noise
also had high Fs-to-enter, but these variables correlated with the
variables chosen and, hence, were not themselves chosen.

The combination of small P3s and more variable RTs suggests
that perhaps latency variability of P3 in individual trials led to
reduced amplitudes in a stimulus-synchronized average.  Kutas et
al. (1977) found P3 latency to vary with RT by analyzing their data
with the adaptive filter invented by Woody (1967).  We applied
this filter to the P3 to infrequents and found that P3 amplitude
increased more in schizophrenics than in controls after application
of the filter but that schizophrenics still had significantly smaller P3s.  Furthermore response-synchronized averages showed just as

great a P3 difference between groups as did the original stimulus-
synchronized average.  These results imply that latency variability
does not completely explain the P3 amplitude differences and, in
fact, the greater gain in schizophrenics' P3 amplitudes with the
adaptive filter may be due to more noise in the schizophrenics' EEG.

Diminished P3s in schizophrenics has been reported from other
laboratories (Levit et al., 1973; Shagass et al., 1977, 1978; Verleger and Cohen, 1978).  The Bleulerian characteristic of schizophrenic autism would be expected to result in small or absent P3s
since P3 amplitude depends on information being taken in from the
external environment (Ruchkin and Sutton, 1978).  Either schizophrenics fail to perceive that information is being delivered such
as might occur if their subjective probability estimates were faulty,
or they fail to react to such information in the same way as they
tend to lack orienting responses.

NORMAL AGING

One of the greatest problems in doing research in aging is
that with age comes disease.  Diagnosed or undiagnosed disease can
cause performance deficits that should be attributed to more specific pathological processes than the more general variable of age.
In the study conducted under the direction of Dr. J.M. Ford, we
recruited women older than 70 years who were subjectively and by
history and physical examination in good health.  None had active
symptoms of cardiovascular, neurological, respiratory, renal, gastro-
intestinal or endocrine disease.  Audiometry excluded subjects with
sensation levels above 30 dB SPL at 500 c/sec.  Thirteen elderly
women between 74 and 87 years (mean (80.2) were compared with thirteen similarly healthy women between 20 and 29 years (mean 22.9).
The mean raw IQ scores on the Wechsler Adult Intelligence Scale
(WAIS) was 109 for the old and 145 for the young.  If age adjusted,
these scores would be 124 for the old and 121 for the young women.
Mean years of education were 16.6 for the old and 15.8 for the young.

These subjects were tested on a battery that included the following paradigms:

(1)  Tone intensities:  As described above.

(2)  Selective attention:  This paradigm was based on the work
of Hillyard and his students (Hillyard et al., 1973; Schwent et al.,
1976a; Schwent et al., 1976b).  Thirty dB SL 50 msec tone pips were
presented at ISIs varying from 200-800 msec.  Tones presented to the
right ear were 800 or 840 c/sec presented randomly in a ratio of
10:1, and to the left ear 1500 or 1560 c/sec presented randomly in
the same ratio.  Subjects listened to the sequence of tones twice,
once counting infrequent stimuli in the right ear and once counting

infrequent stimuli in the left ear.  Fig. 2 shows sample waveforms
for this paradigm for frequent stimuli in attended and nonattended
ears.  Amplitude and latency of N1 were analyzed in averages of
400 frequent trials for a given ear.  P3 was measured for averages
of 40 trials of the infrequent stimulus.

        (3)  Memory retrieval:  This paradigm uses the task developed
by Sternberg (1966) to measure the speed of retrieval of items from
short-term memory.  The ERPs that accompany normal performance of
this task had been investigated in our laboratory previously (Roth
et al., 1975; Roth et al., 1977; Roth et al., 1978b).  Target and
probe stimuli were the digits 0-9 presented for 1 sec on an oscil-
loscope.  In each trial 1 to 4 target digits were presented consec-
utively with a 1 sec interval between them.  The digits define a
memory set with 1, 2, 3 or 4 members.  One second after the memory
set was ended a 0.5 sec warning tone (60 dB SL, 1000 c/sec) came on.
One second after the warning tone went off the probe digit appeared.
Subjects then pushed one of two telegraph keys to indicate if the
probe was in or out of the memory set.  Eight averages could be
formed as defined by memory set size and whether the probe was in
or out of the set.  Each average was comprised of about twenty-two
trials, only correct trials being included.  Fig. 2 shows ample ERPs
for in-set trials with set sizes of 1 and 4.  N1, P2 and P3 to the
warning tone were measured as were the CNV prior to, and the P3
following the probe.  The last peak was located by computer as the
maximum positive peak between 200 and 800 msec.

        Old and young women differed on all three paradigms.  The most
striking finding from the tone-intensities paradigm was that the
SP was much smaller in old than young (p < .001) in an analysis of
variance with Fz, Cz and Pz).  N1 amplitude was the same in both
groups, P1 amplitude was larger in the elderly and P2 amplitude
increased with intensity for the young but decreased or did not
change with intensity for the old.  This combination of findings
cannot be explained by a nonspecific decrease in ERP amplitude with
age.  Pfefferbaum et al. (1978a) speculated that the SP decline in
these old subjects corresponds to the loss of dendritic mass in the
prefrontal cortex of aged brains that can be observed histopatho-
logically.

        The selective attention paradigm showed an N1 effect that was
not statistically different in young and old subjects.  This was
true even though the counting of targets was less accurate in the
old.  P3 to the targets was significantly later in old (482 msec)
than in young (402 msec) subjects [F(1,22) = 11.70; p < .01].  Ford
et al. (1978a) took this as an indication that the cognitive deficit
of old subjects in this task was not an attentional deficit but a
slowness in reacting to relevant information.

        The memory retrieval paradigm yielded a wealth of ERP and

behavioral data.  RT was a linear function of memory set size for
both in-set and out-of-set probes.  According to Sternberg's model,
the intercept of this function represents the sum of time to encode
the probe and the time to make the motor response.  The slope of
this function represents the time to scan memory for a single digit.
In our subjects the RT slope was greater in old (55 msec/digit) than
in young (35 msec/digit) as had been reported previously (Anders
and Fozard, 1973).  RT intercepts were also greater in old (1028
msec) than young (720 msec).  The latency of P3 to the probe did
not follow the same pattern, however.  The table in Ford's abstract
in this volume lists these data.  P3 latencies did increase with set
size, but the slope of this increase was the same for young (27 msec/
digit) and old (29 msec/digit).  The intercepts were larger for old
(448 msec) than young (369 msec) but were in both cases much shorter
than RT intercepts.  Dr. Ford postulated (Ford et al., 1978b) that
P3 latency intercept represents encoding time and that the intercept of the difference between RT and P3 latency is a measure of
motor time alone.  If motor time were constant for each set size the
slope of the RT-P3 latency vs. set size would be zero.  In fact,
the slope of this function is 46 msec/digits for old and 14 msec/
digits for young.  This greater gap between P3 and RT for greater
set sizes in the elderly may represent a slowness in responding
after a more difficult decision.  Subjects are less confident of
their decision when the memory set is larger.  There were more
errors when memory sets were larger which complicates interpretations of the dissociation between P3 latency and RT as being a
manifestation of different speed vs. accuracy trade-offs (Kutas et
al., 1977).  For smaller set sizes there was both more accuracy and
less dissociation, but task difficulty was less as well.

     In summary, our general conclusions from this study were that
old subjects moved much more slowly than young, encoded somewhat
more slowly, scanned memory at the same speed but were considerably
less confident about more difficult decisions.


                          PSYCHOACTIVE DRUGS

     A number of psychoactive substances have been investigated in
our laboratory using versions of the paradigms described above.
Roth et al. (1977) tested the effects of marijuana and ethanol with
this memory-retrieval paradigm, Hink et al. (1978) tested the effects of methylphenidate on a selective attention task and Pfefferbaum et al. (1978b) tested the effects of ethanol and meperidine
with the tone-intensities paradigm.  A version of the RT paradigm
has been used both to test for acute effects of ethanol (Roth et al.,
in prep.) and to try to distinguish abstinent chronic alcoholics
from controls (Pfefferbaum et al., 1978c).  This version of the RT
paradigm delivers three pitches of tone in random order.  One pitch
occurs frequently and two pitches infrequently.  One of the infre-

quent pitches is the target for a button press and the other is not.
The properties of this paradigm have been explored in normals (Roth
et al., 1978c).

In the Pfefferbaum study ten chronic alcoholics and ten age-
and sex-matched controls were tested.  Alcoholics had a ten year or
more history of drinking and met the Research Diagnostic Criteria
for alcoholism.  Subjects with neurological disease were excluded.
All subjects had been abstinent from alcohol for at least two weeks
and off psychotropic medications for at least one week at the time
of testing.  RTs were not significantly different between alcoholics
(289 msec) and controls (272 msec).  Neither were there significant
P3 amplitude differences between groups for either target or nontarget infrequents.  P3 latencies for targets were also comparable
for the two groups, but the latencies of P3 to nontargets were less
than 400 msec in all controls and greater than 400 msec in all of
the alcoholics.  This P3 latency measure was more sensitive than the
Halstead-Reitan battery in distinguishing the groups:  only three
of the alcoholics had "definite" cognitive abnormality while one
other was classified as "borderline".  We have no ready explanation
for these unexpected findings.  In dementia, P3 latency is greater
(Goodin et al., 1978), but why is latency greater only for nontarget P3s?  We plan to continue these investigations and hope to ascertain among other things if this difference is irreversible or if
it disappears after a longer period of abstinence.


RESEARCH GOALS

The main clinical use of electricity in psychiatry today is
electroconvulsive therapy.  Electrodiagnosis has not yet reached
the point of usefulness.  Yet our results indicate that ERP measures
may be sensitive enough to distinguish schizophrenics from controls
to a clinically useful extent.  Now the specificity of these measures must be established.  Would patients with affective disorders
show similar changes?  Since affective disorders are treated with
medications different from those used in schizophrenia, distinguishing between the two is of practical importance.  For ERPs to be useful they must be more accurate or more inexpensive than other methods
for deciding which treatment a patient should receive, or evaluating
the effectiveness of that treatment.  Theoretical insights about cognitive peculiarities of schizophrenics that might be gained through
ERP research are of much less interest to the clinician.

Studies of aging have different goals since there is little
hope of reversing the nonspecific aging process with a particular
treatment.  Deviations from normal aging, however, may indicate the
presence of specific and treatable disease, and so understanding
of normal aging can provide a baseline for abnormality.  Although
another averaging technique, computerized axial tomography, can

tell us about structural alterations in the brain, more subtle functional alterations are more likely to show up with ERP testing. We plan to test this idea by using both methods in a new group of elderly people.

The acute effects of psychoactive drugs can be tested in a research design in which the subject is his own control. This is especially advantageous when measuring components that are very variable between individuals. ERPs can be the best indication that a drug is affecting the brain since biochemical evidences of drug effects require more invasive techniques. The difficulty with human ERP studies is that the establishment of dose-response and time-action curves requires many data points, each comprised of many trials. Unless such curves are established it is impossible to know whether differences between drugs are qualitative or quantitative differences. Chronic effects of psychoactive substances have not been the subject of ERP research previously because of the belief that ERPs had no particular advantage over other forms of cognitive testing. Now it is apparent that ERPs supplement RT and other measures of psychological function in an important way.

SUMMARY

Our laboratory has applied event related potential (ERP) techniques in three main clinical areas: psychopathology, normal aging and drugs of abuse. For the sake of efficiency, multiple paradigms have been administered to a single group of subjects. We recently compared schizophrenics and controls using paradigms that elicit auditory short (brain stem), middle and long latency potentials. Certain middle and long latency potentials differed markedly in latency or amplitude between the groups. In another study we compared healthy elderly women with healthy young women using a test battery that included a dichotic listening task and a Sternberg memory retrieval task. The pattern of ERPs elicited during these challenging tasks helped delineate specific cognitive deficits associated with aging. Several of our paradigms have also been sensitive to acute and chronic effects of psychoactive substances. In certain cases, our ERP findings apparently provide information about the human brain that cannot be obtained by other methods. Such unique information is the final justification for using ERP techniques in clinical areas.

ACKNOWLEDGEMENTS

This research was supported by the Veterans Administration Medical Research Service, NIMH Specialized Research Grant MH30854 and NIA Postdoctoral Fellowship AG 05018.

REFERENCES

Anders, T.R. and Fozard, J.L.   Effects of age upon retrieval from
    primary and secondary memory.   Develop. Psychol., 1973, 9,
    411-416.

Dubrovsky, B. and Dongier, M.   Evaluation of event related poten-
    tials in selected groups of psychiatric patients.   In W.C.
    McCallum and J.R. Knott (Eds.), The Responsive Brain, Bristol:
    John Wright, 1976.

Floris, V., Morocutti, G., Amabile, G., Bernardi, G. and Rizzo, P.
    Recovery cycle of visual evoked potentials in normal, schizo-
    phrenics and neurotic patients.   In N.S. Kline and E. Laska
    (Eds.), Computers and Electronic Devices in Psychiatry, New
    York: Grune and Stratton, 1968.

Ford, J.M., Roth, W.T., Kopell, B.S. and Dirks, S.J.   Evoked res-
    ponse correlates of signal recognition between and within
    modalities.   Science, 1973, 181, 465-466.

Ford, J.M., Roth, W.T. and Kopell, B.S.   Auditory evoked potentials
    to unpredictable shifts in pitch.   Psychophysiol., 1976a, 13,
    32-39.

Ford, J.M., Roth, W.T. and Kopell, B.S.   Attention effects on audi-
    tory evoked potentials to infrequent events.   Biol. Psychol.,
    1976b, 4, 65-67.

Ford, J.M., Hopkins, W.F. III, Roth W.T., Pfefferbaum, A. and Ko-
    pell, B.S.   Age effects on event related potentials in a selec-
    tive attention task.   Submitted for publication.

Ford, J.M., Roth W.T., Mohs, R.C. Hopkins, W.F. III and Kopell,
    B.S.   The effects of age on event related potentials in a
    memory retrieval task.   Submitted for publication.

Goodin, D.S., Squires, K.C. and Starr, A.   Long latency event re-
    lated components of the auditory evoked potential in dementia.
    Brain, in press.

Hillyard, S.A., Hink, R.F., Schwent, V.L. and Picton, T.W.   Electri-
    cal signs of selective attention in the human brain.   Science,
    1973, 182, 177-180.

Hink, R.F., Fenton, W.H. Jr., Tinklenberg, J.R., Pfefferbaum, A.
    and Kopell, B.S.   Vigilance and human attention under condi-
    tions of methylphenidate and secobarbital intoxication:   An
    assessment using brain potentials.   Psychophysiol., 1978, 15,
    116-125.

Kutas, M. McCarthy, G. and Donchin, E.  Augmenting mental chrono-
    metry:  The P300 as a measure of stimulus evaluation time.
    Science, 1977, 197, 792-795.

Levit, A.L., Sutton, S. and Zubin, J.  Evoked potential correlates
    of information processing in psychiatric patients.  Psychol.
    Med., 1973, 3, 487-494.

Pfefferbaum, A., Ford, J.M., Roth, W.T., Hopkins W.F. III and Kopell,
    B.S.  Event related potential changes in healthy aged females.
    Electroenceph. Clin. Neurophysiol., in press.

Pfefferbaum, A., Roth, W.T., Tinklenberg, J.R., Rosenbloom, M.S.
    and Kopell, B.S.  The effects of ethanol and meperidine on
    auditory evoked potentials.  Submitted for publication.

Pfefferbaum, A., Horvath, T.B., Roth, W.T., Clifford, S.T. and
    Kopell, B.S.  The effects of chronic alcoholism on the late
    event related potentials.  Presented at Fourth Bienniel Inter-
    national Symposium on Biomedical Research in Alcohol, Zurich,
    Switzerland, June 1978c.

Roth, W.T.  Auditory evoked responses to unpredictable stimuli.
    Psychophysiol., 1973, 10, 125-138.

Roth, W.T. and Cannon E.H.  Some features of the auditory evoked
    response in schizophrenics.  Arch. Gen. Psychiat., 1972, 27,
    466-471.

Roth, W.T., Kopell, B.S., Tinklenberg, J.R., Darley, C.F., Sikora,
    R. and Vesecky, T.B.  The contingent negative variation during
    a memory retrieval task.  Electroenceph. Clin. Neurophysiol.,
    1975, 38, 171-174.

Roth, W.T., Ford, J.M., Lewis, S.J. and Kopell, B.S.  Effects of
    stimulus probability and task relevance on event related poten-
    tials.  Psychophysiol., 1976a, 13, 311-317.

Roth, W.T., Krainz, P.L., Ford, J.M., Tinklenberg, J.R., Rothbart,
    R.M. and Kopell, B.S.  Parameters of temporal recovery of the
    human auditory evoked potential.  Electroenceph. Clin. Neuro-
    physiol., 1976a, 40, 623-632.

Roth. W.T., Tinklenberg, J.R. and Kopell, B.S.  Ethanol and mari-
    juana effects on event related potentials in a memory retrie-
    val paradigm.  Electroenceph. Clin. Neurophysiol., 1977, 42,
    381-388.

Roth, W.T., Horvath, T.B., Pfefferbaum, A., Tinklenberg, J.R.,
    Mezzich, J.R. and Kopell, B.S.  Late event related potentials

and schizophrenia. In H. Begleiter (Ed.), Evoked Brain Potentials and Behavior, New York: Plenum, in press.

Roth, W.T., Rothbart, R.M. and Kopell, B.S. The timing of CNV resolution in a memory retrieval task. Biol. Psychol., 1978b, 6, 39-49.

Roth, W.T., Ford, J.M. and Kopell, B.S. Long latency evoked potentials and reaction time. Psychophysiol., 1978c, 15, 17-23.

Roth, W.T., Pfefferbaum, A., Ford, J.M. and Kopell, B.S. Effects of ethanol on human evoked potentials, in prep.

Ruchkin, D.S. and Sutton, S. Equivocation and P300 amplitude. In D.A. Otto (Ed.), Multidisciplinary Perspectives in Event Related Brain Potential Research, Washington, D.C.: U.S. Government Printing Office, in press.

Schwent, V.L., Hillyard, S.A. and Galambos, R. Selective attention and the auditory vertex potential. I: Effects of stimulus delivery rate. Electroenceph Clin. Neurophysiol., 1976a, 40, 604-614.

Schwent, V.L., Hillyard, S.A. and Galambos, R. Selective attention and the auditory vertex potential. II: Effects of signal intensity and masking noise. Electroenceph. Clin. Neurophysiol., 1976b, 40, 615-622.

Shagass, C. Evoked Brain Potentials in Psychiatry, New York: Plenum Press, 1975.

Shagass, C., Straumanis, J.J., Roemer, R.A. and Amadeo, M. Evoked potentials of schizophrenics in several sensory modalities. Biol. Psychiat., 1977, 12, 221-235.

Shagass, C., Roemer, R.A., Straumanis, J.J. and Amadeo, M. Evoked potential correlates of psychosis. Biol. Psychiat., 1978, 13, 163-184.

Speck, L. Dim, B. and Mercer, M. Visual evoked responses of psychiatric patients. Arch. Gen Psychiat., 1966, 15, 59-63.

Sternberg, S. High speed scanning in human memory. Science 1966, 153, 652-654.

Timsit-Berthier, M., Delaunoy, J., Koninckx, N. and Rousseau, J.C. Slow potential changes in psychiatry. I. Contingent negative variation. Electroenceph. Clin. Neurophysiol., 1973, 35, 355-361.

Verleger, R. and Cohen, R.  Effects of certainty, modality shifts, and guess outcome on evoked potentials and reaction times in chronic schizophrenics.  Psychol. Med., 1978, 8: 81-93.

Woody, C.D.  Characterization of an adaptive filter for the analysis of variable latency neuroelectric signals.  Med. Biol. Eng., 1967, 5, 539-553.

SPATIAL DISTRIBUTION OF SENSORY EVOKED POTENTIALS IN PSYCHIATRIC

DISORDERS

C. Shagass, R.A. Roemer, J.J. Straumanis and M. Amadeo

Eastern Pennsylvania Psychiatric Institute

Temple University, Philadelphia, Pennsylvania

The topographic dimension has received little attention in evoked potential (EP) investigations of psychiatric patients. Although EPs have been recorded most often from a single lead derivation, some studies involving recordings from more than one site have yielded findings which suggest that the spatial distribution of EPs may be of psychiatric interest. For example, Rodin et al. (1968) in a study of visual evoked potentials (VEPs) observed that assessments of psychopathology in schizophrenics were more often correlated with right than with left hemisphere VEP characteristics. Perris (1974) found that amplitudes of VEPs from the left occiput were lower than those from the right in psychotic depressives while they were ill. Buchsbaum et al. (1977) reported that, in a rapidly cycling manic-depressive patient, a VEP wave was decreased in amplitude at the vertex and increased at the occiput with mania and conversely with depression. Such observations encourage further exploration of EP topography with respect to possible psychiatric correlates.

In recent years we have been using a comprehensive EP recording procedure which was designed to accomplish several purposes; a principal goal was to obtain information about topography in relation to psychiatric criteria. In this procedure recordings were made from fifteen locations, and four kinds of stimuli in three sensory modalities are presented in one experimental session. We have already reported a number of positive findings (Shagass et al., 1977, 1978; Roemer et al., 1978). These can be summarized as follows: 1) In overtly psychotic patients of both schizophrenic and affective type, events occurring more than 100 msec poststimulus were of lower than normal amplitude in EPs of all modalities and in most lead

locations. 2) EPs of nonpsychotic patients and schizophrenics of the
latent subtype were not grossly different from normal. 3) Chronic
schizophrenics (paranoid and undifferentiated) differed from those
of other subtypes with respect to a negative somatosensory EP (SEP)
peak occurring at 60 msec poststimulus (N60); N60 was more negative
posteriorly in the chronic patients. 4) Schizophrenics of all subtypes showed less waveshape stability than normal in VEPs recorded
from the left hemisphere.

We employed a completely objective, automatic computer technique to evaluate EP differences between groups (Shagass et al.,
1977, 1978). Mean EPs were obtained for each group and t-tests
were computed for consecutive corresponding data points; the t-
values were displayed as displacements from a horizontal line when
they were significant (Fig. 1). The drawback of this method is
that it cannot distinguish between effects resulting from differences in amplitude and those due to latency differences. This drawback can be particularly important if one wishes to evaluate group
differences in the topography of EP events since apparent reductions
in amplitude of a peak can result when the latency varies between
subjects. Consequently, although the automatic method has provided
some interesting topographic results, as in the case of the N60 wave,
we found it necessary to use a technique based on visual detection
of peaks in order to obtain more interpretable information about
spatial distribution. The possible problems resulting from the subjective aspects of detecting peaks visually were mitigated by the
fact that the results provided by the objective automatic method
were also available; when the findings yielded by the two methods
converged, they could be accepted with confidence.

We present here the results obtained by comparing several groups
of psychiatric patients and nonpatient control subjects with respect
to the spatial distributions of somatosensory, visual and auditory
EPs. The patients included schizophrenics of several subtypes,
psychotic depressives and nonpsychotics with neuroses and personality
disorders.


METHODS

As the basic recording procedures and the subject groups have
been described in full elsewhere (Shagass et al., 1977, 1978; Roemer
et al., 1978), only an outline will be given here.


Subjects

Data are presented for eighty-eight psychiatric inpatients and
thirty-three paid volunteer nonpatients. These subjects were all of
those from a larger pool who could be matched for age and sex to

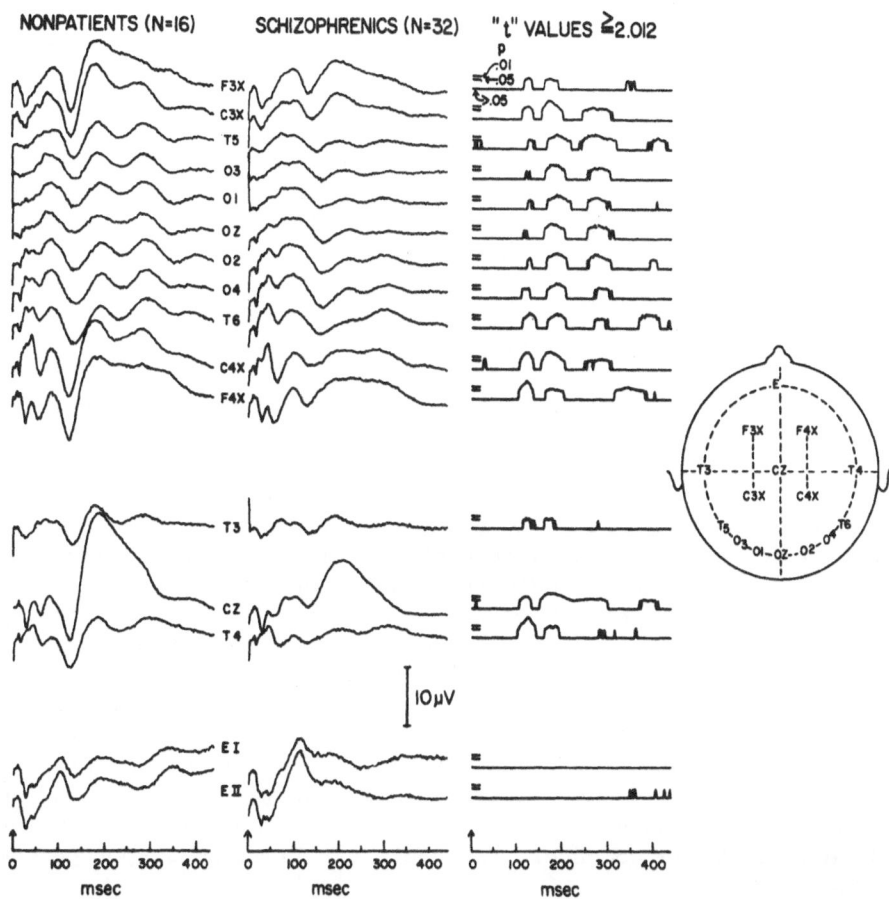

Fig. 1.   Left and center columns:   mean SEPs to left median nerve
stimuli of sixteen nonpatients and thirty-two schizophrenic patients.
All leads referenced to linked ears; scalp positivity gives upward
deflection.   Right column indicates results of 2-tailed t-tests performed on data points corresponding in time to those in EP tracings;
t-values under 2.012 (p=.05) were kept at baseline in t-curve while
values of 2.012 or greater were plotted according to magnitude starting at an arbitrary level above baseline (from Shagass et al., 1977).

provide the following comparisons:   a) chronic schizophrenics (N=26)
vs nonpsychotics (N=26) vs controls (N=25); there were nineteen men
in the control group and twenty in each patient group; ages were
about the same; b) latent schizophrenics vs "other" schizophrenics
vs controls (N=12 each);   c) psychotic depressives vs controls (N=12
each).   Some controls were used in more than one comparison.   Patients in the chronic schizophrenic group were subtyped as follows:

chronic undifferentiated, 14; chronic paranoid, 11; simple, 1. Subtypes included under "other" were: catatonic, 4; schizo-affective,
5; acute, 3. Latent schizophrenics conformed to criteria for pseudoneurotic schizophrenia (Hoch and Polatin, 1949). Nonpsychotics
included eleven neuroses and fifteen personality disorders. At time
of testing, patients had been unmedicated for a median period of ten
days. Diagnoses were made independently by at least two senior
psychiatrists; excluding latent schizophrenia, 86% of the diagnoses
met the relevant research diagnostic criteria of Feighner et al.
(1972) to a definite or probable level.

## Procedures

     Recording leads are indicated in the head diagram of Fig. 1;
the 10-20 system was followed with these exceptions: F3X, F4X, C3X
and C4X were 2 cm posterior and 1 cm lateral to the standard position; O3 and O4, respectively, were midway between O1 and T5 and
O2 and T6. Lead E was used to monitor EOG. All recordings were
monopolar to the ears linked through a 22 Kohm resistor. Two montages were used; each included three pairs of homologous lateral
leads, e.g., T3, T4, either Oz or Cz, and the EOG lead. Stimuli
were: electrical pulses (0.1 msec duration, 10 ma above sensory
threshold) applied percutaneously over left and right median nerves;
a checkerboard pattern flashed briefly on a television (TV) screen;
binaural auditory clicks 50 db above white noise level in earphones.
Order and timing of stimuli was pseudo-randomized; mean interstimulus interval was 1.75 sec. There were 192 stimuli of each kind for
each montage; averages (512 data points, 1 msec each) were summed
on-line in a PDP-12 computer. Subjects sat fixating a spot on the
TV screen.

## Treatment of Data

     Consecutive peaks were detected by visual inspection of select-
ed leads for each type of EP, as displayed on the PDP-12 cathode
ray tube. The leads were C4X and C3X for SEPs to left and right
median nerve, respectively, Oz for VEPs, and Cz for auditory EPs
(AEPs). A program was used to record time in the record at which
a cursor spot was placed on a peak. Utilizing the convention of
designating peaks by polarity and usual latency, the following peaks
were detected: a) SEPs - P15, N18, P30, P45, N60, P90, N130, P185,
P290; b) VEPs - N75, P90, N120, P200, P300; c) AEPs - P30, P50,
N75, P90, N110, P180, P360. These peaks correspond well to those
detected in group mean EPs of nonpatients (Shagass et al., 1977,
1978); Fig. 2 shows labelled examples of records in key leads. The
latencies of these peaks in recordings derived from key leads were
then used to make automatic measurements of amplitude at the same
times in the records from all leads for EPs of a given type for each

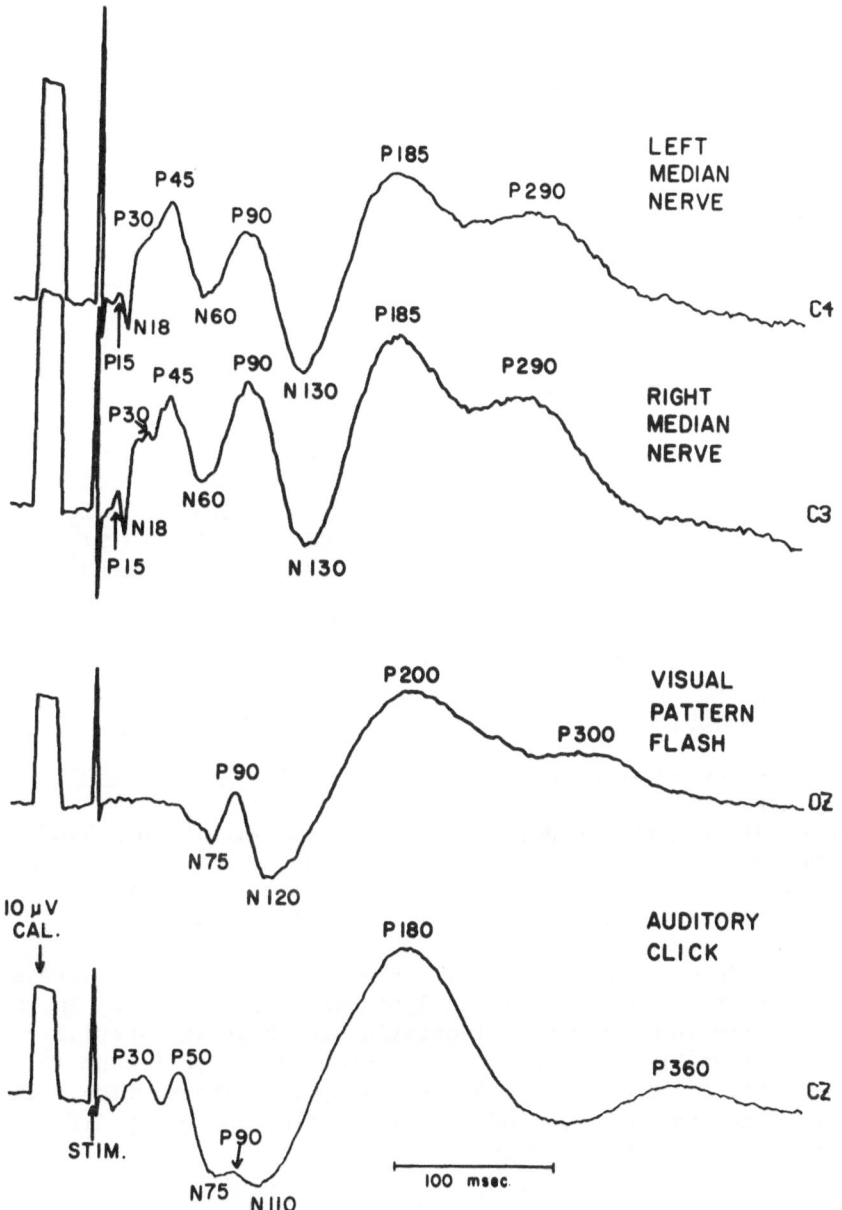

Fig. 2. EPs from key leads for visual detection of designated peaks; C4X (C4) for left median nerve SEP; C3X (C3) for right median nerve SEP; Oz for VEP; Cz for AEP. EPs are group means of twenty-five nonpatient subjects.

Table 1

SEPs - Left Median Nerve Stimulus
Results of Multivariate Profile Analyses Comparing
26 Chronic Schizophrenics (CS), 26 Nonpsychotics (NP)
and 25 Controls (C)

Mean Amplitude (μV)

| Peak | 14 Leads | | | 6 Contralateral Leads | | |
|------|------|------|------|------|------|------|
|      | CS | NP | C | CS | NP | C |
| P15 | 0.64 | 0.92 | 0.51 | 0.74 | 1.02 | 0.55 |
| N18 | -0.35 | -0.36 | -0.40 | -0.78 | -0.82 | -0.75 |
| P30 | -0.03 | 0.52 | 0.14a,d | 1.03 | 2.23 | 1.44b,e |
| P45 | 1.47 | 1.34 | 1.24d | 3.08 | 2.52 | 2.47 |
| N60 | -0.11 | 0.58 | 0.42 | -1.37 | -0.16 | -0.10a |
| P90 | 2.59 | 3.68 | 3.02d | 2.35 | 4.23 | 3.31a |
| N130 | 0.29 | -2.06 | -2.42b,d | 0.04 | -2.22 | -3.21c |
| P185 | 4.22 | 5.24 | 5.13 | 3.97 | 4.45 | 4.57 |
| P290 | 2.26 | 3.76 | 3.85 | 2.61 | 4.05 | 3.86 |

a, b, c - p for means, respectively, < .05, < .01, < .001
d, e    - p for diagnosis x lead interactions, respectively,
          < .05, < .01

subject.  A second version of the program allowed for latency variation by using the detected latency as the center of a time window
extending 5% on either side; maxima or minima within this window
were then detected for measurement.  As results for the two procedures, i.e., absolute latency and ± 5% variation, were very similar,
only the absolute latency data will be presented here.

Amplitude measurements for a given peak across leads were subjected to multivariate profile analysis (Morrison, 1967).  In this
analysis differences between diagnostic groups in the spatial distribution of an EP peak would be reflected by a significant (p = .05)
profile F-ratio, indicating a diagnosis by lead interaction.  In
addition, the analysis yielded F-ratios reflecting group differences
in mean amplitude across leads.

RESULTS

Chronic Schizophrenics vs Nonpsychotics vs Controls

SEP.  Multivariate profile analyses of the SEP data were performed in two ways:  a)  utilizing all fourteen scalp leads; b)

utilizing only the six leads on the hemisphere contralateral to the
stimulated nerve, as the earlier SEP peaks are lateralized (Fig. 1).
Table 1 summarizes the results for SEPs to left nerve stimuli.  Mean
amplitudes of P30 and N130 differed between groups across the fourteen leads; P30 amplitude was greater in the nonpsychotics than in
the other groups, while N130 amplitude was lower in the chronic
schizophrenics.  The data for the six contralateral leads yielded
mean amplitude differences for P30, N60, P90 and N130; P30 and P90
were highest in nonpsychotics; N60 was most and N130 least negative
in chronic schizophrenics.  Topographic differences between groups
were indicated by significant diagnosis by lead interactions for
P30, P45, P90 and N130 (fourteen leads); the six contralateral leads
gave an interaction for P30.

Fig. 3 (right) shows the distribution of P30 and N60 amplitudes
for five of the six contralateral leads (T4 was omitted because it
is not aligned with the other leads).  It will be seen that the
highest amplitude of P30 was at lead O4 in the chronic schizophrenics, at T6 in the controls and at C4X in the nonpsychotics.  The N60
distributions show about equal amplitudes for all three groups in
the frontal lead; in the posterior leads negativity was greater in
the chronic schizophrenics, being greatest at lead C4X.  Fig. 4 displays distributions for P90 and N130; the T3, Cz, T4 leads are plotted separately because of their alignment in the coronal plane.  P90

Table 2

SEPs - Right Median Nerve Stimulus
Results of Multivariate Profile Analyses Comparing
26 Chronic Schizophrenics (CS), 26 Nonpsychotics (NP)
and 25 Controls

Mean Amplitude (μV)

| | 14 Leads | | | 6 Contralateral Leads | | |
|---|---|---|---|---|---|---|
| Peak | CS | NP | C | CS | NP | C |
| P15 | 0.76 | 0.69 | 0.64 | 0.94 | 0.88 | 0.84 |
| N18 | -0.55 | -0.67 | -0.36a | -0.83 | -1.06 | 0.62a |
| P30 | 0.14 | ·0.44 | 0.49 | 1.14 | 1.98 | 1.58d |
| P45 | 1.57 | 1.61 | 1.68 | 3.05 | 2.78 | 2.82 |
| N60 | 0.29 | 1.46 | 1.57b | -1.01 | 0.47 | 1.01c,d |
| P90 | 3.69 | 4.94 | 4.30d | 3.21 | 5.28 | 4.51a,d |
| N130 | -0.10 | -2.17 | -2.36a | -0.42 | -2.37 | -2.66a |
| P185 | 3.42 | 5.82 | 5.52b | 3.29 | 5.32 | 4.88a,e |
| P290 | 2.48 | 4.05 | 4.61a,d | 2.50 | 4.35 | 4.40a |

a, b, c - p for means, respectively, < .05, < .01, < .001
d, e    - p for diagnosis x lead interactions, respectively,
          < .05, < .01

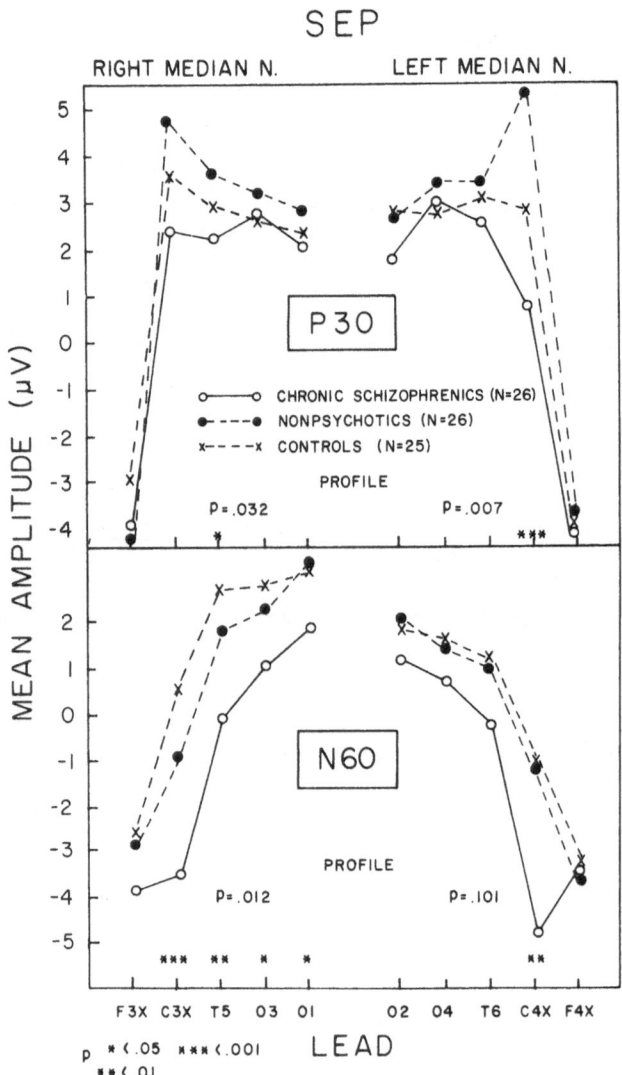

Fig. 3. Spatial distributions for chronic schizophrenics, nonpsychotics and controls of P30 and N60 in SEPs from hemispheres contralateral to stimulated nerves. Leads as in Fig. 1. Values for T3 and T4 not plotted. In this and subsequent figures asterisks indicate significant univariate F ratios; these are shown only when multivariate profile analysis was significant.

amplitude was greatest in the nonpsychotics in anterior leads, particularly in the right (contralateral) hemisphere. Chronic schizophrenics had the lowest P90 amplitude. The distributions for N130
clearly demonstrate the maximum negativity of this peak at leads
around the vertex (Cz, C3X, F3X, C4X, F4X) for controls and nonpsychotics; in the schizophrenics there was very little negativity.

Table 2 summarizes the results for SEPs to right nerve stimuli.
The groups differed with respect to mean amplitude for peaks N18,
N60, N130, P185 and P290 in both sets of analyses; the data for
the six contralateral leads showed an additional amplitude difference for P90. These amplitude findings indicate three trends: a)
N18 was greater (more negative) in the nonpsychotics; b) N60 was
more negative in the chronic schizophrenics; c) peaks from P90 on
were of lower amplitude in the schizophrenics.

The profile analyses for right nerve SEP data indicated group
differences in topography for P90 and P290 with fourteen leads and
in P30, N60, P90 and P185 with only the contralateral leads. The
left half of Fig. 3 shows the distributions for P30 and N60 in SEPs
to right nerve stimuli; in general these are approximate mirror
images of those obtained with left nerve SEPs. Maximum amplitude
of P30 occurred more anteriorly in the SEPs of nonpsychotics than
in those of schizophrenics. N60 peaks were more negative posteriorly in the schizophrenics than in other groups. Fig. 5 shows the
distributions for peaks P90 and P290. As with the left nerve stimuli, P90 amplitude of nonpsychotics was greater in anterior leads
and particularly on the contralateral side; also, although P90
amplitude of controls was like that of nonpsychotics in most leads
it dropped to the level of the schizophrenics in the two frontal
leads. P290 amplitude was greatest at vertex (Cz) in all groups
and decreased more or less symmetrically with increasing distance
from Cz. Controls had the highest and chronics schizophrenics the
lowest P290 amplitudes. The significant interaction for P290 seems
attributable to the variations between leads in the magnitude of
differences between groups (Fig. 5).

VEP. Profile analysis of the VEP results yielded only one
statistically significant finding; the distribution of P300 differed
between groups. Fig. 6 (top) indicates the nature of the topographic differences. VEP P300 amplitude was greatest in controls in the
coronal plane leads, particularly at Cz, while it was highest in
nonpsychotics at most other leads; it was generally low in chronic
schizophrenics.

AEP. Most of the significant AEP findings indicated group differences in mean amplitude. AEP peaks N75, P90 and N110 were generally less negative in the chronic schizophrenics, reflecting low
amplitude of the component often designated as N1 which would include
all three peaks. P180 was of greatest amplitude in the nonpsychotics.

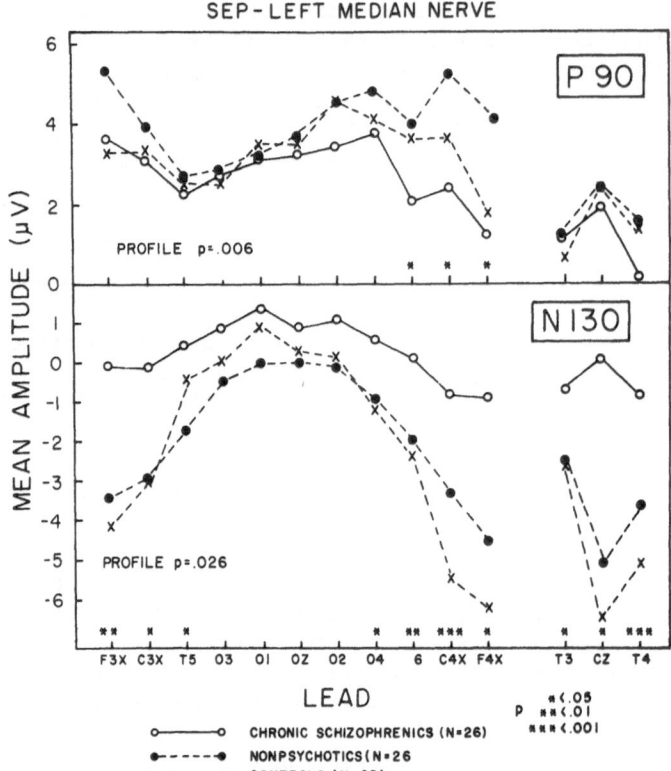

Fig. 4. Spatial distributions of peaks P90 and N130 in SEPs (left median nerve) of chronic schizophrenics, nonpsychotics and controls.

Topographic effects were demonstrated for P180 and P360. Fig. 6 (bottom) shows the P180 distributions; the amplitude of this peak was maximum at vertex in all groups and decreased symmetrically with distance from Cz. The topographic differences seemed to result from variations between leads in the magnitude of group differences. The P360 effect was of similar nature.

### Latent Schizophrenics vs "Other" Schizophrenics vs Controls

Because the small number of subjects imposed constraints upon the number of variables that could be handled at once, the multivariate profile analyses for this set of comparisons were performed separately for the three coronal leads and the remaining eleven leads. The analyses involving eleven leads yielded only one significant difference; mean amplitude of peak P15 in the right nerve SEP was lower for the latent schizophrenics than for the other two groups.

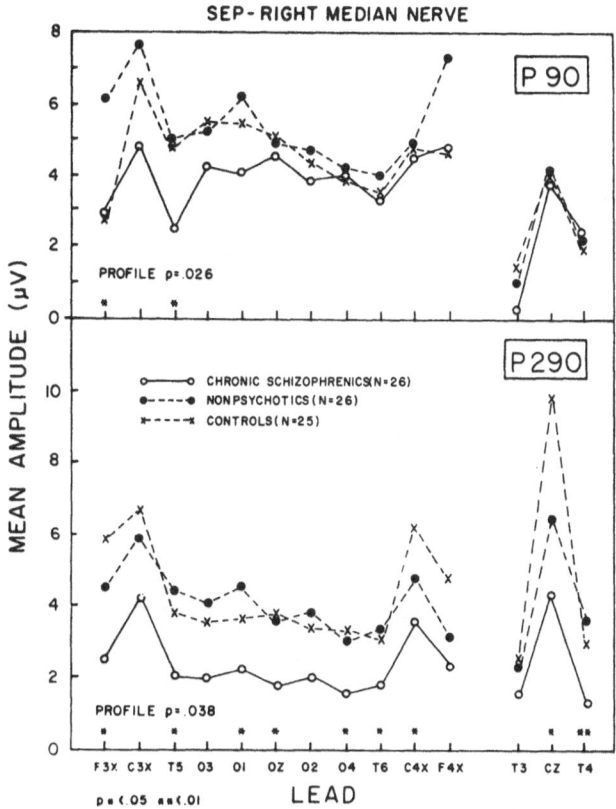

Fig. 5.  Spatial distributions of peaks P90 and P290 in SEPs (right
median nerve) of chronic schizophrenics, nonpsychotics and controls.


        Eleven analyses involving the coronal leads yielded significant
findings.  For left nerve SEPs N18, P45, N60 and P290 differed between groups in mean amplitude; amplitudes of the "other" schizophrenics were lower than those of latent schizophrenics and controls for N18, N60 and P290 and higher for P45.  P90 and P290 gave
distribution differences that appeared to result from relatively
low amplitudes at lead Cz in the "other" schizophrenics, while the
group means were more similar at the T3 and T4 leads.  For right
nerve SEPs, mean P15 amplitude of the latent schizophrenics was
relatively low, and mean P290 amplitude of the "other" schizophrenics was less than that of latents and controls.  P15, P30 and P290
gave distribution effects and only that for P290 seemed clearly
describable.  As with left nerve SEP, it appeared to result from
very low P290 amplitude at Cz in the "other" schizophrenics.  The
distributions of two VEP peaks (N75 and P200) and one AEP peak
(P180) differed between groups.  These effects could be attributed
to greater negativity at Cz for VEP peak N75 in the "other" schizophrenics, greater positivity of VEP peak P200 at Cz in the latent

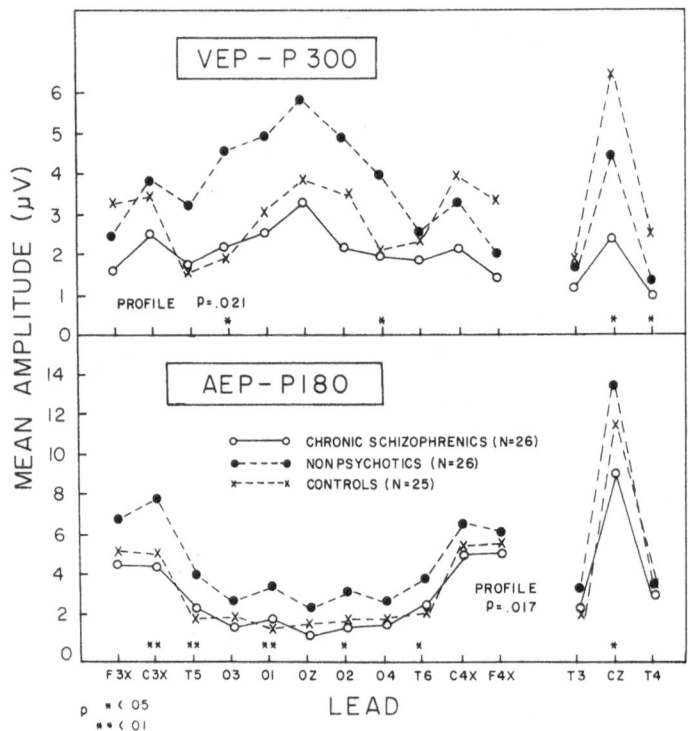

Fig. 6.  Spatial distributions of VEP peak P300 and AEP peak P180 of chronic schizophrenics, nonpsychotics and controls.


schizophrenics and lower amplitude of AEP peak P180 at Cz in the "other" schizophrenics.

### psychotic Depressives vs Controls

These analyses were also performed separately for the three coronal and the remaining eleven leads.  The analyses involving eleven leads showed that the mean amplitudes of right nerve SEP peak P185 and AEP peak N110 were lower in depressives than in controls. Topography differences were found for right nerve SEP peak P290 and AEP peak P190.  The SEP P290 effect seemed due to a reduction at T5 and T6 of the difference in amplitude at all other leads, that of controls being greater.  For AEP P180 maximal amplitudes were more posterior in controls (at leads C3X and C4X) than in depressives (leads F3X and F4X).  The analyses involving the three coronal leads yielded four group differences in mean amplitude – SEP N130 (both nerves), AEP P90 and N110 amplitudes were lower in psychotic depressives than in controls.  An interaction for left nerve SEP peak N130 resulted from virtual absence of this peak in the depressives.

## DISCUSSION

The data revealed a number of differences between the comparison groups with respect to both mean amplitudes of EP peaks and
their spatial distributions.  It seems pertinent to first consider
the amplitude results because of their methodological relevance for
the topography data.  Convergence between the data yielded by the
present method of detecting peaks visually and those provided by
the previously used fully automatic technique (Shagass et al., 1977,
1978) would augment confidence in the reliability of the topographic
data.

A main finding in our previous reports was that EPs of overtly
psychotic patients differed from normal, particularly in events
100 msec or more poststimulus, while those of nonpsychotic patients
and latent schizophrenics did not.  Present results generally replicate this finding.  In chronic schizophrenics amplitudes were lower
than those of nonpsychotics or normals in SEP peaks P90 to P290
(Tables 1 and 2), VEP peak P300 and AEP peaks N75, P90, N110 and
P180.  Amplitudes of later EP events also tended to be lower in
the group of "other" overt schizophrenics than in controls and latent schizophrenics and lower than normal in psychotic depressives.
In addition previous evidence of greater SEP N60 amplitude in chronic schizophrenics was confirmed here (Tables 1 and 2).  There was
thus a degree of convergence between the results yielded by the two
methods of measurement, allowing greater confidence in the topography findings than one might have if the automatically obtained
data were not available.

SEP peaks P30 and N60 provided the topographic differences
between clinical groups of greatest interest (Fig. 3).  The P30
differences were surprising to us.  Our impression from years of
recording SEPs in all kinds of subjects was that P30 distribution
was relatively constant, with maximum positivity at leads near the
postcentral gyrus hand area (C3X, C4X).  However, nearly all of our
localization experience was with bipolar leads.  While present data
for nonpsychotic patients agreed with our expectations, those for
chronic schizophrenics did not, and many controls exhibited a P30
amplitude maximum that was more posterior than anticipated, particularly in the right hemisphere (Fig. 3).

The topography results suggest that the P30 generator is more
anteriorly located in nonpsychotic patients than in chronic schizophrenics.  Although not statistically reliable, there was also a
trend for P30 to peak more anteriorly in latent than in the "other"
schizophrenics.  The explanation for the posterior distribution of
P30 in overt schizophrenics is not readily forthcoming.  Although
an anatomical difference in the orientation of the probable source
in the posterior bank of the postcentral gyrus (Goff et al., 1977)
is theoretically possible, one would be more comfortable with a

functional explanation.  The topographic differences could result
if there were multiple generators for P30 and if the relative bal-
ance of activity in these generators differed between groups.

The N60 peak is the last SEP event restricted to the contralateral hemisphere (Fig. 1); it appears to be part of the "primary"
complex, like P30.  Since N60 was also distributed more posteriorly
in chronic schizophrenics than in nonpsychotics or normals (Fig. 3),
one may ask to what extent P30 and N60 may reflect the same process.
They are probably independent events; their spatial distributions
differ (Goff et al., 1977), and we found low correlations between
our P30 and N60 measurements.  Furthermore although P30 tended to
be posteriorly located in the "other" schizophrenic group, that
group differed from chronic schizophrenics with respect to N60
(Shagass et al., 1977).  This suggests that the diagnostic correlates of P30 and N60 topography are not identical and that there
may be some specificity.  The findings for psychotic depressives,
which revealed no differences from normal in P30 and N60 topography,
provide additional evidence favoring diagnostic specificity for the
deviant distributions of these peaks.

The results indicating that both P30 and N60 are more posteriorly distributed in chronic schizophrenia may be related to the
findings provided by measurements of regional cerebral blood flow
(RCBF).  Ingvar and Franzen (1974), using intracarotid radioactive
isotope injection, and Jacquy et al. (1976), using rheoencephalography, both reported that RCBF was reduced anteriorly and increased
posteriorly in chronic schizophrenics.  The higher posterior lead
amplitudes of P30 and N60 in chronic schizophrenics may thus be
paralleled by increased RCBF.  This apparent correlation requires
experimental confirmation.  If one accepts Ingvar's (1975) interpretation of the RCBF differences as indicative of a functional
disorder, confirmation of a correlation between RCBF and EP distributions would tend to favor the functional rather than anatomical
interpretation of deviant EP topography.

The distributions of SEP peak P90 are of interest in relation
to the report by Goff et al. (1977) that this peak (designated by
them as P100) appears to consist of a frontal myogenic fraction
and a posterior neurogenic fraction.  The rather complex distribution patterns found for P90 (Figs. 4 and 5) seem congruent with the
idea of two generators and suggest that both the myogenic and neurogenic fractions could have contributed to differences between groups
in P90 topography.

The diagnosis by lead interactions found for several later
peaks such as SEP N130 (Fig. 4) pose an interpretive problem, as
they seem due mainly to low amplitudes at or near the vertex in
schizophrenics rather than to clear distribution differences.  The
statistical topographic effects for these peaks may thus be "artifi-

facts" of amplitude differences. In contrast, the results for VEP peak P300 (Fig. 6) represent a true group difference in spatial distribution. The greatest amplitude of VEP P300 occurred at vertex in controls and at Oz in nonpsychotics and schizophrenics, indicating a more posterior midline distribution in the patients.

Finally, it should be emphasized that this is an initial study and that the specific results require confirmation. However, they indicate that the topographic dimension of EPs merits further investigation.

## SUMMARY

This study attempted to determine whether the spatial distributions of somatosensory, visual and auditory EPs differ in relation to psychiatric illness. EPs to intermingled left and right median nerve shocks, checkerboard pattern flashes and binaural clicks were recorded from one EOG lead and fourteen scalp leads in undrugged psychiatric patients and nonpatients. Various age and sex matched clinical groups were compared. To assess topographic differences consecutive peaks in EPs of each type were first detected by visual inspection (cursor program) of certain key leads, and the latencies of the peaks for each subject were then used to measure automatically the amplitudes of events at these times in all leads. To assess group differences in topography, amplitude measurements across leads were subjected to multivariate file analysis. The largest number of topographic differences involved comparisons between chronic schizophrenics, nonpsychotic patients and nonpatients. The distributions of SEP peaks P30, N60, P90, N130 and P180 differed between groups, P30 and N60 being maximal at more posterior locations in the schizophrenics. P300 in the VEP was maximum at the vertex in controls and near Oz in both nonpsychotic and schizophrenic patients.

## ACKNOWLEDGEMENTS

This research was supported in part by USPHS Grant MH12507. We thank the following for their assistance: S. Dinsmore, I.C. Hung, J. Kline, A. McGrath, A. McLean, T. McLean, W. Nixon, J. Pressman, S. Slepner.

## REFERENCES

Buchsbaum, M., Post, R. and Bunney, W.E., Jr. Average evoked responses in a rapidly cycling manic-depressive patient. Biol. Psychiat., 1977, 12, 83-99.

Feighner, J.P., Robins, E., Guze S.B., Woodruff, R.A., Winokur, G. and Munoz, R. Diagnostic criteria for use in psychiatric research. Arch. Gen. Psychiat., 1972, 26, 57-63.

Goff, G.D., Matsumiya, Y., Allison, T. and Goff, W.R. The scalp topography of human somatosensory and auditory evoked potentials. Electroenceph. Clin. Neurophysiol., 1977, 42, 57-76.

Hoch, P. and Polatin, P. Pseudoneurotic forms of schizophrenia. Psychiat. Quart., 1949, 23, 248-276.

Ingvar, D.H. Brain work in presenile dementia and in chronic schizophrenia. In D.H. Ingvar and N.A. Lassen (Eds.) Brain Work: The Coupling of Function, Metabolism and Blood Flow in the Brain, Munksgaard: Copenhagen, 1975.

Ingvar, D.H. and Franzen, G. Distribution of cerebral activity in chronic schizophrenia. Lancet, 1974, ii, 1484-1485.

Jacquy, J., Wilmotte, J., Piraux, A. and Noel, G. Cerebral blood flow patterns studied by rheoencephalography in schizophrenia. Neuropsychobiology, 1976, 2, 94-103.

Morrison, D.F. Multivariate Statistical Methods, McGraw-Hill: New York, 1967.

Perris, C. Averaged evoked responses (AER) in patients with affective disorders. Acta Psychiat. Scand., 1974 Suppl., 89-98.

Rodin, E., Grisell, J. and Gottlieb, J. Some electrographic differences between chronic schizophrenic patients and normal subjects. In J. Wortis (Ed.), Recent Advances in Biological Psychiatry, Vol X., Plenum Press: New York, 1968.

Roemer, R.A., Shagass, C. Straumanis, J.J. and Amadeo, M. Pattern evoked potential measurements suggesting lateralized hemispheric dysfunction in chronic schizophrenics. Biol. Psychiat., 1978, 13, 185-202.

Shagass, C., Roemer, R.A., Straumanis, J.J. and Amadeo, M. Evoked potential correlates of psychosis. Biol. Psychiat., 1978, 13, 163-184.

Shagass, C., Straumanis, J.J., Jr., Roemer, R.A. and Amadeo, M. Evoked potentials of schizophrenics in several sensory modalities. Biol. Psychiat., 1977, 12, 221-235.

CONTRAST EVOKED POTENTIALS AND PSYCHOPHYSICS IN MULTIPLE SCLEROSIS

PATIENTS

H. Spekreijse, A.L. Duwaer and F.E. Posthumus Meyjes

Netherlands Ophthalmic Research Institute and
Department of Neurology, Wilhelmina Gasthuis, Amsterdam;
Laboratory of Medical Physics, University of Amsterdam

Visual evoked potentials (VEPs) have become widely accepted in recent years in diagnostic schemes for the assessment of multiple sclerosis (MS). It has been shown that for this purpose a deviation in latency is a better criterion than a deviation in amplitude, since amplitude varies widely among subjects, whereas EP latency, especially with contrast stimulation, remains restricted to a rather narrow range. The latency of the EP to stimulation with a reversing checkerboard pattern appears to be increased in 268 out of 393 (= 68%) MS patients (Halliday et al., 1973: 49/51 = 96%; Asselman et al., 1975: 34/51 = 61%; Mastaglia et al., 1976: 34/68 = 50%; Regan et al., 1976: 6/13 = 46%; Lowitsch et al., 1976: 98/135 = 73%; Hennerici et al., 1977: 35/57 = 61%; Duwaer and Spekreijse, 1978: 12/18 = 67%). However, latency increases are not specific for multiple sclerosis since they have also been observed in patients with a variety of other pathologies (Assesman et al., 1975; Halliday et al., 1976). Furthermore, an increased EP latency cannot always be ascribed to an increased conductance time due to demyelination of the optic nerve fibers since a variety of modifications in the stimulus situation - modifications which might also be induced by the presence of pathologies in the subject - may result in an increased EP latency (Duwaer and Spekreijse, 1978). Some examples are given in Fig. 1.

The responses in Fig. 1A show that nonoptimal optical correction can increase the latency of the contrast EP without affecting the shape of the response. This condition mimics what may happen in subjects with lower visual acuity. Furthermore, a reduction of contrast (Fig. 1B) or reduction of the mean luminance level of the checkerboard pattern (Fig. 1C) - conditions which both may simulate

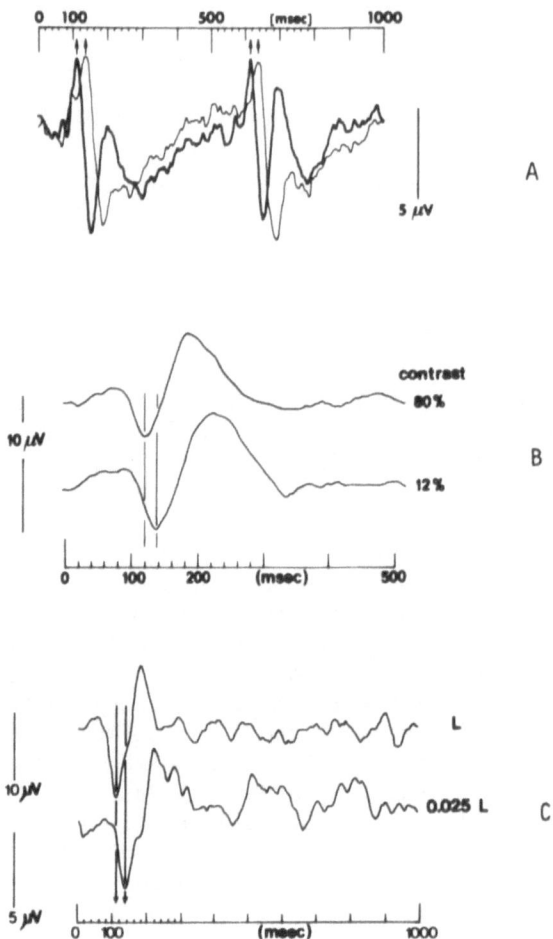

Fig. 1.   Examples of peak latency increases and broadening of the
contrast EP by manipulation of stimulus parameters.   A:   Transient
(inion-vertex) EPs to pattern reversal (mean luminance 150 asb) in
a healthy emmetropic subject with (thin line) and without (heavy
line) a cylindrical lens of +3D inserted to blur the horizontal
edges of the checks.   The binocularly presented checkerboard with
15' checks and 80% contrast reversed with a repetition period of
500 msec.   Although the shapes of the responses are rather similar,
the latency appears to increase by 25 msec when the lens is inserted.
B:   Transient (inion-vertex) EPs of a healthy subject to the appearance of a checkerboard (mean luminance 150 asb) with 10' checks at
80% contrast (upper trace) and 12% contrast (lower trace).   The
checks were presented for 40 msec with a repetition period of 520
msec.   The EP obtained at 12% contrast has an 18 msec longer latency
than the EP obtained at 80% contrast.   C:   Transient (inion-vertex)
EPs of a healthy subject to the appearance of a checkerboard with

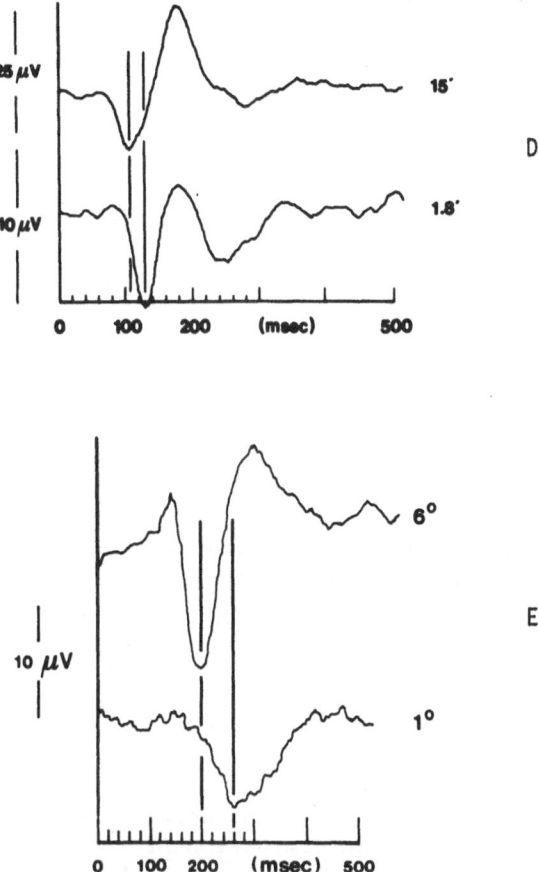

20' checks at 80% contrast and a mean luminance of 200 asb (upper
trace) and 5 asb (lower trace), respectively. The checks were presented monocularly once per sec for 40 msec. The low luminance
contrast EP has a 25 msec longer latency. D: Transient (inion-
vertex) EPs to the appearance of a monocularly presented checkerboard of 80% contrast and checks of 15' (upper trace) and 1.8' (lower
trace), respectively. The pattern with a mean luminance of 150 asb
was presented for 40 msec with a repetition period of 520 msec. The
EP to 15' check presentation has a 20 msec longer latency than the
EP obtained with 1.8' checks. E: Transient (inion-vertex) EPs to
the appearance of a checkerboard pattern with checks of 15' and 10%
contrast. The checkerboard with a mean luminance of 2000 asb was
presented for 250 msec with a repetition period of 500 msec. The
peak latency of the EP obtained with a stimulus field diameter of
$1^{o}$ has a 40 msec longer peak latency than the $6^{o}$ field diameter EP.
Note the broadening of the response with reduction of stimulus field
diameter.

lowered sensitivity - can result in latency increases of the same
order as in positive classification of MS patients.  The same happens
when check size (Fig. 1D) is reduced, a simulation of the situation
in amblyopes since mean receptive field diameter varies with eccentricity.  Finally, reduction of stimulus field size, simulating
visual field defects (Fig. 1E), can cause broadening of the waveform
of the contrast EP and a substantial increase of its peak latency.
These examples illustrate directly that there can be many causes for
the increase of the contrast EP latency and/or broadening of the
waveform of the response.  Although it cannot be said beforehand
whether, in the presence of pathologies in the visual system, broadening of the response or solely a shift in latency will occur, it is
our finding that near psychophysical threshold broadening of the
response nearly always predominates.

     Since contrast EP latency increases can apparently be due to
many causes, it might be expected that part of the EP latency
increase in MS patients can be attributed to causes other than
increased conductance time in optic nerve fibers.  Many of these
causes can also be detected with other, nonspecific visual tests
such as acuity, static perimetry and CFF, as has, in fact, been
demonstrated by Lowitsch et al. (1976).  It has, therefore, become
important to evaluate whether contrast EPs can provide additional
information for the diagnosis of multiple sclerosis and to establish
whether contrast EP tests can be made more specific for multiple
sclerosis by considering features of the response other than latency
alone.

     In a previous paper (Duwaer and Spekreijse, 1978) we recommend-
ed, for MS diagnosis, (a) determination of the apparent latency from
the phase spectrum of the responses to checkerboard reversal at
repetition rates between 5 and 20 Hz, since in that frequency range
the failure rate was found to be minimal, and (b) investigation of
the waveform of the transient EP obtained at a low reversal rate.
In the present paper we will discuss whether the specificity of the
apparent latency data can be improved by also taking into account
the shape of the amplitude characteristic obtained with these reversal stimuli.  For this purpose, and for an evaluation of additional
information provided by EP data, psychophysical data, such as flicker
fusion curves (De Lange curves) and perimetric sensitivity profiles,
will also be considered.


                              METHODS

     A TV screen (Sony CVM-1810 E, 50 Hz) subtending $8^{\circ}$ x $6^{\circ}$ was
used to display at a mean luminance of 150 asb a black and white
checkerboard pattern of 90% contrast with checks ranging from 15'
to 55'.  The subjects were asked to fixate upon a pink square of
10', which was positioned approximately in the center of the screen.

The EPs were derived from 2 Ag-AgCl electrodes positioned on
the midline at respectively 1 cm and 10-14 cm above the inion, and
from a third electrode placed on the right mastoid.  An electrode
half way between the two midline electrodes served as patient ground.
In the text only inion-vertex recordings will be shown.  The first
mentioned electrode location is the positive one, and the polarity
convention adopted in the figures is positive upwards.  The bandwidth of the EEG amplifiers was set at 0.5 - 75 Hz; the EP latencies
and amplitudes were corrected for the phase shift and amplitude
reduction introduced by the low pass fourth order Butterworth filter
(Barr and Strout EF 14; cut-off frequency 75 Hz).  An HP-2100 computer was used to average the pattern EPs and to determine the phase
and amplitude of the first harmonic component in the EPs to checkerboard reversal.  Depending on the stimulus condition 40 to 300 EPs
were averaged; the reversal rates were fixed by the 25 Hz frame
frequency of the TV stimulator at 5.6, 6.2, 7.1, 8.3, 10.0, 12.5,
16.7 and 25 rev/sec.  The apparent latency of the EPs to pattern
reversal was calculated from the slope of the phase spectrum according to:

$$\text{apparent latency } \tau = (\frac{\text{phase difference in degrees}}{\text{frequency interval in Hz}}) \text{ x } \frac{1000}{360} \text{ msec}$$

The stimulus for the flicker fusion curves was generated by circular
fluorescent lamps.  The circular sine wave modulated stimulus field
of $1^{0}$ diameter had a mean luminance of 2000 asb and was surrounded
by a $25^{0}$ steady field of 10 times lower luminance level.  The visual
field plots of the multiple sclerosis patients were determined with
the Friedmann analyser (flash duration 300 μsec) and the Tubinger
perimeter (flash duration 500 msec).


RESULTS AND DISCUSSION

Fig. 2 presents some typical amplitude characteristics obtained
in three healthy subjects to monocular presentation of the pattern
reversal stimulus.  Note the substantial interindividual variability
in the shape of these characteristics.  To compare the amplitude
characteristics of healthy subjects and MS patients, the high frequency attenuation was determined for reversal frequencies at 8.3
and 16.7 rev/sec.  It was not possible to estimate attenuation over
a higher frequency octave since, at the highest reversal frequency
of 25 rev/sec that could be produced by our TV stimulator, only rarely could a reliable reversal EP be recorded.  Furthermore, the responses at reversal rates of 10 and 12.5 rev/sec had to unfortunately
be ignored since these responses can show substantial scatter due
to contamination by α-activity.  The attenuations determined over
the frequency octave from 8.3 to 16.7 rev/sec are presented along
the vertical axis in Fig. 3.  Along the horizontal axis in this
figure the corresponding apparent latencies, estimated over the
same frequency trajectory of the phase characteristic, are presented.

In the healthy subjects the mean apparent latency amounts to 109 +
9 msec.  Both the mean and the standard deviation of the apparent
latency are somewhat higher than reported in a previous study (105
+ 7 msec; Duwaer and Spekreijse, 1978), since the responses obtained
in the frequency trajectory from 5.6 to 8.3 rev/sec were not considered in the present study.  With the criterion that apparent
latencies can be classified as abnormal when they exceed 3 SD, i.e.,
reach a value of $\bar{\tau} + 3\alpha_{\tau}$, the EPs in sixteen out of twenty-three
MS patients were classified as deviating.  This detection rate of
70% agrees quite well with those reported in literature for non-
selected MS patients, classified according to McAlpine's criteria
(see introduction).  Inspection of Fig. 3 shows, furthermore, that
attenuation per se seems to be of no use in clinical diagnosis.
Although the scatter is substantial, the data in Fig. 3 show a relation between apparent latency and attenuation.  The regression lines
in Fig. 3 have a correlation coefficient of 0.4 (p < 0.1%, t-test)
and slopes of 0.08 dB/msec and 2.2 msec/dB, respectively.  This
significant correlation between high frequency attenuation and ap-

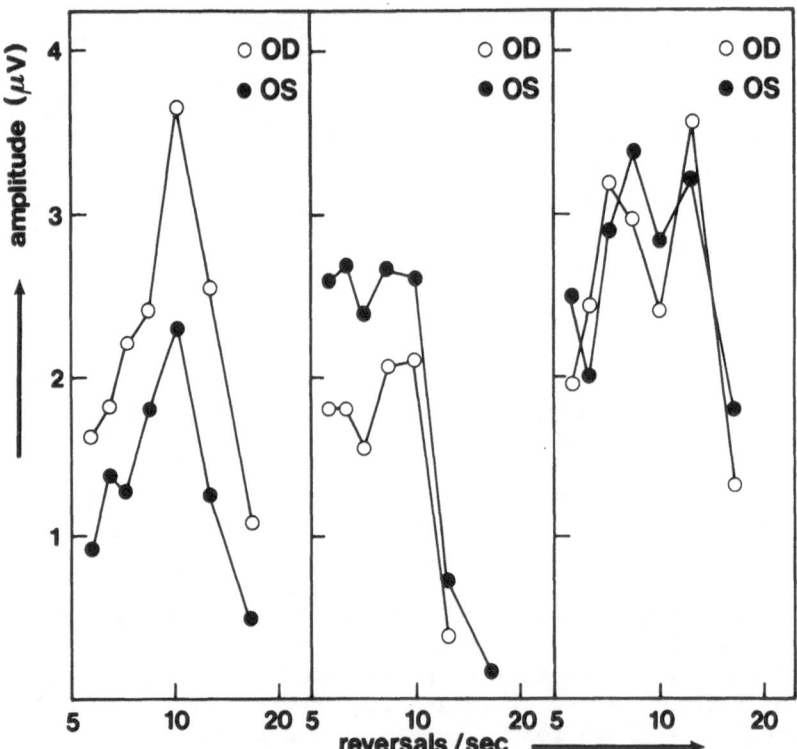

Fig. 2.  Amplitude of the first harmonic component in the inion-
vertex EP of three healthy subjects as a function of the reversal
frequency of a monocularly presented checkerboard with 20' checks
of 90% contrast.  Note the large interindividual variability.

parent latency suggests that it cannot be excluded that part of the
apparent latency increase in MS patients is due to an increase in
high frequency attenuation.  It should be noted that this can be
caused by either a lowering of the cut-off frequency and/or a steep-
ening of the high frequency slope of the amplitude characteristic.

To illustrate how profound the effect of a change in dynamics
can be on the apparent latency of the contrast reversal responses,
reversal EPs were recorded in four healthy subjects at four levels
of mean luminance, ranging from 200 asb to as low as 0.5 asb (intensity range of 2.6 log units).  These data, which are presented in
Fig. 4, show that a reduction of mean luminance level has a strong
effect on both the attenuation and the apparent latency of the reversal EP.  Since reduction of luminance results mainly in dynamical
changes at distal retinal levels, whereas the pathology in the visual
system of MS patients is most likely located in the optic nerve,
this result indicates that reduced high frequency sensitivity is not
necessarily characteristic for MS.

On the other hand, latency increases can by themselves result
in high frequency attenuation.  If by progressive demyelination the
conduction of times of those optic nerve fibers that serve as input
channels for the contrast EP vary substantially, then the steady
state EP may be attenuated and the waveform of the transient EP
broadened.  If for the sake of simplicity the assumption is made
that the conduction time across the optic nerve fibers follows a
Gaussian distribution, then the frequency components in the contrast
EP are attenuated according to:

$\exp\{-\frac{\omega^2\alpha^2}{2}\}$, in which $\alpha$ is the spread in latency in sec, and $\omega=2\pi f$

with f the frequency in Hz.  Since conduction time increases due to
demyelination of optic nerve fibers can be at most 30 msec (Ogden
and Miller, 1966; McDonald and Sears, 1969, 1970; Rasminsky and
Sears, 1972), $\alpha$ is not likely to exceed 10 msec.  With $\alpha$ = 10 msec
the high frequency attenuation over the frequency trajectory from
8.3 to 16.7 Hz is increased by a factor of only 1.5 (3.5 dB).  So,
conduction time jitter is not likely to explain the frequently observed high frequency attenuation in MS patients.  However, increase
of conduction time is not the only cause for latency jitter.  If,
for example, the overall sensitivity is reduced and hence the contrast stimulus closer to psychophysical threshold, then the waveform
of the contrast EP generally broadens by much more than 30 msec
(see for example Fig. 1E).  So, latency jitter cannot, therefore,
be excluded as a major cause of increased high frequency attenuation
in MS patients.

Due to the large interindividual variability, the shapes of
the amplitude characteristics obtained with contrast reversal cannot
be used as an interindividual criterion that will be conclusive in

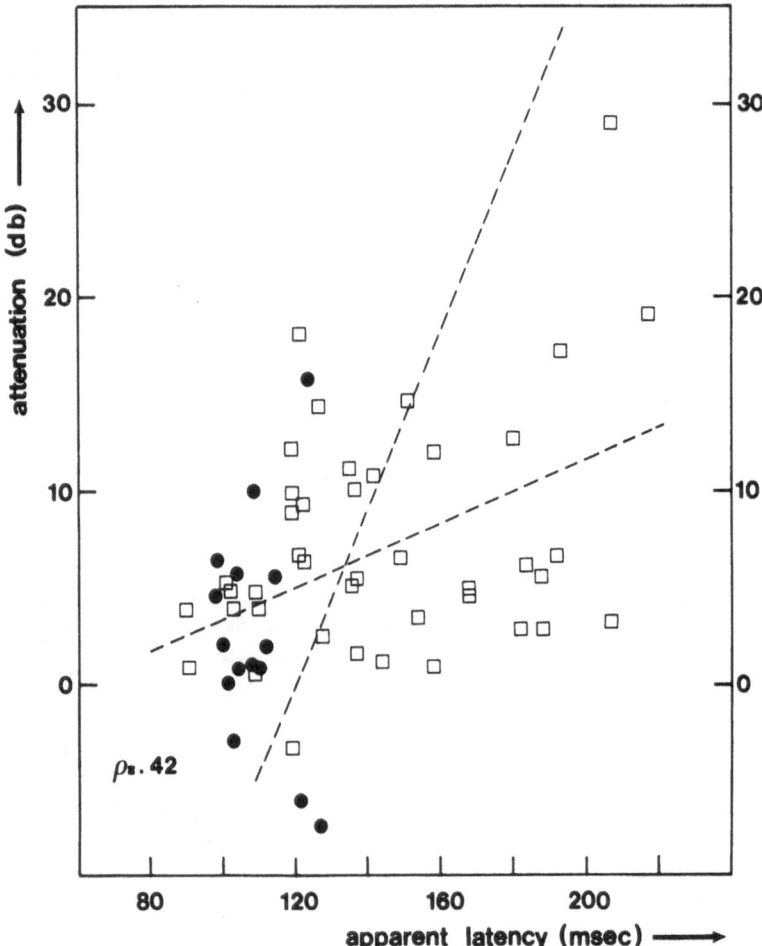

Fig. 3.  Amplitude attenuation of inion-vertex EPs to checkerboard
reversal is plotted versus the apparent latency of these EPs, which
were obtained in eight healthy subjects and twenty-three MS patients.
The monocularly presented checkerboard of 8° X 6° consisted of 20'
checks at 90% contrast.  Amplitude attenuation was calculated from
8.3 to 16.7 rev/sec according to A = 20 log A16.7/A8.3 dB, in which
A16.7 and A8.3 represent the amplitudes of the first harmonic component of the contrast EP to 16.7 and 8.3 rev/sec, respectively.
Apparent latencies were calculated from the slope of the phase
characteristic of the first harmonic component in the EP to 8.3, 10,
12.5 and 16.7 rev/sec, respectively.  The attenuation was plotted
in decibels (dB) along the vertical axis and the apparent latency in
milliseconds (msec) along the horizontal axis.  The data for healthy
subjects are indicated by filled circles; those of MS patients by
open squares.  The regression lines through all data points have
the slopes of 0.08 dB/msec and 2.2 msec/dB, respectively.  The correlation coefficient amount of 0.42 (p < 0.1%, t-test).

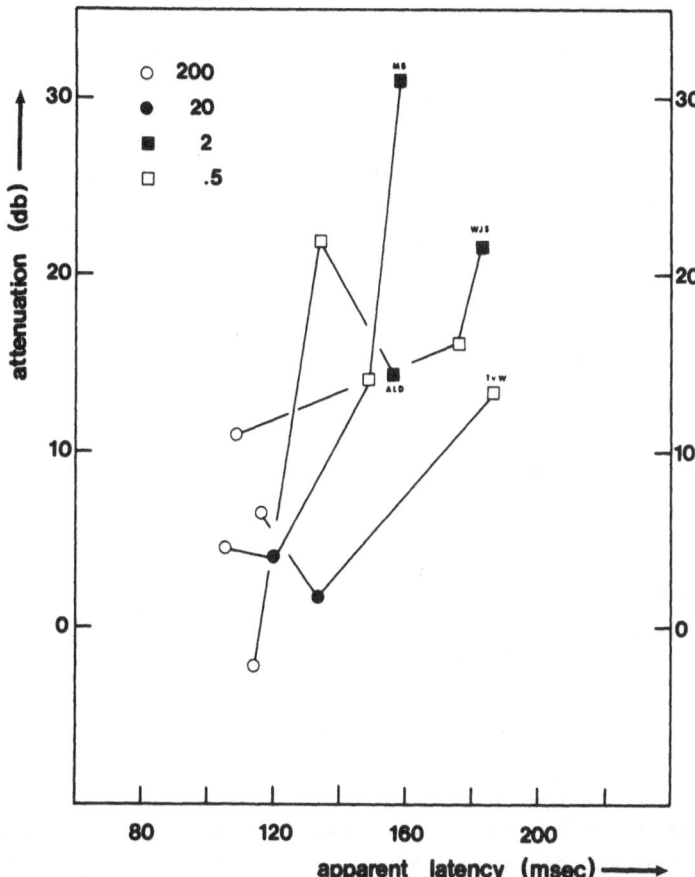

Fig. 4. High frequency amplitude attenuation of inion-vertex EPs to
checkerboard reversal is plotted versus the apparent latency of
these responses, which were recorded from four healthy subjects.
The mean luminance of the monocularly presented checkerboard (20'
checks; 90% contrast) was set at four levels of 200 asb (open circles), 20 asb (filled circles), 2 asb (filled squares) and 0.5 asb
(open squares), respectively. Throughout the experiments an arti-
ficial pupil of 3 mm diameter was used.


attributing latency increases to reduction in high frequency sensi
tivity. However, inspection of the monocular amplitude characteristics (see Fig. 2) shows that the intraindividual variability is
much weaker. So the attribution of latency increases to changes in
amplitude characteristics (and vice versa) should be inferred from
intraindividual comparison of contrast reversal characteristics.
Such an approach may become even more conclusive when psychophysical
data such as flicker fusion curves (De Lange curves) and perimetric-
ally determined sensitivity profiles are also taken into consideration.

With regard to the interpretation of the visual field profiles determined with brief flashes (the Friedmann perimeter uses flashes with a duration of 0.3 msec), it should be noted that a reduced sensitivity for these brief flashes can point to both a loss in overall sensitivity (i.e., a reduced gain irrespective of frequency) and to reduced high frequency sensitivity. On the other hand, visual field plots determined with the Tubinger perimeter will be less influenced by sole reduction of high frequency sensitivity, since the Tubinger perimeter employs flashes of 500 msec which contain less high frequencies than brief flashes. So not only can reduced high frequency sensitivity be detected by means of the flicker fusion curves but also by comparison of results obtained with the Friedmann and Tubinger perimeters.

The additional information for the diagnosis of MS that can be gained from considering not only the EP latency but also the contrast EP amplitude characteristic, flicker fusion curve and visual field profile will be exemplified by results obtained in three MS patients.

The first case is a definite MS patient according to McAlpine's criteria. Stimulation of the left eye of this patient gives a deviating flicker fusion curve (Fig. 5A). Not only is the overall sensitivity reduced by about a factor of 5, but there is also a substantial loss of high frequency sensitivity. Furthermore, the peak latency of the transient reversal EP upon stimulation of the left eye is increased (interocular latency difference of 44 msec; Fig 5B), and also the apparent latency is abnormal (interocular latency difference of 71 msec, Fig. 5C). Finally, the amplitude characteristic upon reversal stimulation of the left eye shows pronounced loss of high frequency sensitivity (interocular attenuation difference from 8.3 to 16.7 rev/sec amounts to 19 dB; Fig. 5D). From these data it is evident that the latency increase of the left eye contrast EP is at least partly due to increased high frequency attenuation. Further inspection of the flicker fusion curves reveals an interocular attenuation difference of about 3 dB in the frequency range from 4 to 8 Hz and of about 15 dB over the trajectory from 8 to 16 Hz. The latter attenuation difference is more compatible with the interocular attenuation difference of the EP amplitude characteristic than the former one. This suggests that the pathology in the visual system of this patient operates upon the reversal frequency instead of the luminance modulation frequency of the individual checks in the reversing checkerboard. Since this patient had suffered from left eye optic neuritis, the origin of the increased high frequency attenuation is most likely the optic nerve. This implies that an analysis of signal processing in the optic nerve to a reversal stimulus should be based upon the dynamics at contrast frequencies.

The second case is a definite MS patient whose right eye has an abnormal sensitivity profile with scotoma in separate segments of

the visual field (Fig. 6A).  Also the peak latencies of the right
eye transient reversal EPs are abnormal (for checks of 55' the interocular latency difference amounts to 40 msec; Fig. 6D).  However,
the apparent latencies derived from high reversal rate EPs are normal
(right eye 119 msec; left eye 121 msec; Fig. 6C), and the corresponding amplitude characteristics have the same slope (Fig. 6B).  So,
on the sole basis of apparent latency of the reversal EPs this patient would have been classified as normal.  However, inspection of
the amplitude characteristics shows that at progressively lower
reversal rates the interocular amplitude difference gradually disappears.  This suggests that the optic nerve fibers that transmit
the signals which finally result in the contrast EP can be roughly
divided into two populations: one with normal conduction time and
high frequency sensitivity and the other with increased conduction
time and reduced high frequency sensitivity.  At low reversal rates
both populations contribute to the response, resulting in a broadening of the transient contrast EP and roughly similar EP amplitudes.
At high reversal rates only the normal population initiates the
contrast EP resulting in normal apparent latency and normal high
frequency attenuation, although, of course, the amplitude of the
response is smaller.  This hypothesis is supported by the sensitivity
profile of the right eye of this patient which, indeed, shows patchy
scotomata in the central $8^0$ of the visual field, i.e., the retinal
region from which contrast EPs can be recorded.

The third case is a probable MS patient whose flicker fusion
curves (Fig. 7A) and EP amplitude characteristics (Fig. 7B) seem
rather similar for stimulation of either eye.  Yet the apparent
latencies (left eye 207 msec; right eye 188 msec; Fig. 7C) and the
peak latencies of the transient reversal EPs (left eye 177 msec;
right eye 158 msec; Fig. 7D) are quite abnormal.  So, this patient
seems to be one of the rare cases in which latency increase is not
accompanied by a loss in high frequency sensitivity.

The above results show that part of the latency increases of
the contrast EPs in multiple sclerosis patients are accompanied by
reduced sensitivity and increased high frequency attenuation.  A
latency increase of contrast EPs seems, therefore, to imply deviating results in standard methods of testing visual functioning, in
particular static perimetry.  This has been confirmed in twelve MS
patients by direct comparison of EP latency and sensitivity profiles
obtained with static perimetry.  In all patients with increased EP
latency (eight out of twelve), sensitivity appears to be reduced
in the central $10^0$ of their visual field.  In nine out of eleven
eyes with increased contrast EP latency, sensitivity was also reduced
outside the central $10^0$ region.  In one patient with normal EP
latency, sensitivity was reduced in the central $10^0$.  Comparison of
the results obtained with the Friedmann perimeter (pulse width 300
msec) and those obtained with the Tubinger perimeter (pulse width
0.5 sec) shows that in these patients abnormalities are always de-

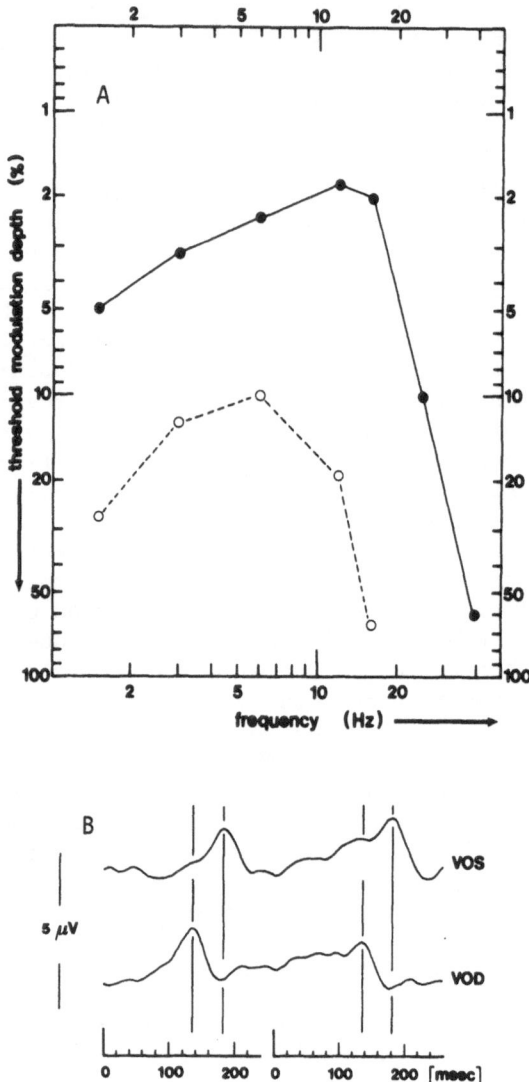

Fig. 5.  Psychophysics and electrophysiology of a definite MS patient.
A:   Threshold modulation depth is plotted as a function of the frequency of a sinusoidally modulated, homogeneously illuminated test
field with a diameter of 1° and a mean luminance of 2500 asb.   The
left eye flicker fusion curve (open circles, dashed line) has a
lower sensitivity and cut-off frequency than the "normal" right eye
curve (filled circles, solid line).   B:   Inion-vertex EPs to monocular stimulation with 20' checks at 90% contrast reversing at a rate
of 3.85 rev/sec.   The peak latency of the first positive component
in the left eye EP (upper trace) amounts to 180 msec and that of the
right eye EP is 136 msec (lower trace).   C:   Phase lag of the first
harmonic component in the inion-vertex EP as a function of the re-

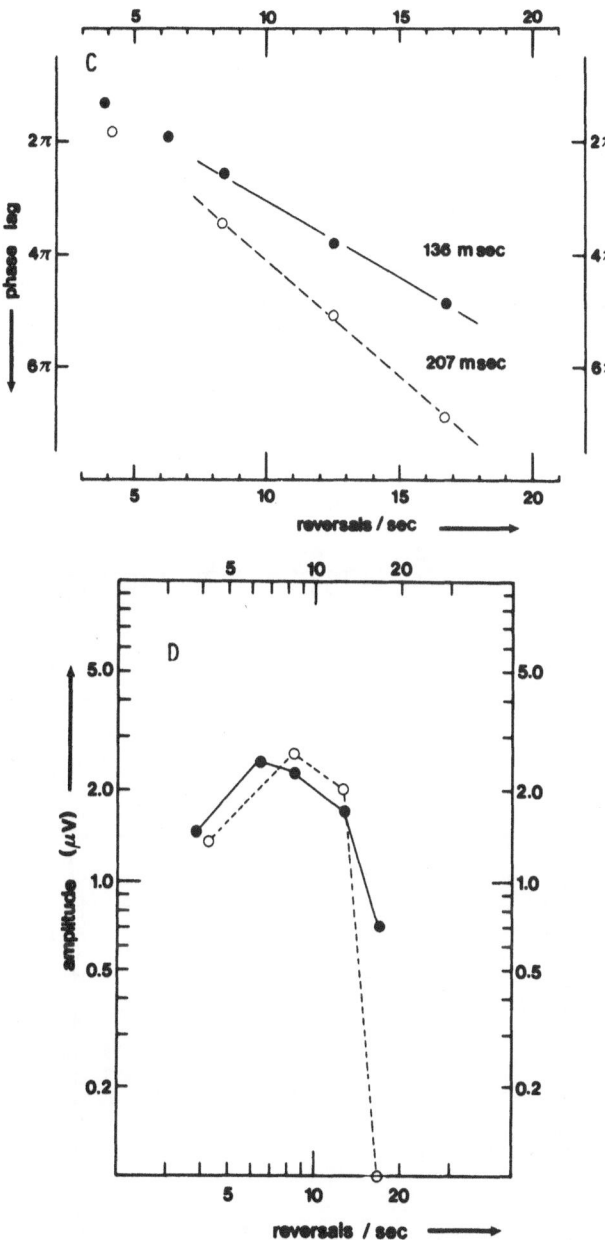

versal frequency of a monocularly presented checkerboard with 20'
checks at 90% contrast. The slope of the right eye phase characteristic (solid line) gives an apparent latency of 136 msec, that of
the left eye (dashed line) of 217 msec. D: Amplitude of the first
harmonic component of the inion-vertex EPs is plotted versus the
reversal frequency of a monocularly presented checkerboard with 20'
and 90% contrast. The amplitude attenuation between 8 3 and 16.7
rev/sec amount to 29 dB for the left eye (dashed line) and 10 dB
for the right eye (solid line).

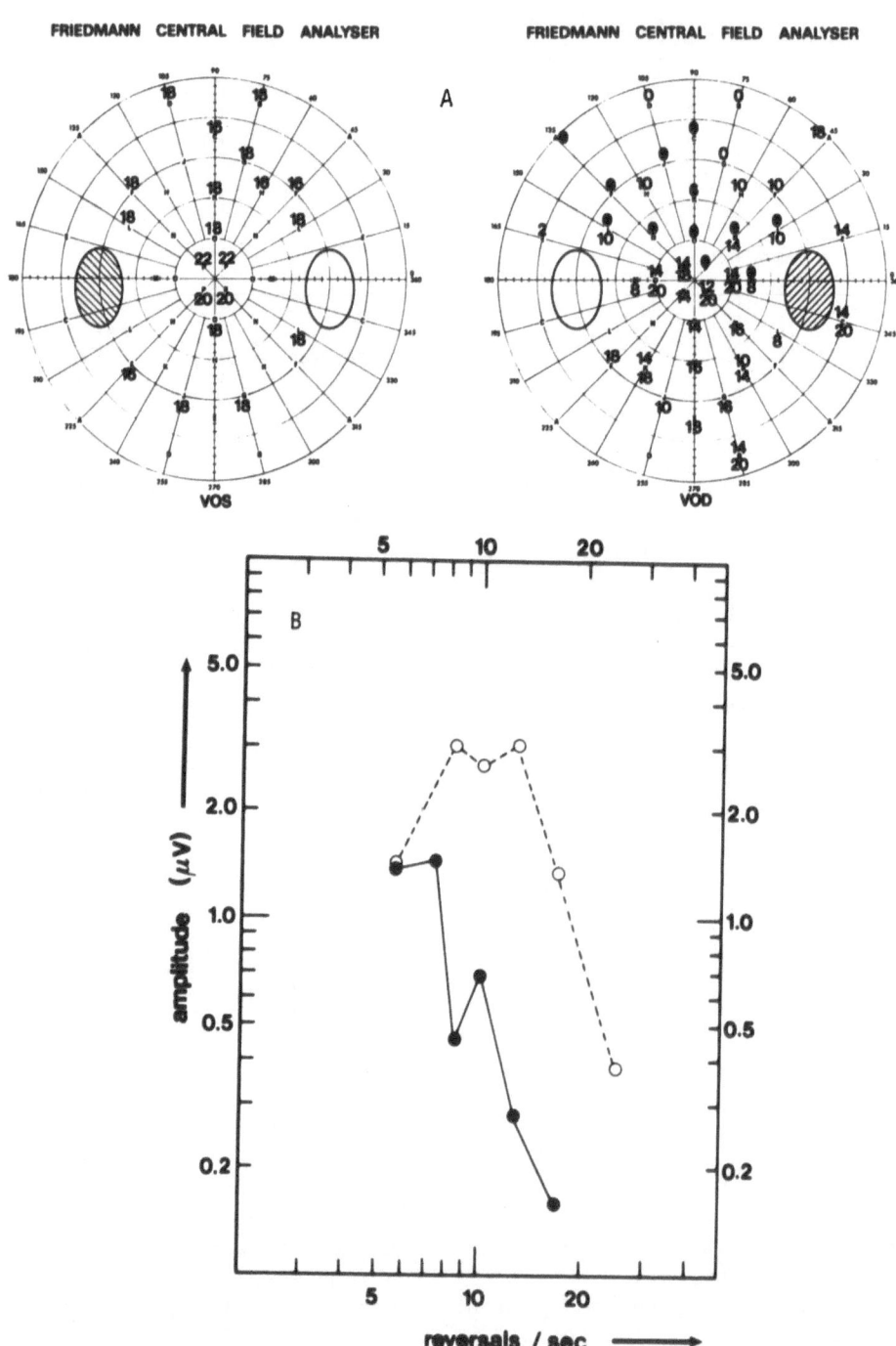

Fig. 6.  Psychophysics and electrophysiology of a definite MS patient.  A:  The visual field plots were determined with the Friedmann analyzer.  The numbers are a measure for sensitivity in log
units (e.g., 2.0, 1.8, 0.8).  B:  Amplitude characteristics of inion-
vertex EPs to monocular checkerboard reversal (stimulus conditions

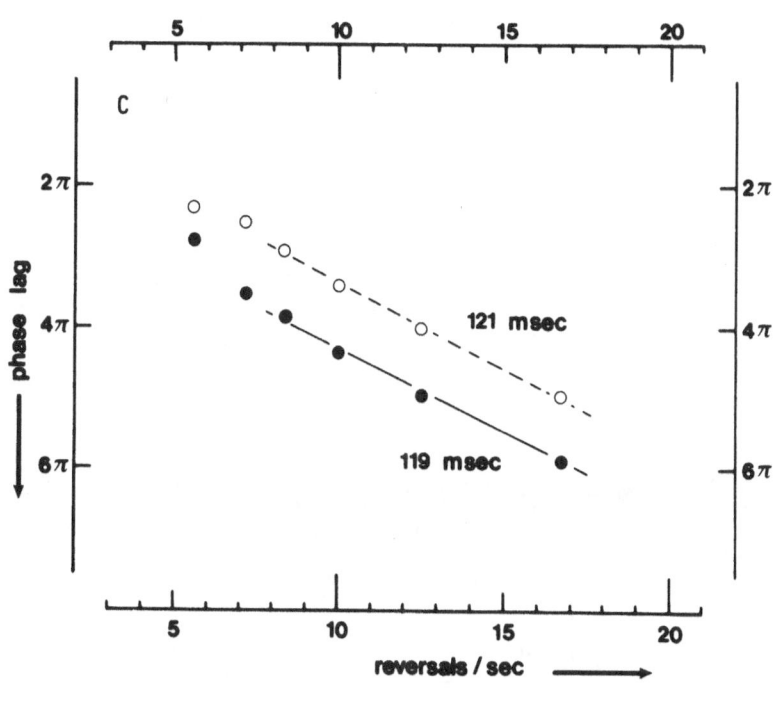

55´ checks

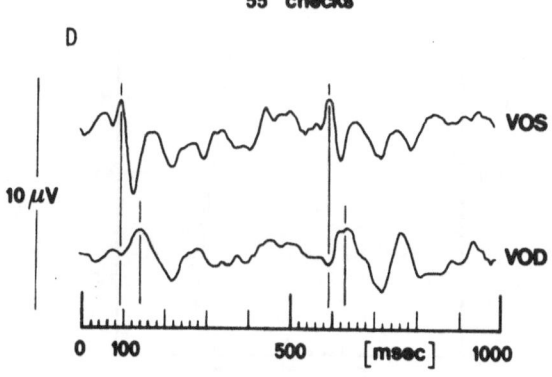

as in Fig. 5D). The amplitude attenuation between 8.3 and 16.7
rev/sec amounts to 6.3 dB and 8.9 dB for left eye and right eye,
respectively. C: Phase characteristics of inion-vertex EPs to
monocular checkerboard reversal (stimulus conditions as in Fig. 5C).
Apparent latencies amount of 119 msec and 121 msec for right and
left eye, respectively. D: Inion-vertex EPs to monocular stimulation with 55' checks at 90% contrast, reversing at a rate of 2 rev/
sec. The peak latency of the first positive component in the left
eye EP amounts to 90 msec; that of the right eye EP is 135 msec.

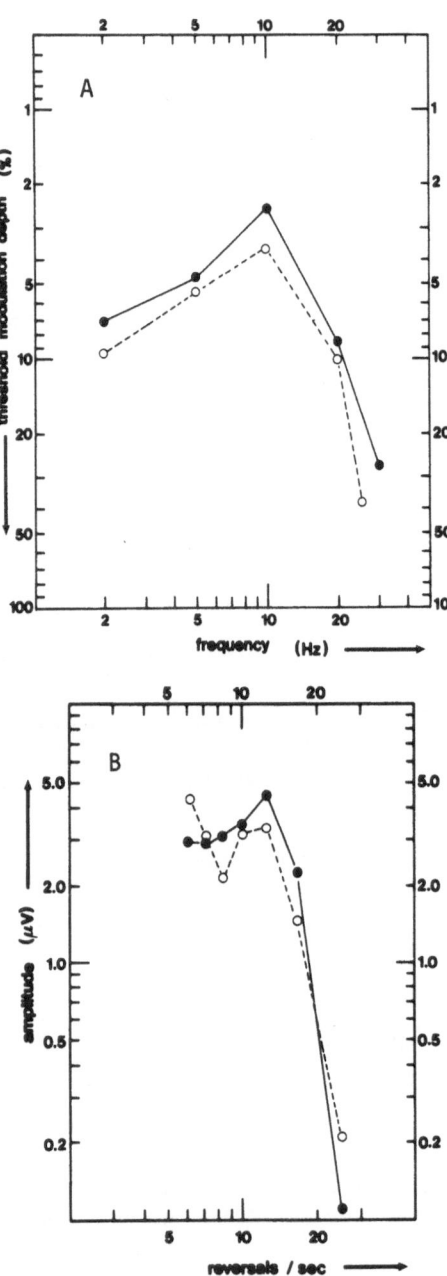

Fig. 7.   Psychophysics and electrophysiology of a probable MS patient.   A:   Flicker fusion curves to separate stimulation of right
(filled circles and solid line) and left eye (open circles and
dashed line).   For stimulus conditions, see Fig. 5A.   B:   Amplitude
characteristics of inion-vertex EPs to monocular checkerboard reversal.   For stimulus conditions, see Fig. 5D.   The amplitude attenuation between 8.3 and 16.7 rev/sec amounts to 3.3 dB and 2.9 dB
for left and right eye, respectively.   C:   Phase characteristics

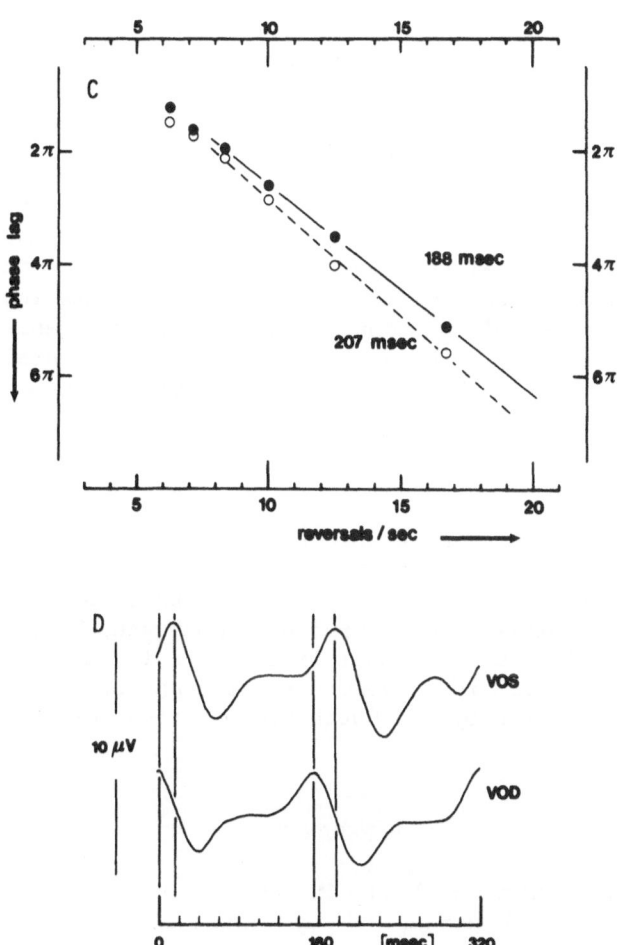

of inion-vertex EPs to monocular checkerboard reversal. For stimulus
conditions, see Fig. 5C. Apparent latencies amount to 188 msec and
207 msec for right and left eye EPs, respectively. D: Inion-vertex
EPs to monocular stimulation with 20' checks at 90% contrast, reversing at a rate of 6.25 rev/sec. The peak latency of the first positive component in the left eye EP (upper trace) amounts to 177 msec
and that of the right eye EP (lower trace) is 159 msec.

tected with both perimeters.  This suggests that for the multiple
sclerosis patients studied, increased high frequency attenuation
only rarely occurs without a reduced overall sensitivity.  Similar
results have been described by Lowitsch et al. (1976).  In their
study, sixty-four out of seventy-one MS patients with abnormalities
in Goldmann perimetry showed increased contrast EP latency.  Their
publication does not provide the combined detection rate of Friedmann and Goldmann perimetry.  Their data do show, however, that the
detection rate on the basis of contrast EP latency (98 out of 135)
is only slightly higher than the combined detection rate of other,
nonspecific methods of testing visual functioning (95 out of 135).

## SUMMARY

Our data indicate that additional information can be gained
for the diagnosis of MS by considering not only the apparent latency
of the contrast reversal EPs, but also their amplitude characteristics.  Results obtained from twenty-three MS patients indicate that
the latency increase of the contrast EP may be accompanied by increased high frequency attenuation or by a reduced overall sensitivity.  The latter has been confirmed in another group of twelve
MS patients of whom all eight with increased contrast EP latency
had a lower sensitivity in static perimetry.

## ACKNOWLEDGEMENTS

We are grateful to Dr. H.F.E. Verduyn Lunel, Eye Clinic, for
ophthalmological examinations; Mrs. H. Groothuyse, Perimetry Department, for determination of visual field plots in multiple sclerosis
patients; Dr. D. Reits for development of computer software.  This
research was supported by the Dutch Organization for Health Research
(TNO).

## REFERENCES

Asselman, P., Chadwick, D.W. and Marsden, C.D.  Visual evoked res-
     ponses in the diagnosis and management of patients suspected
     of multiple sclerosis.  Brain, 1975, 98, 261-282.

Duwaer, A.L. and Spekreijse, H.  Latency of luminance and contrast
     evoked potentials in multiple sclerosis patients.  Electroen-
     ceph. Clin. Neurophysiol., 1978, 45, 244-258.

Halliday, A.M., Halliday, E., Kriss, A., McDonald, W.I. and Mushin,
     J.  The pattern evoked potential in compression of the anterior
     visual pathways.  Brain, 1976, 99, 357-374.

Halliday, A.M., McDonald, W.I. and Mushin, J.  Visual evoked res-
     ponse in the diagnosis of multiple sclerosis.  Brit. Med. J.,
     1973, IV, 661-664.

Hennerici, M., Wenzel, D. and Freud, H.J.  The comparison of small
     size rectangle and checkerboard stimulation for the evaluation
     of delayed visual evoked responses in patients suspected of
     multiple sclerosis., Brain, 1977, 100, 119-136.

Lowitsch, K., Kuhnt, U., Sakmann, Ch., Maurer, K., Hopf, H.C.,
     Schott, D. and Tater, K.  Visual pattern evoked responses and
     blink responses in assessment of MS diagnosis.  (A clinical
     study of 135 Multiple Sclerosis patients.)  J. Neurol., 1976,
     213, 17-32.

Mastaglia, F.L., Black, J.L. and Collins, D.W.K.  Visual and spinal
     evoked potentials in diagnosis of multiple sclerosis.  Brit.
     Med. J., 1976, VI, 732.

McAlpine, E., Lumsden, C.E. and Acheson, E.D.  Multiple Sclerosis,
     Edinburgh: Livingstone, 1965.

McDonald, W.I. and Sears, T.A.  Effect of demyelination on conduc-
     tion in the central nervous system.  Nature, 1969, 221, 182-
     183.

Ogden, T.E. and Miller, R.F.  Studies of the optic nerve of the
     rhesus monkey: Nerve fiber spectrum and physiological proper-
     ties.  Vis. Res., 1966, 6  455-506.

Rasminsky, M. and Sears, T.A.  Internodal conduction in undissected
     demyelinated nerve fibers.  J. Physiol., 1972, 227, 323-350.

Regan, D., Milner, B.A. and Heron, J.R.  Delayed visual perception
     and delayed visual evoked potentials in the spinal form of
     multiple sclerosis and in retrobulbar neuritis.  Brain, 1976,
     99, 43-46.

EVENT RELATED POTENTIALS IN DEVELOPMENT, AGING AND DEMENTIA


Kenneth Squires, Douglas Goodin and Arnold Starr

University of California, Irvine

Irvine, California 92717


An abnormal response to sensory information can result from
deficits in sensory transmission, cognitive processing or response
production.  Recently it has become feasible to comprehensively
evaluate sensory transmission using event related potentials (ERPs).
With ERP techniques the functioning of the afferent pathways can
now be reliably determined, and lesions in the pathways can, in
many instances, be precisely localized (see Starr, 1978 for review).
Among neurological patients, however, the problem often lies at
one of the two remaining stages about which ERP procedures currently
in clinical use provide little information.  Among these patients,
differentiating those with real deficits in cognitive function
from those who are unable to interact with the examiner due to
motor or language deficits, or who are unwilling to cooperate, is
often a difficult and subjective task.  Direct recording of brain
activity in the form of ERPs is one way to overcome such obstacles
of communication and cooperation since it requires no overt response
on the part of the patient and only a modicum of cooperation.  Also,
since certain "endogenous" components of the ERP have been unequiv-
ocally associated with cognitive activity in a wide variety of
studies (see Donchin et al., in press, and Tueting, in press, for
reviews), it is now possible to unobtrusively monitor cognitive
activity as well as sensory function.  The purpose of the studies
described here was to determine the feasibility of utilizing the
endogenous components of the ERP as an objective measure of mental
function in neurological diseases which produce cognitive deficits.


AGE AND ERPS

In the early stages of this work it became evident that age

has significant effects on the endogenous components. Similar
observations have recently been made by others, both with respect
to aging in adults (Brent et al., 1976; Ford et al., in press;
Marsh and Thompson, 1972; Pfefferbaum et al., in press) and with
respect to development in children (Courchesne, 1977; Karrer and
Ivins, 1976; Shelburne, 1973), though age effects have not been
systematically studied across the complete lifespan.

In order to evaluate the effects of age on both the exogenous
and endogenous components of the ERP, forty-seven normal subjects
between the ages of 6 and 76 years were tested (Goodin et al., 1978).
Trains of tonal stimuli (60 dB SL) were presented through earphones.
Eighty-five percent of the tones had a frequency of 1000 Hz, and
15% had a frequency of 2000 Hz; the subjects were asked to count
the occurrences of the rare tones. ERPs were averaged separately
for the rare and frequent tones in each condition.

The ERPs of one subject are shown in Fig. 1. All waveforms
were characterized by the exogenous N1 and P2 components of the
auditory "vertex" potential. The rare tone was also associated
with a prominent endogenous P3 component, reflecting the differential cognitive processing of that tone. In Fig. 2 the rare tone

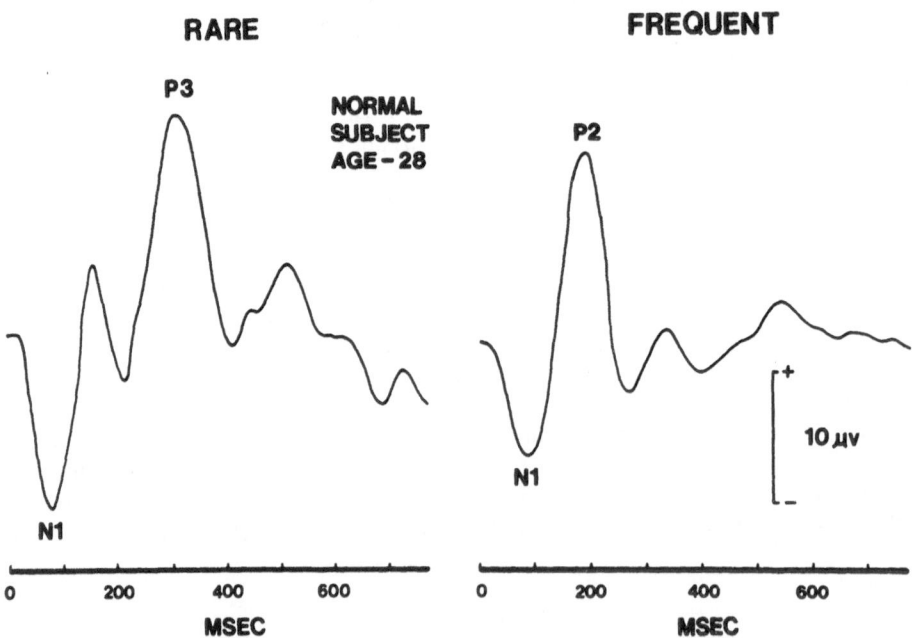

Fig. 1. ERP waveforms for one subject (Cz-linked mastoids) for
the rare and frequent tones.

waveforms are shown for six adult subjects.   These data illustrate
one of the primary results of the study.   For adults there was a
systematic shift of the P3 component to longer latencies (p < .001)
with increasing age (top to bottom).   The P3 latency for young

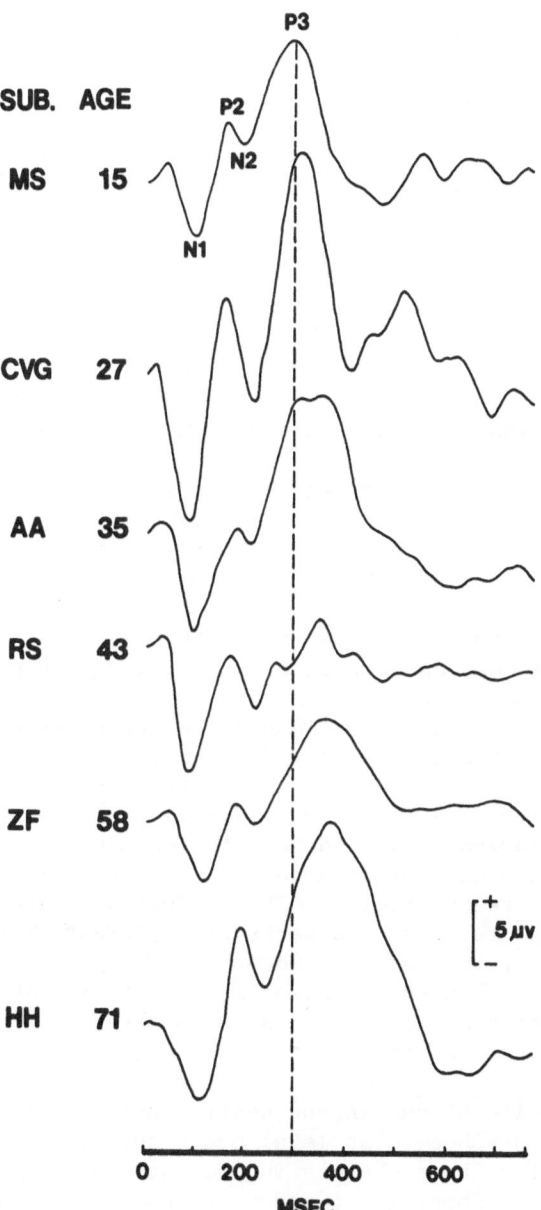

Fig. 2.   Rare tone ERPs for six subjects shown in the order of increasing age (top to bottom).

adults (15 to 20 years) was approximately 300 msec, but it increased to 400 msec or more by the seventh decade. The effects of age
on the latencies of all components are shown in Fig. 3. Significant increases in latency with increasing age were also found for
the N2 (p < .001) and P2 (p < .001) components of the ERP, though
the magnitude of the age related latency increase diminished for
successively earlier components. The N1 component, in fact, showed
only a nonsignificant trend toward longer latencies with increasing
age.

Quite a different picture of the effects of age on the latencies of ERP components emerged for the subjects between the ages of
6 and 15 years (also shown in Fig. 3). The latency of the P3 component decreased markedly with age (p < .001), as did the latency
of the N2 component (p < .05). The combined result of the developmental and aging effects on these components was that the minimum
N2 and P3 latencies were recorded from subjects in their mid- to
late teens. Developmental changes in the N1 and P2 latencies were
not significant, though such effects cannot be ruled out because
of the small number of young subjects in the study.

The increases in the N2 and P3 latencies with increasing age
in adults were paralleled by a significant (p < .01) decrease in
the peak-to-peak N2-P3 amplitude. There was also a significant
decrease (p < .05) in the N1-P2 amplitude with age in adults.

In summary, age change was found to have significant effects
on the latencies and amplitudes of the various ERP components. The
most dramatic changes were in the latencies of the endogenous N2
and P3 components. During childhood the latencies of the N2 and
P3 components decreased markedly (at a rate of 12.3 and 18.4 msec/
year, respectively). This result is consistent with those reported
by Courchesne (1977) and Shelburne (1973). The latency decreases
for N2 and P3 during childhood were followed by gradual increases
in N2 and P3 latencies with increasing age (at a rate of 0.79 and
1.64 msec/year, respectively). This effect of aging is also consistent with the results of other studies (Brent et al., 1976; Ford
et al., in press, this volume; Marsh and Thompson, 1972). The particular value of this study, however, is that a common procedure
was used to test subjects of all ages so that the biphasic nature
of the age related latency changes were clearly evident.

Numerous alterations in the central nervous system at the
tissue level and subcellular level occur over the lifespan which
might account for these changes in the latency of neural events
(see Terry and Gershon, 1976, and Ordy and Brizzee, 1975, for
reviews). Unfortunately a correlation between effects on scalp
recorded events and changes at the cellular level or even in the
cortical mantle is a step which cannot be made. It is, however,

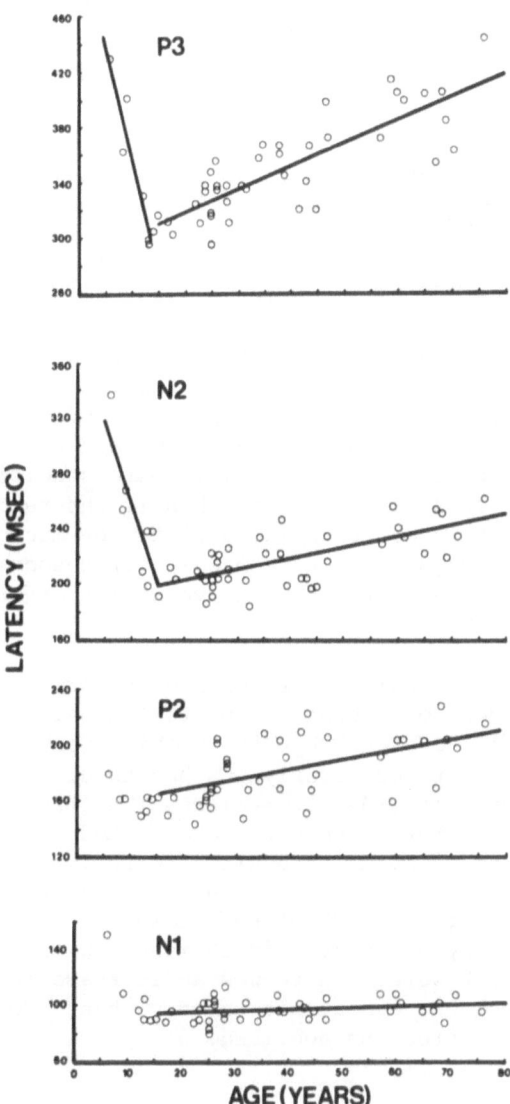

Fig. 3. Latencies of ERP components as a function of age. Regression lines were calculated separately for subjects less than and greater than 15 years of age. The N2 and P3 latencies were derived from the rare tone ERP waveform. The N1 and P2 latencies were measured from the frequent tone ERP waveform.

possible to relate the age related latency changes in the endogenous potentials to functional changes in the relative timing of cognitive processes.

Correlations between P3 latency and decision latencies, as assessed by behavioral reaction time measures, have been reported on several occasions (Kutas et al., 1977; Ritter et al., 1972; Roth et al., 1978; N. Squires et al., 1977). The extension of that relationship to the data of this study would suggest that a decrease in the speed of cognitive processes occurs with advancing age in adults. This suggestion has been made on the basis of reaction time data alone (see Botwinik, 1973, for a review), and Ford et al. (in press) have discussed the issue in relation to age related changes in both the P3 and reaction time latencies in a memory retrieval task. Choice reaction times for children are also reported to decrease with age in a manner similar to the latency decreases of the N2 and P3 potentials reported here (Hohle, 1967). Moreover, in cases where P3 and reaction time latencies are not perfectly correlated it appears that the P3 latency is more specifically related to the timing of cognitive activity than is the reaction time since the latter measure is additionally affected by many variables, only some of which are cognitive in nature (e.g., response selection) while others are related to physical variables affecting the motor pathways (Ford et al., in press).

The slowing of cognitive processing in normal aging is presumed to be independent of decreased auditory sensitivity with age (Corso, 1971). All of the subjects in this study reported that they could hear the tones clearly and had no difficulty discriminating their pitches. In order to evaluate the effects of stimulus intensity, however, three subjects were tested in a series of conditions in which the stimulus intensities were lowered in 10 dB steps. The result was that the P3 latency remained constant until the tone intensities were within 15 dB of threshold, at which time the P3 latency increased by an average of 15 msec. With the decrease in signal intensity, however, there was an increase in the N1 latency of nearly 40 msec. No comparable latency change for N1 was found as a function of increasing age (Fig. 3).

## MENTAL FUNCTION AND ERPS

Two groups of patients were tested in order to determine whether the P3 latency might be useful as an objective measure of mental function in neurological disease (Goodin et al., in press). The first group of patients consisted of thirty-two individuals ranging in age from 25 to 84 years who were diagnosed as having decreased mental functioning (dementia). Their mental function was further quantified with the Mini-Mental Exam (Folstein et al., 1975). The

diagnoses and mental status examination scores for these patients
are shown in Table I. The mean score for the demented patients was
20.7 out of the possible 30 points on the examination. For comparison normal subjects usually scored either 29 or 30 points on the
test.

The second group of patients consisted of thirty-one individuals ranging in age from 19 to 78 years with no discernible deficits
in mental function. The diagnoses and mental status scores for
this group are shown in Table II.

The testing procedure was the same as used for the normal subjects. While the task was not difficult for most subjects, some
demented patients had to be frequently reminded of the task, and
their counts were not accurate. These reminders seemed adequate
since the patients were cooperative and eager to please. From an

Table I.  Diagnoses and mental status examination scores of the
          demented patients.

|                                    | Number | MMS     | $\Delta P3(\sigma)$ |
|------------------------------------|--------|---------|----------|
| Senile and Pre-Senile Dementia     | 10     | 19.4**  | +2.58*** |
| Metabolic Encephalopathy*          | 6      | 21.5    | +3.71*** |
| Hydrocephalus                      | 6      | 21.1    | +2.93    |
| Cerebro-Vascular Disease           | 2      | 21.5    | +3.06    |
| Brain Tumor                        | 1      | 17.0    | +4.00    |
| Herpes Simplex Encephalitis        | 1      | 20.0    | -0.29    |
| Uncertain Etiology                 | 6      | 21.8**  | +4.64    |
| Mean                               | 32     | 20.7    | +3.23    |

*   Hypothyroidism, alcoholic with severe electrolyte disturbances,
    anoxia, steroid encephalopathy.

**  One patient could not be tested and is not included in the
    calculations.

*** One patient could not be assigned a P3 latency and is not
    included in the calculations.

Table 2.   Diagnoses and mental-status examination scores of the
           non-demented patients.

| | Number | MMS | ΔP3(σ) |
|---|---|---|---|
| Multiple Sclerosis | 5 | 29.0 | +0.39 |
| Depression | 5 | 28.6 | -0.36 |
| Cerebrovascular Disease | 3 | 28.7 | -0.26 |
| Parkinson's Disease | 4 | 29.5 | +0.76 |
| Schizophrenia | 3 | 27.5** | +0.50 |
| Hydrocephalus | 1 | 29.0 | -0.93 |
| Porencephalic Cyst | 1 | 30.0 | +0.83 |
| Miscellaneous* | 9 | 29.4 | +0.03*** |
| Mean | 31 | 28.8 | +0.14 |

*     Diabetic neuropathy, casalgia, bilateral subdural hematoma,
      diffuse cortical atrophy, anosmia with left arm weakness,
      gait apraxia, vertigo, Huntington's Chorea.

**    One patient could not be tested and is not included in the
      calculations.

***  One patient could not be assigned a P3 latency and is not
      included in the calculations.

operational point of view the task appeared to have the desired
effect.  Namely, it induced the patients to attend to the auditory
stimuli and elicited differential processing of the rare and frequent tones (as indicated by the presence of P3 components).

     The P3 latencies of all of the patients are shown in Fig. 4.
The data for the normal subjects (greater than age 15) tested previously are represented by regression lines and lines indicating
one and two standard deviations from normal which are superimposed
on the data for the demented patients (top) and non-demented patients (bottom panel).

It should be noted that of the fifty-nine patients tested, a reliable measure of the P3 latency was impossible for only three patients: two demented patients and one non-demented patient.  One of the demented patients would not remain still during the test. Consequently the waveforms were contaminated by muscle artifact. For the other two patients, the ERP waveform consisted of the N1

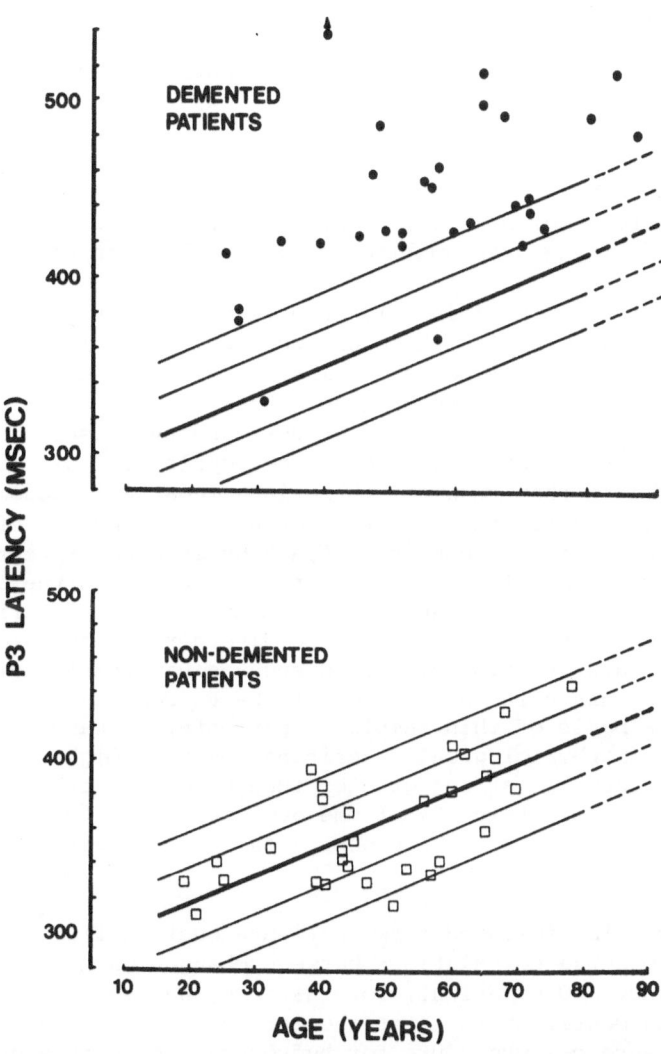

Fig. 4.  Latency of the P3 component as a function of age for demented patients (top) and non-demented patients (bottom).

and P2 potentials followed by a broad positivity between 300 and
500 msec without any clear peak.

The distribution of P3 latencies for the non-demented patients
and the normal subjects were essentially identical.  For the
demented patients, however, the P3 latencies were uniformly long
relative to normal.  The average P3 latency for the demented patients exceeded the latency derived from the normal regression line
by 3.23 standard deviation units.  Of the thirty demented patients
with definable P3 components, twenty-five (or 83%) had P3 latencies that exceeded the norm by 2 or more standard deviations.  This
occurred only once among the non-demented patients, which would be
expected on statistical grounds.  The mean P3 latency deviations
from normal for the various subgroups of patients are presented in
Tables I and II.

The amplitude of the P3 component for the demented patients
was also found to be significantly (p < .05) smaller than normal.
The mean difference, however, relative to the normal variability
of the P3 amplitude, was small compared to that for the P3 latency.

The patients tested in this study were pre-screened only to
the extent of eliminating those who were sufficiently uncooperative
to submit to testing or had gross involuntary movements which might
have interfered with the recordings.  Thus the composition of patients in the various diagnostic groups, and the results for each,
can be considered representative of the population that might be
encountered.  In that respect, there is a remarkable consistency
among the results for the demented patients, regardless of etiology.
Apparently a slowing of cognitive function is a consistent effect
of most of the dementing processes studied here.  On the other hand,
in cases where there were apparent, but not actual, deteriorations
in mental function due to psychiatric disorders (such as depression
or schizophrenia or motor disorders such as Parkinson's disease),
there was no change in the latency of the P3 component (see Table
II).  On the basis of this sample of patients, a reasonable criterion for electrophysiologically defining dementia might be a P3 latency 2 standard deviations greater than normal.  With such a
criterion, approximately 80% of the demented patients would be
correctly classified with an expected false alarm rate of about
5%.

We have also followed a few patients over sufficient periods
of time to observe correlations between changes in mental function
and P3 latency.  One patient, for instance, has shown a marked improvement in mental status over the period of a year following a
successful surgical procedure for hydrocephalus, with a corresponding shift in the P3 latency from late to within the normal range.
There have likewise been instances of a decline in mental function
associated with an increase in P3 latency, or even the disappear-

ance of the component.

There remain a number of questions regarding the five patients in this study who were clinically demented but who fell within the normal range according to the measure of P3 latency.  No consistent pattern of etiology or test scores was found that could categorize these patients.  This lack of correspondence between the test score and the electrophysiological measure probably reflects a weakness in the brief procedure for testing mental status which might be eliminated by a more comprehensive mental status test.  Clearly all aspects of mental function cannot be covered by a thirty-point test.  This was quite evident in the case of the nearly pure amnestic syndrome found in the one patient who had experienced an episode of herpes simplex encephalitis.  This patient (age 31) had a normal latency P3 component, as shown in Fig. 4 and Table I.  Quite significantly, this patient also had no difficulties with the processing of information as long as a memory component was not involved.  In such a case a speed measure of cognitive activity such as P3 latency apparently does not reveal the patient's deficit in mental function.

It should be recognized that the distinctions made here, at least for individual patients, were not possible based upon analysis of the exogenous components of the ERP.  There were no differences in the N1 or P2 amplitudes or latencies among the groups.  In many cases of dementia the sensory pathways are relatively unaffected.  In any case, it seems most reasonable to test mental function with a procedure that challenges the patient's mental capabilities and, as a result, elicits endogenous potentials.

The results of these two studies suggest a variety of applications of the endogenous ERP components to the assessment of mental function.  During childhood there is a sufficiently rapid decrease in P3 latency that relatively fine distinctions regarding the course of an individual child's development might be possible.  Such a measure could supplement the standard psychometric tests of development and may be particularly useful in difficult patients with language or motor deficits.  Some applications of similar procedures to mental retardation are discussed elsewhere in this volume (N. Squires et al.).

The procedures described here are only a first attempt to use endogenous potentials to evaluate mental function in a clinical situation.  It can reasonably be expected that more nearly optimum conditions might be found that would decrease the reliability and sensitivity of the procedure.  In addition, higher levels of mental function may be accessible for testing if linguistic stimuli, rather than simple tones, are used since normal subjects are able to categorize rare and frequent stimuli on the basis of their linguistic attributes, thus producing P3 results similar to those shown here (Kutas et al., 1977). It is thus foreseeable that a battery of tests might be developed around a common basis of rare and frequent events to evaluate successively higher cognitive functions.

## SUMMARY

The feasibility of using event related potentials to provide an objective means for assessing normal and abnormal changes in cognitive function associated with development and aging is examined. Of the numerous waveform amplitude and latency measures obtained, the latency of the P3 component (latency 300-500 msec) was found to be the most sensitive to variations in age. The shortest P3 latencies were found for subjects in their late teens with a sharp decrease in latency between ages 6 and 15 followed by a more gradual increase in latency with increasing age beyond age 15. For demented patients the P3 latency substantially exceeded the normal value for their age in more than 80% of the cases. The P3 latency recorded from the patients without dementia, however, did not differ significantly from the normal values. The latencies of the earlier, stimulus related components did not differentiate either patient group from normal.

## ACKNOWLEDGEMENTS

This research was supported by USPHS Grant NS11876.

## REFERENCES

Botwinik, J. Aging and Behavior, New York: Springer-Verlag, 1973.

Brent, G., Smith, D., Michalewski, H. and Thompson, L. Differences in evoked potentials in young and old subjects during habituation and dishabituation procedures. Psychophysiol., 1976, 14, 96-97.

Corso, J.F. Sensory processes and age effects in normal adults. J. Gerontol., 1971, 26, 90-105.

Courchesne, E. Event related brain potentials: Comparison between children and adults. Science, 1977, 147, 589-592.

Donchin, E., Ritter, W. and McCallum, W.C. Cognitive psychophysiology: The endogenous components of the ERP. In E. Callaway, P. Tueting and S. Koslow (Eds.), Event Related Brain Potentials in Man, New York: Academic Press, 1978.

Ford, J., Roth, W., Mohs, R., Hopkins IV, W. and Kopell, B.   The
    effects of age on event related potentials in a memory re-
    trieval task.   In press.

Ford et al., this volume.

Goodin, D., Squires, K. and Starr, A.   Long latency event related
    components of the auditory evoked potential in dementia.
    Brain, in press.

Goodin, D., Squires, K., Henderson, B. and Starr, A.   Age related
    variations in evoked potentials to auditory stimuli in normal
    human subjects.   Electroenceph. Clin. Neurophysiol., 1978, 44,
    447-458.

Hohle, R.   Component process latencies in reaction times of children
    and adults.   In L.P. Lipsitt and C.C. Spiker (Eds.), Advances
    in Child Development and Behavior, New York: Academic Press,
    1967.

Karrer, R. and Ivins, J.   Steady potentials accompanying perception
    and response in mentally retarded and normal children.   In R.
    Karrer (Ed.), Developmental Psychophysiology of Mental Retarda-
    tion, Springfield: Thomas, 1976.

Kutas, M., McCarthy, G. and Donchin, E.   Augmenting mental chronom-
    etry:   The P300 as a measure of stimulus evaluation.   Science,
    1977, 792-795.

Marsh, G. and Thompson, L.   Age differences in evoked potentials
    during an auditory discrimination task.   Gerontol., 1972, 12,
    44.

Ordy, J. and Brizzee, K.   Neurobiology of Aging, New York: Plenum,
    1975.

Picton, T., Hillyard, S., Krausz, H. and Galambos, R.   Human audi-
    tory evoked potentials.   I:   Evaluation of components.   Elec-
    troenceph. Clin. Neurophysiol., 1978, 36, 179-190.

Pfefferbaum, A., Ford, J.M., Roth W., Hopkins IV, W. and Kopell, B.
    Event related potential changes in healthy aged females.
    Electroenceph. Clin. Neurophysiol., in press.

Ritter, W., Simson, R. and Vaughan Jr., H.   Association cortex
    potentials and reaction time in auditory discrimination.
    Electroenceph. Clin. Neurophysiol., 1972, 33, 547-555.

Roth, W., Ford, J. and Kopell, B.   Long latency evoked potentials
    and reaction time.   Psychophysiol., 1978, 15, 17-23.

Shelburne, S.  Visual evoked repsonses to language stimuli in normal
    children.  Electroenceph. Clin. Neurophysiol., 1973, 34, 135-
    143.

Squires, N., Donchin, E., Squires, K. and Grossberg, S.  Bisensory
    stimulation:  Inferring decision related processes from the
    P300 component.  J. Exp. Psychol. HPP., 1977, 3, 299-315.

Squires, N., Galbraith, G. and Aine, C.  Event related potential
    assessment of sensory and cognitive processes in the mentally
    retarded.  This volume.

Starr, A.  Sensory evoked potentials in clinical disorders of the
    nervous system.  Ann. Rev. Neurosci., 1977, 1, 103-127.

Terry, R. and Gershon, S.  Aging III: Neurobiology of Aging, New
    York: Raven Press, 1976.

Tueting, P.  Event related potentials, cognitive events and infor-
    mation processing.  In D. Otto (Ed.), Multidisciplinary Pers-
    pectives in Event Related Potential (ERP) Research, Washington
    D.C.: U.S. Government Printing Office, in press.

# EVENT RELATED POTENTIAL ASSESSMENT OF SENSORY AND COGNITIVE

# DEFICITS IN THE MENTALLY RETARDED

N.K. Squires, G.C. Galbraith and C.J. Aine

University of California Neuropsychiatric Institute

Pomona, California 91766

The application of event related potential (ERP) techniques to the mentally retarded presents a somewhat different challenge to the electrophysiologist than does the application of ERPs to other clinical populations. In particular, while differential diagnosis is of major interest in the investigation of such problems as minimal brain damage (MBD), schizophrenia and dementia, diagnosis is of less importance in mental retardation. What is important is to differentiate among the different types of information processing deficits occurring in the retarded so that educational remediation may be designed on an individual basis to compensate for sensory and intellectual inadequacies.

Recent advances in our understanding of the determinants of the human ERP suggest that electrophysiological techniques may be useful in untangling the web of cognitive and perceptual problems exhibited in the retarded population. The ERP consists of a series of components that reflect the successive activation of different neural generators. Some of these components, such as the auditory far field response, are primarily sensitive to variations in stimulus parameters and have thus been labeled "exogenous" components. These components have proven to be well suited for the assessment of basic sensory function (e.g., Picton et al., 1977) and in the identification of localized brain lesions (Sohmer et al., 1974; Starr and Hamilton, 1976; Sohmer and Student, 1978). Other components, termed "endogenous", have been shown to depend primarily on the meaning the stimuli have for an individual (Tueting, in press; Donchin et al., in press). Experimental studies in normal adults suggest that the endogenous components may be useful in the assessment of attention, memory and perception.

The major advantage ERP techniques have over more traditional methods of assessing mental functions in the retarded is twofold. First, since retarded individuals are likely to suffer from multiple deficiencies, including problems of motor control, it is difficult to identify a behavioral deficit with a particular processing stage. Most ERP components are independent of motor output variables and, within certain broad limits, are also independent of each other, making it possible to tap into single information processing stages. Second, since problems with speech reception and production are almost universal in the retarded, traditional testing techniques which rely heavily on verbal instruction and verbal report are unsuitable while ERP measurement requires only a minimum of verbal interaction.

In our laboratory we are investigating a variety of ERP components in the severely and profoundly retarded in order to develop a battery of ERP assessment techniques that may be useful in evaluating a broad range of sensory and cognitive functions in the retarded. Two of those experiments will be reported here.

### EXPERIMENT I:  BRAIN STEM AND CORTICAL ERPS TO MONAURAL AND BINAURAL AUDITORY STIMULATION

The first seven vertex positive waves of the human auditory evoked response occur within 10 msec following a brief auditory stimulus (Sohmer and Feinmesser, 1967; Jewett et al., 1970; Jewett and Williston, 1971). The evidence increasingly supports the conclusion that these waves reflect the activation of successive brain stem auditory nuclei (Jewett, 1970; Lev and Sohmer, 1972; Buchwald and Huang, 1975). Since brain stem structures have been implicated in retardation on both neuroanatomical and neurological grounds, abnormalities in these potentials in retarded individuals might be useful in localizing their problems to particular brain locations. The current experiment sought to make this comparison under conditions in which the potentials would be likely to reflect a fundamental aspect of auditory information processing, the integration of binaural information.

Interactions in the acoustic input from the two ears have been demonstrated at widespread levels of the brain stem auditory pathway, including the superior olive (e.g., Galambos et al., 1959) and the inferior collicullus (e.g., Erulkar, 1959). At each level these interactions may be either excitatory or inhibitory. Recent evidence suggests that binaural auditory experience early in life is essential for the development of normal binaural processing in the rat (Silverman and Clopton, 1977; Clopton and Silverman, 1977). On the basis of the latter data, the retarded might be expected to have a higher incidence of acquired as well as congenital defects of binaural processing.

Two experiments in the cat (Jewett, 1970; Huang and Buchwald,
1978) have reported indications of binaural interactions in the
surface recorded potentials.  In both cases the amplitude of wave IV
was reduced during simultaneous stimulation of both ears compared
to the algebraic summation of the potentials to left and right ears
when stimulated separately.


## Method

Seventeen institutionalized Down's syndrome individuals were
brought to the laboratory for evoked response assessment.  Four
proved uncooperative, and two were subsequently deleted from the
study due to probable left/right hearing asymmetries (defined as a
wave V latency difference greater than .5 msec between the two ears)
This left eleven subjects with usable data.  The mean age of the
Down's syndrome subjects was 28 years (range 21-38), and their mean
IQ was 28 (range 9-64).

Twenty-two control subjects also participated.  Two gave brain
stem recordings of unacceptable quality and one was rejected on the
basis of left/right hearing asymmetry.  The control group thus consisted of nineteen individuals drawn from UCLA students, hospital
staff and volunteers.  Their mean age was 28 (range 16-56).

Clicks (0.1 msec duration, 65 dB HL) were delivered through
TDH-39 headphones.  Stimulus repetition rate was 1/sec for the cortical ERPs and 20/sec for the brain stem ERPs.  Blocks of 128 (cortical) or 2048 (brain stem) stimuli were delivered to left, right or
both ears.  With the exception of one Down's syndrome individual,
it was possible to complete two repetitions of each stimulus condition.  The EEG was recorded from a vertex electrode referred to the
left mastoid.  The ground electrode was on the forehead.  Interelectrode resistance was generally below 5K Ohms.  EEG signals were
conditioned by Grass P511 amplifiers.  Cortical EEG activity from
1-100 Hz (3 dB down) was amplified with a gain factor of 50K; brain
stem activity between 30 and 3 K Hz was amplified by 200 K.  During
the recording the subjects reclined on a bed located inside a sound
attenuating room.  An attendant remained with hospital residents at
all times.  Signals were averaged on line by means of a Nicolet 1170
computer.  An averaging epoch of 500 msec was used for cortical recordings and an epoch of 10 msec for the brain stem recordings.

The main comparisons between the ERPs in the binaural condition and the sum of the ERPs in the monaural left and monaural right
conditions (L + R).  Latencies were measured for the N1, P2 and N2
components of the cortical response and for waves I-VI of the brain
stem response.  Waves IV and V were frequently difficult to separate
so the IV-V "complex" was considered as one component.  Amplitudes

were obtained for N1-P2 and P2-N2 of the cortical response. Amplitudes of the brain stem responses were measured from the peak waves
I, II, III and IV-V to the immediately following trough, from the
trough following wave III to the peak of IV-V and from the trough between waves V and VI to the peak of wave VI    Average values for the
two replicates were analyzed by means of a 2 X 2 (retarded vs. nonretarded X binaural vs. monaural) repeated measures analysis of
variance computed separately for each component and independent t-
tests.


## Results

       The waveforms of one normal subject are shown in Fig. 1 for the
short latency (A) and long latency (B) potentials.  As illustrated
here, certain components in each latency region were smaller in
amplitude in the binaural than in the summed monaural conditions.
Table I compares the mean amplitudes for each peak in the binaural
and monaural conditions (upward arrows code amplitude measurements
from trough to peak, downward arrows from peak to trough).  The brain
stem potentials showed a significant within-subjects effect ($F$ =
30.29, df = 1, 28, $p < .01$) for the amplitude measured from the
trough following wave III to the peak of wave IV-V.  Similar patterns
were observed for the N1-P2 ($F$ = 31.39) and P2-N2 ($F$ = 43.79) amplitudes.  In no case was there a significant group X condition interaction.  Hence the normal and Down's syndrome groups showed similar
patterns of larger ERP amplitudes for the left-plus-right than for
the binaural stimulation.  Also shown in Table I is the percentage
increase of (L + R)/B for each ERP component.  Overall, cortical
ERPs show larger increases than brain stem ERPs.

       Table II compares the peak latencies and amplitudes of the two
groups under binaural stimulation.  All the brain stem potentials
had shorter latencies in the Down's syndrome group but the differences were significant only for waves II ($p < .05$) and III ($p < 01$).
The cortical data, however, showed significantly longer N1 latencies
for the Down's syndrome group ($p < .05$).  The amplitudes of the retarded subjects were smaller for waves II ($p < .05$).  The amplitudes
of the retarded subjects were smaller for waves II ($p < .01$), III
($p < .01$) and V ($p < .05$).


## Discussion of Experiment I

       The comparison of the groups under binaural stimulation showed
that the Down's syndrome individuals had brain stem latencies for
waves I and II that were significantly shorter than the normal group.
In addition, the Down's syndrome subjects had significantly smaller
brain stem amplitudes for waves II, III and IV-V.  These results are

TABLE I.   COMPARISON OF BINAURAL AND LEFT

PLUS RIGHT AMPLITUDES (in μV)

|  | I↓ | II↓ | III↓ | ↑V** | V↓ | ↑VI | $N_1-P_2$** | $P_2-N_2$** |
|---|---|---|---|---|---|---|---|---|
| NORMALS: B | .19 | .12 | .27 | .76 | .83 | .15 | 2.26 | 2.95 |
| L + R | .18 | .12 | .30 | .91 | .89 | .22 | 3.40 | 4.32 |
| % (L + R)/B | (−5) | (0) | (+11) | (+20) | (+7) | (+47) | (+50) | (+46) |
| DOWN'S: B | .17 | .05 | .13 | .62 | .77 | .12 | 2.38 | 3.04 |
| L + R | .13 | .05 | .14 | .72 | .80 | .14 | 3.67 | 4.49 |
| % (L + R)/B | (−24) | (0) | (+8) | (+16) | (+4) | (+17) | (+54) | (+48) |

TABLE II.   COMPARISON OF BINAURAL ERPs FOR NORMAL (N=19)
AND DOWN'S SYNDROME (N=11) SUBJECTS.

A.   LATENCY (in msec)

|  | I | II* | III** | V | VI | $N_1$* | $P_2$ | $N_2$ |
|---|---|---|---|---|---|---|---|---|
| NORMALS | 1.77 | 2.93 | 3.90 | 5.86 | 7.50 | 87.6 | 151.0 | 248.9 |
| DOWN'S | 1.67 | 2.79 | 3.69 | 5.69 | 7.30 | 101.4 | 161.4 | 250.9 |

B.   AMPLITUDE (in μV)

|  | I↓ | II↓** | III↓** | ↑V* | V↓ | ↑VI | $N_1-P_2$ | $P_2-N_2$ |
|---|---|---|---|---|---|---|---|---|
| NORMALS | .19 | .12 | .27 | .76 | .83 | .15 | 2.26 | 2.95 |
| DOWN'S | .17 | .05 | .13 | .62 | .77 | .12 | 2.38 | 3.04 |

* p< .05

**p< .01

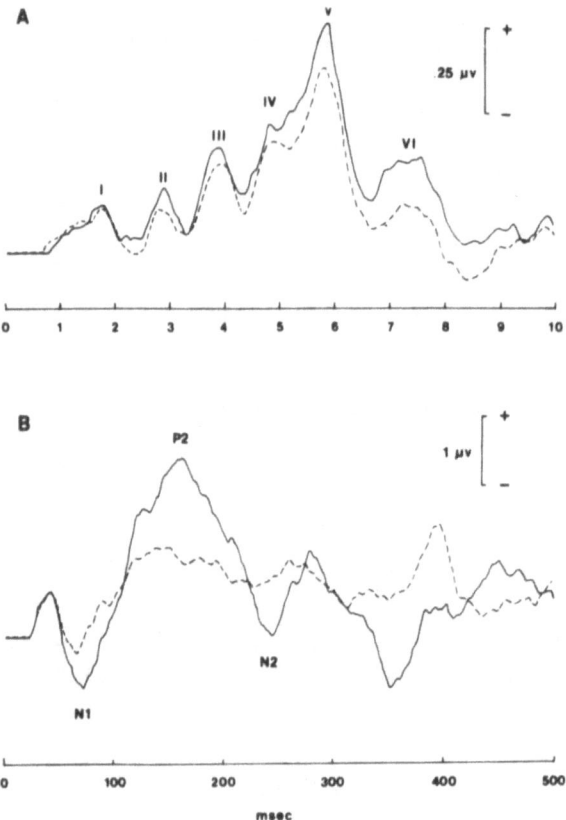

Fig. 1.  Auditory evoked response of one normal subject to binaural
(dashed line) and L + R monaural (solid line) stimuli.  A.  Short
latency brain stem ERP.  B.  Long latency ERP.

similar to findings reported previously in our laboratory (Galbraith
et al., in press), although in the present study significant effects
were found for fewer waves.

The cortical ERPs showed a significantly longer N1 latency in
the Down's syndrome group but no differences in amplitude.  Several
studies have previously reported longer evoked response latencies in
Down's syndrome individuals (Bigum et al., 1970; Marcus, 1970; Gliddon et al., 1975).  However, studies of Down's syndrome subjects also
typically report significantly larger amplitudes as well (Barnet and
Lodge, 1967; Bigum et al., 1970).  Gliddon et al. (1975) showed that
large evoked response amplitudes in Down's syndrome individuals occur
primarily at higher stimulus intensity levels (in the visual system

at least). The lack of an amplitude differential in the current
results might reflect the difference in stimulus modality or the
lack of an optimal stimulus intensity. In view of the growing literature on the effects of attention on the amplitude of the vertex
potential (Hillyard and Picton, 1978), it is also possible that previous reports reflect differential attention between the two groups
as a function of stimulus intensity. Such effects are less likely
in the auditory system since peripheral adjustment of the sensory
mechanisms is not a factor. Comparisons of these late potentials
are probably best made under conditions where independent information
is available on the subject's psychological state (Sutton, 1969).

While binaural interactions might have been expected at the
level of the superior olive (wave III) on the basis of the neurophysiological literature, the restriction of these effects to wave
IV-V in both groups of adults studied here is consistent with previous investigations of the surface potentials in cats (Jewett,
1970; Huang and Buchwald, 1978).

The cortical data showed a significant binaural occlusive effect for both amplitude measures (N1-P2 and P2-N2). However, the
size of the effect (in terms of the L + R/B ratio) was larger in the
cortical ERPs than in the brain stem. It thus appears that the
binaural occlusion increases from the level of the inferior collicullus (the probable generator of wave V) to the cortex. The amplitudes of wave VI are in line with this trend (Table I) although the
difference between conditions was not significant at this level.

Despite the fundamental differences in the latency and amplitude characteristics of the ERP between the Down's syndrome and
normal groups at all levels, the ERP reflections of binaural processing were nearly identical for the two groups. To the extent
that the processes reflected here are involved in binaural analyses
such as lateralization and localization, the data suggest that those
aspects of information processing are essentially normal in the
Down's syndrome individuals. This conclusion would be consistent
with recent behavioral assessments of localization in the retarded
(Heffner, 1977).

## EXPERIMENT II: VISUAL ERPS
### AND PERCEPTUAL AND DECISION PROCESSES

As one proceeds to successively longer latency components, the
dependence on stimulus parameters is reduced. Thus while the auditory far field responses are entirely stimulus bound, the N1-P2
component of the vertex potential is affected both by stimulus and
cognitive variables, and the endogenous components N2 and P3 are
almost completely dependent on the subject's psychological reaction

to the stimuli.  This experiment sought to determine whether separate contributions of perceptual and cognitive factors to the visual
ERP would differentiate between retarded and normal adults.

Typically the endogenous components are elicited in tasks that
require the subject to count or otherwise keep track of certain
stimulus events.  Under these conditions unexpected events reliably
evoked endogenous N2 and P3 components in addition to the exogenous
components evoked by all stimuli.  While procedures such as the counting task are simple and effective with normal subjects, they must be
modified to be within the capabilities of our target population.
The procedure we have adopted does not require that the subject make
difficult decisions about the stimuli, or even to discriminate the
different events, and is suitable for all but the very lowest functioning individuals.

## Method

Three visual stimuli occurred in random order in each block
of trials.  One was presented frequently (p = .80) and the other two
were presented rarely (p = .10).  One of the rare stimuli was a red
circle on a white background and was designated as the target.  The
retarded subjects were taught to associate the target stimulus with
a token reward by requiring them to say "token" to each occurrence
of the target if they were verbal or to point to the stimulus if
they were not.  If no response was made the subject was prompted.
Tokens were given for correct response and were exchanged later for
food or other rewards.  Nonretarded subjects tested in the same
procedure pressed a button in response to the target stimulus.  The
purpose of the verbal or nonverbal response to the target was to
keep the subject's attention on the visual display.

The nontarget stimuli, which did not require a response, provided the major experimental data since the ERPs to these stimuli
were free from contamination due to motor responses.  (Since no
emphasis was placed on speed of response and most responses to the
targets occurred beyond the one-second averaging epoch, the target
ERPs were also relatively free of artifact.)  The frequent stimulus
was always a dim flash (1 FtL).  In separate blocks the rare nontarget stimulus was either a small increase in stimulus intensity (11
FtL, the "small increment" condition) or a large increase in intensity (110 FtL, the "large increment" condition).  All nontarget
stimuli were 200 msec in duration.  The target stimuli remained on
the screen until a response was made.  Stimuli were presented via
a Kodak Carousel projector at the rate of one per second in blocks
of 80 stimuli.  Half of the subjects were given the large increment
condition first, and the other half were given the small increment
condition.  Each condition contained three blocks of stimuli.

Thirty retarded subjects of mixed diagnosis and thirteen normal subjects participated in the experiment.  The ages of the retarded subjects ranged from 13 to 53 (mean = 26), and their IQs from 6 to 69 (mean = 35).  The ages of the normal subjects ranged from 19 to 55 (mean = 25).  The normal subjects were non-paid UCLA students and staff volunteers.  The data of one retarded and one normal subject were excluded due to equipment malfunctions.

Electrodes were placed at Fz, Cz and Pz referred to the right mastoid.  The left mastoid was used as ground, and the EOG was measured from above the right eye to the outer canthus.  All trials with large eye movements were excluded from the average.  The data of one retarded subject were excluded due to excessive eye movement. During testing the retarded subject's behavior was monitored, and data from periods of inattention or excessive movement were rejected. For most subjects such periods were rare.  The EEG was amplified with Grass P511 amplifiers (.1-100 Hz), digitized and stored on magnetic tape for off line averaging and analysis.

## Results

Fig. 2 shows the ERPs to the rare and frequent nontarget stimuli for three retarded and three normal subjects in the large increment condition.  For both the retarded and normal subjects the ERPs to the frequent stimuli (solid lines) consist of the N1 and P2 components while the ERPs to the rare stimuli (dashed lines) also contain the endogenous N2 and P3 components.

As would be expected of the exogenous components, N1-P2, amplitude increased as a function of increasing intensity of the three nontarget stimuli ($F = 52.7$, $df = 2,76$, $p < .01$; Fig. 3).  There was no significant difference in the N1-P2 amplitudes of the retarded and normal subjects and no significant interaction with stimulus intensity.

For the N2-P3 component there was no main effect on amplitude of the type of rare stimulus (large increment flashes, small increment flashes and targets);  however, N2-P3 amplitudes were smaller in the retarded (mean = 13.9 $\mu V$) than in the normals (mean = 20.4 $\mu V$; $F = 11.57$, $df = 1,38$, $p < .01$).  There was also a significant interaction between stimulus and group effects ($F = 7.0$, $df = 2,76$, $p < .01$); the N2-P3 amplitude difference between groups was greater for the target stimuli than for either of the other rare stimuli.

Fig. 4 shows the mean latencies of the components averaged across the three types of rare stimuli.  While N1 latency did not differ between the normal and retarded subjects ($F = .1$, $df = 1,38$), significant latency differences were found for P2, N2 and P3 ($F = 14.86$, $22.65$ and $10.53$, respectively, $df = 1,38$ and $p < .01$ in each case).

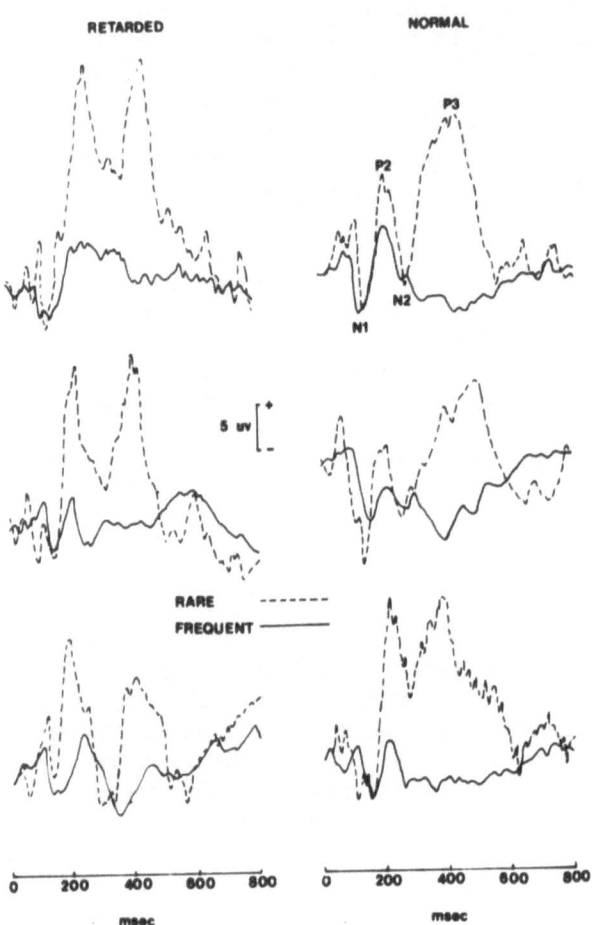

Fig. 2.  Visual evoked responses of three retarded and three normal subjects in the large increment condition.

Although N1 was of normal altency for the retarded group as a whole, one subset from the retarded group did have prolonged N1 latencies.  Eight of the retarded were reported by the direct care staff as having visual difficulties.  Significantly more of these individuals had N1 latencies that were greater than one standard deviation above the mean for the normal subjects ($\chi^2 = 5.62$, $p <$ .01).  Similar analyses of the effect of visual deficits on the latencies of the later peaks showed no significant differences.

The mean latency of the P3 to the nontarget rare stimuli decreased by about 40 msec from the small increment condition to the large increment condition for both the retarded and the normal sub-

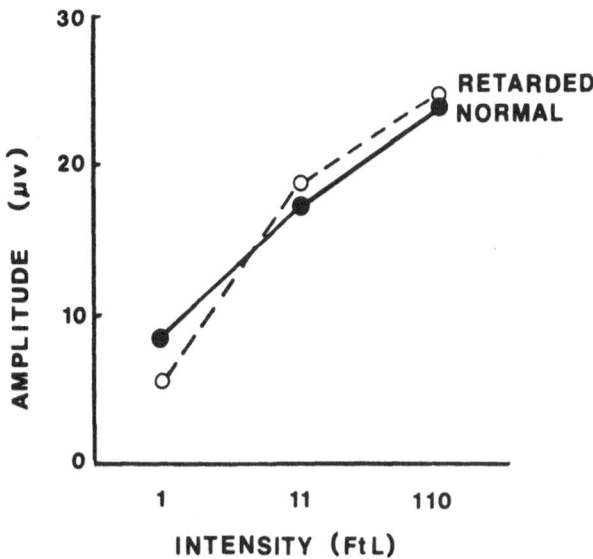

Fig. 3.  N1-P2 amplitude as a function of the intensity of the nontarget stimuli.

jects, and P3 latency was about 50 msec longer in the retarded than
in the normals in each condition (Fig. 5).  The P3 latency of the
retarded to the large increment was thus about the same as the P3
latency of the normals to the small increment.  There were no
significant differences between normal and retarded in the scalp
amplitude distribution of the P3s to any of the rare stimuli.  The
mean amplitudes across all rare stimuli were 12.6, 13.9 and 12.8
µV at Fz, Cz and Pz for the retarded and 16.9, 20.4 and 16.1 µV
for the normal subjects.


Discussion of Experiment II

The main difference in the visual ERPs of the retarded and
nonretarded subjects was in the endogenous components evoked by the
rare events.  These components were of longer latency and smaller
amplitude in the retarded than in the normal subjects.  Since P3
latency primarily indexes the speed of a perceptual decision (Ritter
et al., 1972; Ford et al., 1976; Squires et al., 1972, Kutas et al.,
1977) the latency data suggest that the information processing of
the retarded is characterized by slower perceptual recognition and
decision processes.  Since P3 amplitude is influenced by a subject's
expectancies and by his/her memory for events in the prior sequence
of events (Squires et al., 1976), the smaller than normal P3 amplitudes of the retarded subjects may be the result of deficiences in
expectancy formation or in memory processes, both of which have been
implicated in behavioral studies of retardation (Kirby et al., 1977).

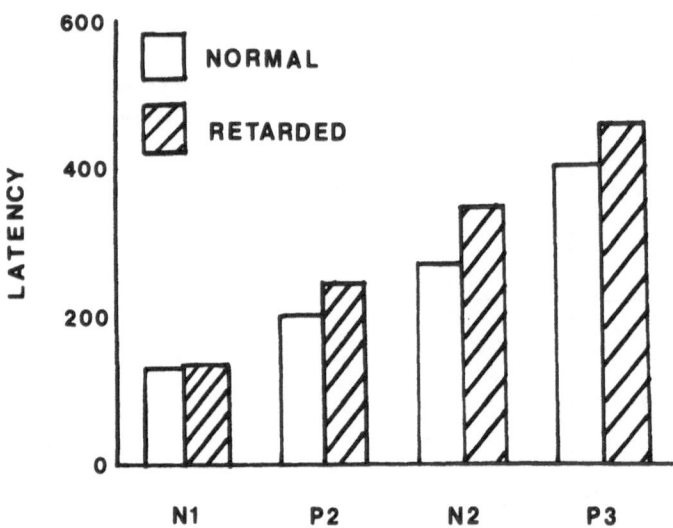

Fig. 4.  Peak latencies of the major ERP components averaged across
the three rare stimuli.


     The ERP differences shown here between the retarded and the
normal subjects cannot be readily attributed to differences in
sensory acuity since the latency and amplitude of the exogenous
N1 component did not differ between the two groups.  The use of
N1 latency as a measure of sensory magnitude is supported by the
delayed N1s found for those retarded subjects with reported visual
problems.  That N1 could be delayed in these individuals without a
concomitant slowing of decision processes, indexed by P3 latency,
is consistent with the data of Squires et al. (this volume) who found
that in normal subjects decreasing the intensity of auditory stimuli produced a delayed N1 but had no effect on P3 until both the
rare and frequent stimuli were within 15 dB of threshold.  Apparently P3 latency is determined by the perceptual recognition of stimulus differences rather than by absolute stimulus intensity.

     As a whole these data suggest that the visual information pro-
cessing of the retarded is characterized primarily by deficits in
the higher cognitive functions reflected in the endogenous potentials.  This pattern of normal exogenous potentials and abnormal
endogenous potentials is typical of populations with diminished mental functions such as the demented and the aged (Squires et al.,
this volume; Goodin et al., in press) as well as the developmentally immature (Squires et al., this volume; Goodin, 1978) and the
hyperkinetic (Prichep et al., 1976).  To determine whether or not
the ERP abnormalities of these groups actually reflect the same
functional deficiences, more detailed experiments need to be performed to parcel out the contributions of short- and long-term

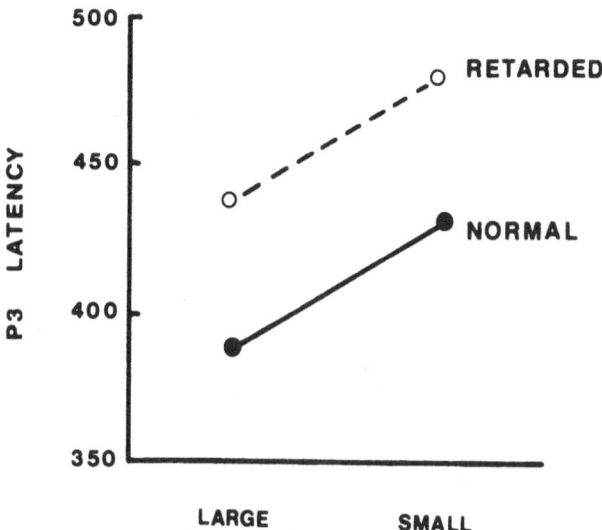

Fig. 5.  P3 latency as a function of the intensity difference between rare and frequent stimuli.

memory, perceptual and other cognitive factors.  Many ERP techniques for making such distinctions have already been developed in research with normal adult subjects and the field is making continuous progress in this direction (Donchin et al., in press).


## CONCLUSION

It is increasingly evident that a high degree of analytical specificity can be obtained from components of the ERP.  Thus the sequence of potentials occurring within 10 msec following a brief auditory stimulus reflect quite specific processes within the auditory relay nuclei and pathways of the brain stem.  Such potentials reflect only stimulus characteristics and are not altered by attention, sleep, etc.  At the other extreme the long latency potentials are known to reflect both endogenous and exogenous factors but more generally at a higher (i.e., cortical) level.  Not surprisingly, the clarification of these endogenous properties often requires special experimental paradigms.

Neuroanatomical and neuropathological studies indicate that mentally retarded individuals suffer from disturbances in neural organization throughout the extent of the brain, from brain stem to cortex.  We sought, therefore, to utilize the ERP as a means of elucidating possible differences in neural organization between mentally retarded and nonretarded individuals.  Our results showed

instances where there were no differences.  However, certain parameters were significantly different in both the brain stem and cortical ERPs.  We feel, therefore, that the ERP has great utility
in providing meaningful information about the functional integrity
of the mentally retarded nervous system.

## SUMMARY

     Both the long- and the short-latency auditory evoked responses
were recorded in a group of Down's syndrome retarded individuals
and in a group of normal controls to assess binaural auditory information processing.  Previous studies in animals and normal humans
show that amplitudes are reduced during binaural stimulation as compared to the sum of monaural left-plus-right ear stimulation.  The
current results showed that Down's syndrome subjects had shorter
BAER latencies and reduced amplitudes.  Their long latency potentials
had normal amplitudes, but longer than normal latencies.  Despite
these differences in the auditory evoked potentials, however, the
degree of amplitude decrement produced by the binaural stimulation
was similar in the Down's syndrome and normal groups.  It, therefore, appears that the processing of simultaneous input from the
two ears is not degraded in Down's syndrome individuals insofar as
that processing is reflected in the potentials investigated.  The
visual evoked responses for a group of retarded adults of mixed
diagnoses were compared to those of a group of normal adults.  The
primary differences in the ERPs of the two groups were found in the
endogenous components, N2 and P3, suggesting diminished perceptual
recognition and decision making processes in the retarded individuals.  The earlier N1 component was abnormal only in a subset of
retarded individuals with known deficits in visual acuity.  The N2
and P3 components of this subset did not differ from the retarded
group as a whole.  These results indicate that the exogenous (N1 and
P2) and endogenous (N2 and P3) components of the visual response
can be used to differentiate between sensory and cognitive deficits
in the visual information processing of the retarded.

## ACKNOWLEDGEMENTS

     This research was supported by USPHS Program Project Grant
HD-5958 and USPHS Fellowship NS05725.

## REFERENCES

Barnet, A.B. and Lodge, A.  Click evoked EEG responses in normal
     and developmentally retarded infants.  Nature, 1967, 214, 252-
     255.

Bigum, H.B., Dustman, R.E. and Beck E.C.  Visual and somatosensory evoked responses from mongoloid and normal children.  Electroenceph. Clin. Neurophysiol, 1970, 28, 576-585.

Buchwald, J.S. and Huang, C.-M.  Origins of the far field acoustic response in cats.  Science, 1975, 189, 382-384.

Clopton, B.M. and Silverman, M.S.  Plasticity of binaural interaction.  II.  Critical period and changes in midline response.  J. Neurophysiol., 1977, 40, 1275-1280.

Donchin, E., Ritter, W. and McCallum, C.  Cognitive psychophysiology: The endogenous components of the ERP.  In E. Callaway, P. Tueting and S. Koslow (Eds.), Event Related Brain Potentials in Man, Academic Press: New York, in press.

Erulkar, S.D.  The responses of single units of the inferior colliculus of the cat to acoustic stimulation.  Proc. Royal. Soc., 1959, 150, 336-355.

Ford, J., Roth, W. and Kopell, B.  Auditory evoked potentials to unpredictable shifts in pitch.  Psychophysiol., 1976, 13, 32-39.

Galambos, R., Schwartzkopff, J. and Rupert, A.L.  Microelectrode study of superior olivary nuclei.  Amer. J. Physiol., 1959, 197, 527-536.

Galbraith, G.C., Squires, N., Altair, D. and Gliddon, J.B.  Electrophysiological assessments in mentally retarded individuals: From brain stem to cortex.  In H. Begleiter (Ed.), Evoked Brain Potentials and Behavior, New York: Plenum Press, in press.

Gliddon, J.B., Busk, J. and Galbraith, G.  Visual evoked responses as a function of light intensity in Down's syndrome and nonretarded subjects.  Psychophysiol., 1975, 12, 416-422.

Gliddon, J.B., Galbraith, G.C. and Busk, J.  Effect of preconditioning visual stimulus duration on visual evoked responses to a subsequent test flash in Down's syndrome and nonretarded individuals.  Amer. J. Mental Def., 1975, 80, 186-190.

Goodin, D.S., Squires, K.C., Henderson, B.H. and Starr, A.  Age related variations in evoked potentials to auditory stimuli in normal human subjects.  Electroenceph. Clin. Neurophysiol., 1978, 44, 447-458.

Goodin, D.S., Squires, K.C. and Starr, A.  Long latency event related components of the auditory evoked potential in dementia.  Brain, in press.

Heffner, R.S.  Neurological evaluation of the auditory system in
    nonverbal severely retarded children.  Paper presented at the
    17th Annual Meeting of the Society for Neuroscience, Anaheim,
    California, 1977.

Hillyard, S.A. and Picton, T.W.  Event related brain potentials
    and selective information processing in man.  In J.E. Desmedt
    (Ed.), Cerebral Evoked Potentials in Man, Oxford University
    Press:  Oxford, 1978.

Huang, C.-M. and Buchwald, J.S.  Factors that affect the amplitudes
    and latencies of the vertex short latency acoustic responses
    in the cat.  Electroenceph. Clin. Neurophysiol., 1978, 44,
    179-186.

Jewett, D.L.  Volume conducted potentials in response to auditory
    stimuli as detected by averaging in the cat.  Electroenceph.
    Clin. Neurophysiol., 1970, 28, 609-618.

Jewett, D.L., Romano, M.N. and Williston, J.S.  Human auditory
    evoked potentials:  Possible brain stem components detected on
    the scalp.  Science, 1970, 167, 1517-1518.

Jewett, D.L. and Williston, J.S.  Auditory evoked far fields aver-
    aged from the scalp of humans.  Brain, 1971, 94, 681-696.

Kirby, N.H., Nettelbeck, T. and Tiggeman, M.  Reaction time in re-
    tarded and nonretarded young adults:  Sequential effects and
    response organization.  Amer. J. Mental Def., 1977, 81, 492-498.

Kutas, M., McCarthy, G. and Donchin E.  Augmenting mental chronome-
    try:  The P300 as a measure of stimulus evaluation.  Science,
    1977, 197, 792-795.

Lev, A. and Sohmer, H.  Sources of averaged neural responses record-
    ed in animal and human subjects during cochlear audiometry
    (electrocochleogram).  Arch. Klin. Exp. Ohr.-, Has.-u. Kehlk.
    Heilk., 1972, 201, 79-90.

Marcus, M.M.  The evoked cortical response:  A technique for assess-
    ing development.  Calif. Mental Health Res. Dig., 1970, 8, 59-
    72.

Picton, T.W., Woods, D.L., Baribeau-Braun, J. and Healey, M.G.
    Evoked potential audiometry.  J. Otolaryngol., 1977, 6, 90-119.

Prichep, L.S., Sutton, S. and Hakerem, G.  Evoked potentials in
    hyperkinetic and normal children under certainty and uncertain-
    ty:  A placebo and methlphenidate study.  Psychophysiol., 1976,
    13, 419-428.

Ritter, W., Simson, R. and Vaughan, J.G. Jr. Association cortex
    potentials and reaction time in auditory discrimination.
    Electroenceph. Clin. Neurophysiol., 1972, 33, 547-555.

Silverman, M.S. and Clopton, B.M. Plasticity of binaural interac-
    tion. I. Effect of early auditory deprivation. J. Neurophysiol.,
    1977, 40, 1266-1274.

Sohmer, H. and Feinmesser, M. Cochlear action potentials recorded
    from the external ear in man. Ann. Otolaryngol., 1967, 76,
    427-436.

Sohmer, H., Feinmesser, M. and Szabo, G. Sources of electrocochleo-
    graphic responses as studied in patients with brain damage.
    Electroenceph. Clin. Neurophysiol., 1974, 37, 663-669.

Sohmer, H. and Student, M. Auditory nerve and brain stem evoked
    responses in normal, autistic, minimal brain dysfunctioned
    and psychomotor retarded children. Electroenceph. Clin. Neuro-
    physiol., 1978, 44, 380-388.

Squires, K.C., Wickens, C., Squires, N.K. and Donchin, E. The
    effect of stimulus sequence on the waveform of the cortical
    event related potential. Science, 1976, 193, 1142-1146.

Squires, N.K., Donchin, E., Squires, K.C. and Grossberg, S. Bisen-
    sory stimulation: Inferring decision related processes from
    the P300 component. J. Exper. Psychol: Human Percept. Per-
    form., 1977, 3, 299-315.

Starr, A. and Hamilton, A.E. Correlation between confirmed sites
    of neurological lesions and abnormalities of far field auditory
    brain stem responses. Electroenceph. Clin. Neurophysiol.,
    1976, 41, 585-608.

Sutton, S. The specification of psychological variables in an
    average evoked potential experiment. In E. Donchin and D.B.
    Lindsley (Eds.), Average Evoked Potentials, NASA SP-191, 1969,
    Washington, D.C.

Tueting, P. Event related potentials, cogntive events and informa-
    tion processing. In D. Otto (Ed.) New Perspective in Event
    Related Potential (ERP) Research, U.S. Government Printing
    Office: Washington, D.C., in press.

ANATOMICAL AND PHYSIOLOGICAL ORIGINS OF AUDITORY BRAIN STEM

RESPONSES (ABR)

Arnold Starr and L. Joseph Achor

University of California, Irvine

Irvine, California 92717

The development of far field recording techniques to measure the activity of the auditory pathway in its course from the cochlea to the cortex has had important clinical applications.  In man there are up to seven vertex positive waves that occur in the first ten msec after a click signal (Fig. 1).  The largest of these components, designated variously as the IV-V complex, 4a and 4b, or N4 and N5, is usually 0.5 µV in amplitude and occurs at a latency of 5.6 - 6.0 msec for a 65 dB (H.L. re normal) click.  Since the components of the auditory brain stem responses (ABR) change in latency in an orderly manner with signal intensity (Fig. 1) the measure can provide objective definition of hearing threshold in difficult-to-test subjects such as newborn infants or mentally impaired patients (Davis and Hirsch, 1977; Hecox and Galambos, 1974; Mokotoff et al., 1977; Shulman-Galambos and Galambos, 1975; Sohmer and Feinmesser, 1973; Starr et al., 1977; Yamada et al., 1975).  The ABR evoked by clicks primarily reflects high frequency hearing capacities since it depends on the activity of the basilar or high frequency end of the cochlea.  However, there are several methods under evaluation that will enable the ABR to serve as a reliable measure of hearing threshold across a wide range of signal frequencies; these include the use of filtered clicks (Davis, 1976) and narrow band masking noise (Don and Eggermont, 1978).

The expectation that each component of the ABR represents the activity of one of the nuclei along the brain stem auditory pathway (Jewett, 1970; Lev and Sohmer, 1970) has obvious relevance for the evaluation of neurological disorders.  A large body of clinical data has now been collected that show correlation between alterations in the ABR and various brain stem lesions (Chiappa et al., in press; Robinson and Rudge, 1977; Starr, 1976, 1977; Starr and Achor

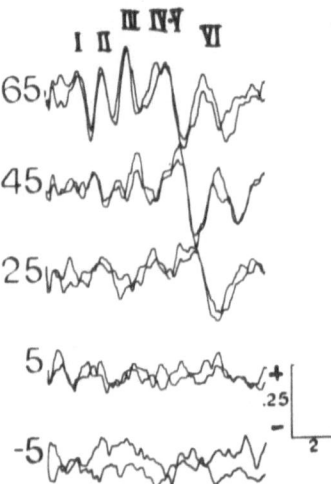

Fig. 1.  Auditory brain stem responses from a normal human adult.
Recording was made between vertex (Cz) referenced to the earlobe
ipsilateral to the click stimulus.  The intensity of the click in
dB H.L. re a jury of normal subjects is to the left of each response.
Duplicate averages were obtained of each intensity.  Note the latency shift of the components as signal intensity is lowered.  This
subject did not show a Wave VII.

1975; Starr and Hamilton, 1976; Stockard et al., 1977; Stockard
and Rossiter, 1977; Thornton and Hawkes, 1976).

     Two types of changes in the ABR occur with central nervous
system lesions in man.  The first is a loss or marked attenuation
of components of the ABR; the second is a prolongation in latency
between the various ABR components, in which case there is abnormal
"central conduction time".  Since absolute amplitudes of the components of the ABR can vary considerably among normal subjects, due
to the low amplitude of the ABR relative to amplifier "noise" or
other biological signals such as the electroencephalogram (EEG) or
electromyogram (EMG), we have suggested that amplitude ratios of
various components can be a useful index of abnormality.  In particular, Wave V is usually larger than Wave I (V/I > 1) to signal
intensities of 60 dB H.L. re normal or less (Chiappa et al., in
press; Rowe, 1973; Starr and Achor, 1975).

     The measure of central conduction times was developed for
neurological evaluations because the absolute latency of all of
the components will be affected by middle ear or cochlear functions,
whereas the interpeak latencies are relatively independent of both

click intensity and hearing loss (Rowe, 1978; Starr, 1977; Stockard, and Rossiter, 1977). The time difference between Waves I and V is commonly employed, and values above 4.4 msec are considered to be abnormal (> 2 S.D. above normal). Variables such as body temperature (Stockard et al., 1978) and depressant drugs (Squires et al., 1978) can prolong central conduction times, but this measure will exceed normal values only when these factors are extreme.

From a survey of the clinical data (Starr, 1978) it appears that lesions of the thalamus or cortex are not associated with changes in the ABR. The report that Waves VI and VII were abolished in a patient with a thalamic tumor (Stockard and Rossiter, 1977) is of limited use since these components may also be absent in normal subjects (Chiappa et al., in press; Rowe, 1978). Lesions of the midbrain are associated with a loss or prolongation in latency of components beginning with Waves IV and V. Lesions of the pons affect the ABR beginning with component III. Lesions of the eighth nerve may be associated with a loss of the entire ABR or prolongation in the latency of components after Wave I. Wave I may also be increased in width with tumors that compress the eighth nerve (Terkildsen et al., 1977). The changes in the ABR in these clinical situations suggest that the generators of the various components of the ABR may be as follows: Wave I - the eighth nerve; Wave III - the pons; Waves IV and V - the midbrain. Waves II, VI and VII occur with sufficient variability in normal subjects making a definition of their generators from clinical-pathological studies uncertain.

The types of lesions encountered in clinical situations usually extend beyond a single auditory structure and, in addition, have remote effects on other parts of the brain stem from pressure or edema. The results of using the ABR in the clinic provides an impetus for further experimental studies in animals to clarify in precise detail the generator sites for the various components.

Two types of experimental studies have been performed in animals to define the anatomical bases of the ABR. The first method relies on a correlation between the latency of evoked potentials or single units recorded in particular brain stem auditory structures with the components of the ABR recorded from the scalp (Achor, 1976; Huang and Buchwald, 1977; Jewett, 1970). The second method relies on changes in the ABR that accompany the destruction of portions of the auditory pathway (Buchwald and Huang, 1975; Lev and Sohmer, 1970). These studies have been interpreted as indicating that certain components of the ABR are generated by a single auditory structure, but there may be disagreement as to the identity of that structure. For instance, Jewett (1970), using depth and surface evoked potentials in the cat, found large amplitude fields in the inferior colliculus at the time of Wave IV, whereas Buchwald and Huang (1975) found that ablation of the inferior colliculus in the cat was not associated with any changes in Wave IV. The study by these last authors, which involved making sequential transections of the brain stem in cats, suggested that Wave I originates from the eighth nerve, Wave II from the cochlear nucleus, Wave III from the superior olive, Wave IV from bilateral pathways in the pons and Waves V and VI (both of which are quite small and variable in the cat) from the inferior colliculus. There are some obvious differences between the clinical material in humans and the results from cats, the major one being the identity of the generators for Waves IV and V.

We have been investigating the origins of the ABR in anesthetized cats using both depth recordings and the effects of discrete brain stem lesions. An examination of the evoked potentials recorded from several of the auditory structures (Fig. 2) shows that each may extend for many msec, and therefore several sites can be active simultaneously. Thus a causal relationship between activity in one brain stem structure and the far field occurrence of one component of the ABR is unlikely.

In our experiments we made a detailed analysis of the evoked potentials every two millimeters throughout the brain stem. This relatively fine-grained analysis provided a detailed spatial estimate of the distribution of potential fields in the brain stem

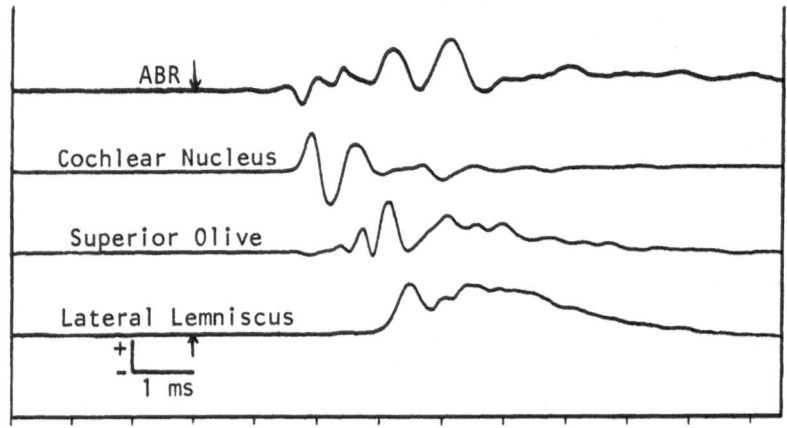

Fig. 2. Auditory brain stem responses (ABR) recorded from the scalp referenced to the neck of an anesthesized cat (top trace) compared with recordings from several auditory brain structures also referenced to the neck. The amplitude calibration for the ABR is 10 µV and for the depth recordings, 500 µV. The click stimulus was presented at the arrow through stereotaxic hollow ear bars. Note that the potentials evoked in the auditory brain stem sites persist for many msec.

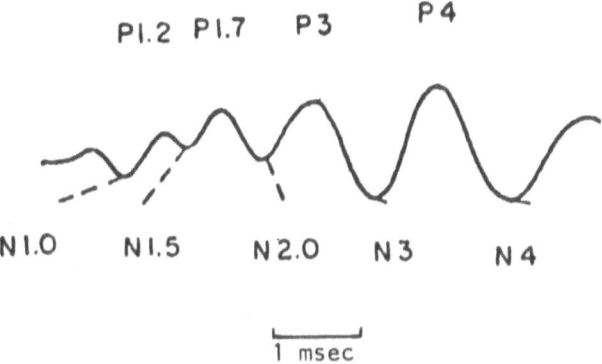

Fig. 3.   Auditory brain stem potentials recorded from the anesthetized cat as in Fig. 2.   The time base has been enlarged and the
components labeled for reference to Tables I and II.

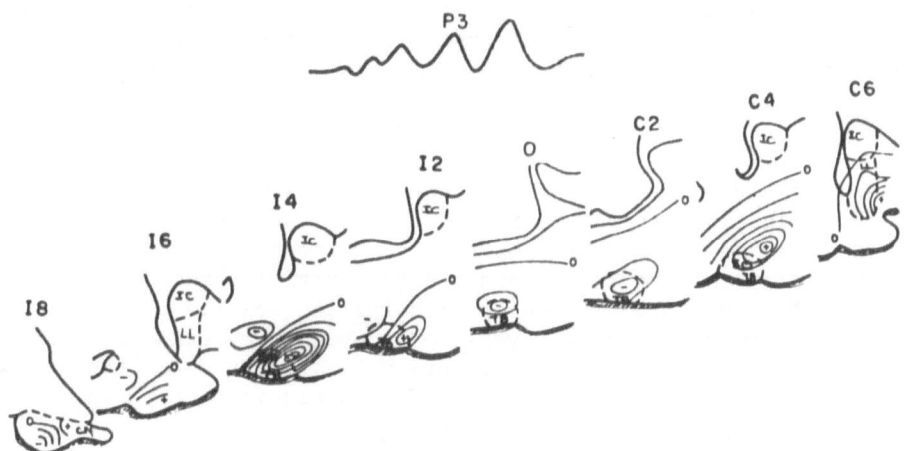

Fig. 4.   An isopotential map of the brain stem of the cat at the
peak of component P3.   There are eight sagittal sections onto which
are traced the isopotential contours.   The sections begin in the
brain stem ipsilateral to the stimulated ear and proceed in 2 mm
steps across the brain stem.   Rostral is to the right of each section.   The letters above each section refer to the plane of the
section (I8 is ipsilatearl 8 mm from the midline, 16 is ipsilateral
6 mm, etc., 0 is the midline and C refers to contralateral sections).
There is no section at C8 because of the absence of any fields in
the contralateral cochlear nucleus.   The zero isopotential plane
(o) is indicated in each section and each line represents a 200 µV
change.   The polarity of the field, i.e., positive (+) or negative
(-) is also indicated.   Note that significant potential fields are
present in almost every section of the brain stem at the peak of
P3.

at the time of occurrence of each peak and trough of the ABR (Fig.
3). Fig. 4 shows one of the isocontour maps that derives from the
analysis of the distribution of potential fields throughout the
brain stem at the time of occurrence of one of the components, P3.
It is obvious that at this instant in time there are high amplitude
fields present throughout the brain stem from cochlear nucleus to
colliculus. These fields, moreover, are not stationary but show
rapid movement through the brain stem within a few hundred micro-
seconds. Fig. 5 includes the potential maps from a single sagittal
section of the brain stem involving the contralateral inferior
colliculus and lateral lemniscus at the peak of P3 and 100 msec
both prior to (-100) and after (+100) its occurrence. Note the
movement of the fields from the pons up to the colliculus in this
short time span.

Quantification of the amplitudes of the potentials in the various auditory nuclei and tracts of the brain stem at the time of
each of the components of AGR revealed that more than one site had
high amplitude fields at the time of each of the components. Table
I contains the results from this analysis in four cats. For each
component of the ABR in each of the cats the amplitude of the potential field in a brain stem auditory structure was expressed as a
percentage of the maximum field found anywhere in the brain stem at
that instant in time. The positive and negative fields were averaged separately, and those fields that were 40% or more of the
maximum field found anywhere are noted by an asterik and arbitrarily
considered a "major" contributor to the ABR component. A single
source (VIII N/CN) can be defined for the initial three components
(N 1.0, P 1.2, N 1.5). Thereafter significant voltage fields
(> 40% of maximum) occur in several of the auditory structures at
the time of each of the ABR components. For instance, at the time
of P 3.0 there are at least four sites with significant potential

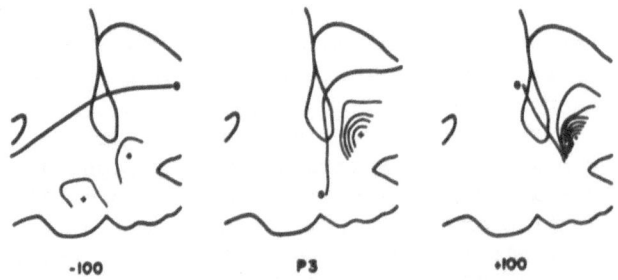

Fig. 5. An isopotential map of one plane of the brain stem of the
cat (contralateral 6) through the inferior colliculus and lateral
lemniscus at the peak of P3 (middle trace) and 100 μsec before
(-100) and after (+100) this component. Note the movement of the
field from the pons up to the inferior colliculus in this short
time span. The description of the contour maps are in Fig. 4.

Table I.  Potential fields in the brain stem auditory pathway expressed as a percent of the maximum field anywhere in the brain stem at the time of occurrence of each of the ABR components (N = 4 cats).

ABR COMPONENT

Positive Fields

|          | N 1.0 | P 1.2 | N 1.5 | P 1.7 | N 2.0 | P 3.0 | N3  | P4  | N4  |
|----------|-------|-------|-------|-------|-------|-------|-----|-----|-----|
| VIII N/CN | 95*  | 80*   | 50*   | 32    | 75*   | 20    | 22  | 15  | 10  |
| (I) SO   | 0     | 0     | 0     | 8     | 60*   | 55*   | 35  | 40* | 7   |
| (I) LL   | 0     | 0     | 0     | 0     | 0     | 0     | 0   | 40* | 0   |
| (I) IC   | 0     | 0     | 0     | 0     | 0     | 0     | 0   | 0   | 0   |
| TB       | 0     | 0     | 10    | 63*   | 65*   | 58*   | 38  | 0   | 15  |
| (C) SP   | 0     | 0     | 0     | 0     | 48*   | 85*   | 45* | 30  | 52* |
| (C) LL   | 0     | 0     | 0     | 0     | 0     | 40*   | 38  | 42* | 8   |
| (C) IC   | 0     | 0     | 0     | 0     | 0     | 0     | 0   | 0   | 15  |

Negative Fields

|          | N 1.0 | P 1.2 | N 1.5 | P 1.7 | N 2.0 | P 3.0 | N3  | P4  | N4  |
|----------|-------|-------|-------|-------|-------|-------|-----|-----|-----|
| VIII N/CN | 15   | 75*   | 95*   | 85*   | 35    | 30    | 8   | 0   | 33  |
| (I) SO   | 0     | 0     | 0     | 7     | 40*   | 38    | 52* | 48* | 5   |
| (I) LL   | 0     | 0     | 0     | 0     | 0     | 0     | 0   | 0   | 47* |
| (I) IC   | 0     | 0     | 0     | 0     | 0     | 0     | 0   | 0   | 0   |
| TB       | 0     | 0     | 7     | 0     | 10    | 0     | 0   | 60* | 0   |
| (C) SO   | 0     | 0     | 0     | 9     | 30    | 43*   | 92* | 85* | 55* |
| (C) LL   | 0     | 0     | 0     | 0     | 21    | 0     | 68* | 24  | 72* |
| (C) IC   | 0     | 0     | 0     | 0     | 0     | 0     | 0   | 0   | 0   |

* denotes fields > 40% of maximum anywhere in brain stem

VIII N/CN   eighth nerve/cochlear nucleus
SO          superior olive nucleus
LL          lateral lemniscus

IC   inferior colliculus nucleus
TB   trapezoid body
(I)  ipsilateral to acoustic stimulus
(C)  contralateral to acoustic stimulus

fields: the ipsilateral and centralateral superior olives, the trapezoid body and the contralateral lemniscus.  There did not appear
to be any regular correlation between the polarity of the brain stem
fields and the polarity of the far field components.  Finally, the
inferior colliculus did not have high amplitude fields at the time
of the occurrence of the ABR through component P4.  Thus the results
of this potential field analysis suggest that for each component of
the ABR (beginning with P 1.7) there is more than one auditory brain
stem structure making a significant contribution to its generation.
Moreover not every auditory structure appears to participate in the
generation of the ABR.

     There are several weaknesses in this type of potential field
mapping study.  First, the definition of a high amplitude field in
the brain stem does not assure that the field is reflected on the
surface.  Second, the mapping does not take into account such variables as "closed" versus "open" fields and inhomogenities in current
movements through the brain.  Finally, the requirements for multiple
electrode penetrations to obtain these maps must have disrupted
"normal" brain stem functions.  However, in spite of these limitations the major conclusion that the generators of most of the ABR
components involve several auditory structures is quite apparent.

     We then carried out a second series of experiments making dis-
crete electrolytic lesions in various auditory brain stem structures
and assessing the changes in the ABR.  The experiments were carried
out in anesthetized cats.  The major effect of these acute electrolytic lesions was to attenuate the amplitude of the ABR and to have
little effect on latency.  Fig. 6 shows that an extensive unilateral
lesion and a smaller contralateral lesion in the central nucleus of
the inferior colliculus has no effect on the ABR.  This result corresponds to the conclusions of the field mapping studies.  In contrast, a lesion in the ventral cochlear nucleus (Fig. 7) affected
all the components beginning with P 1.7.  Table II contains a list
of the changes in the amplitude of the ABR components with lesions
at different levels of the auditory brain stem pathway.  The data
for each level is derived from a single animal and were chosen
because the animal demonstrated maximum effects from the lesion among
the animals studied.

     A complete lesion of the eighth nerve attenuated all neural
components.  The remaining events detected in scalp recordings were
cochlear microphonics.  A lesion of the ventral cochlear nucleus
(VCN) that destroyed approximately 50% of the structure caused an
attenuation of all components of the ABR (40-76%) beginning with
P 1.7 to an ipsilateral stimulus.  A partial lesion of the ventral
acoustic striae (VAS) just medial to the cochlear nucleus attenuated
P3, and P4 and N4 to ipsilateral stimulation.  N3 was not affected.
A lesion of the superior olivary nucleus (SO) that also transected

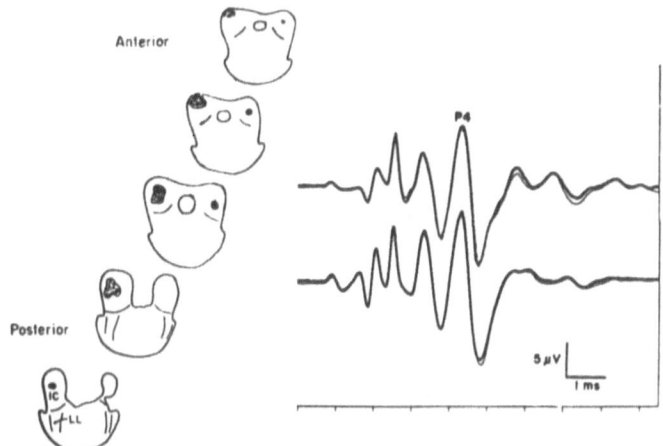

Fig. 6.  Auditory brain stem responses from stimulation of each ear
(top and bottom traces) from a cat before (faint lines) and after
(dark lines) an electrolytic lesion of the inferior colliculus.
The extent of the lesions are shown in the figure.  One of the
lesions destroyed approximately 50% of the nucleus unilaterally.
There was not change in the ABR.

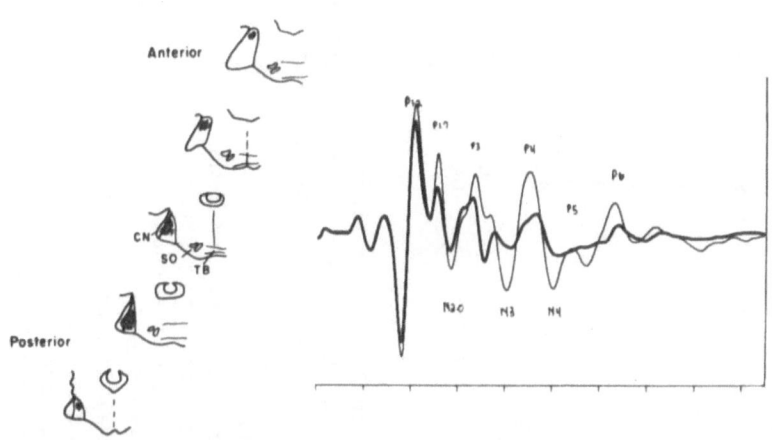

Fig. 7.  Auditory brain stem responses from a cat before (light line)
and after (dark line) a lesion of the ventral cochlear nucleus.
Note that components beginning with P 1.7 are markedly attenuated
without a latency shift.  The amplitude decrements in P 1.2 and N 1.0
are less than 10% and cannot be distinguished from normal variability.
The amplitude scale of the abscissa is 1.0 msec.

Table II. The decrease in amplitude of the ABR components (expressed as a percentage change) with particular lesions.

| | VIII N* | VCN* | VAS* | SO | | TB | | LL** | DCN/DAS/IC | |
|---|---|---|---|---|---|---|---|---|---|---|
| ABR COMPONENT | I | I | I | I | C | I | C | C | I | C |
| P 0.8 – N 1.5 | 100 | 0 | 0 | 0 | 0 | 0 | 0 | 0 | 0 | 0 |
| P 1.7 | 100 | 40 | 0 | 0° | 0° | 20 | 20 | 0 | 0 | 0 |
| N 2.0 | 100 | 48 | 0 | 0° | 0° | 0° | 0° | 0 | 0 | 0 |
| P 3. | 100 | 40 | 38 | 95 | 95 | 36 | 37 | 0 | 0 | 0 |
| N 3. | 100 | 74 | 0 | 90 | 34 | 89 | 78 | 44 | 0 | 0 |
| P 4 | 100 | 76 | 44 | 95 | 42 | 33 | 32 | 0 | 0 | 0 |
| N 4 | 100 | 64 | 22 | 74 | 63 | 50 | 41 | 29 | 0 | 0 |

\* Effect only on ABR to ipsilateral stimulation
\*\* Effect only on ABR to contralateral stimulation
o These components shift in polarity but do not change in amplitude if measured from the peak of P 1.7

VIII N   eighth nerve
VCN      ventral cochlear nucleus
VAS      ventral acoustic stria
SO       superior olive nucleus
TB       trapezoid body
LL       lateral lemniscus
DCN      dorsal cochlear nucleus
DAS      dorsal acoustic stria
IC       inferior colliculus
I        ipsilateral
C        contralateral

50% of the trapezoid body fibers ventral to the nucleus severely
attenuated (> 75%) the components of the ipsilaterally evoked ABR
from P3 on.  While P3 of the contralaterally evoked ABR was almost
totally abolished (95%), the subsequent components (N3, P4, N4) of
the contralaterally evoked ABR were only partially affected (34%,
42% and 63%, respectively).  Thus a unilateral lesion of the superior
olive nucleus (SO) can have equivalent effects on P3 evoked from
stimulating each ear but markedly asymmetrical effects on P4.  The
difficulty with interpreting the superior olivary lesions is that
they also invariably impinged on the trapezoid body (TB).  A lesion
of this latter structure in the midline that did not destroy the
superior olivary had fairly comparable effects on the ABR evoked
from ipsilateral or contralateral stimulation.  The effect began
with P 1.7 but was maximal at N3.  Finally a lesion of the lateral
lemniscus (LL) affected the ABR evoked by contralateral stimulation
but was limited to N3 and N4 and spared P4.

A synthesis of the results from the lesion experiments suggests
that N4 is generated in both the superior olive and the lateral
lemniscus; P4 is generated in bilateral pathways close to the superior olives; N3 is generated in both the lateral lemniscus and the
superior olive; P3 is generated primarily in the superior olives;
N 2.0 and P 1.7 are generated primarily in the cochlear nucleus, and
all other components originate in the eighth nerve.

We emphasize caution in transferring the ABR results derived
from electrolytic lesions in animals to the human clinical experience.
First, in several animals which were allowed to recover after the
lesion the large amplitude changes in the ABR noted acutely were
much less prominent when recordings were made in subsequent weeks.
It is likely that the lesions may have had acute transient effects
on brain stem structures remote from the electrode tip due to physiological factors (diaschisis), or even to vascular or edematous
complications.

The prominent change in central conduction times of the ABR
described in patients with disorders of brain stem function did not
occur with the acute electrolytic lesions in these animal experiments.
Certainly the types of pathological processes in humans (tumors,
demyelinating disorders, edema, infarcts from vascular diseases)
must have vastly different pathophysiological effects on neural
processes than the electrolytic lesions employed here.  Moreover,
we suspect that amplitude changes of up to 40%, as defined in the
ABR in these animal studies, would probably not be discernible as
abnormal in man simply because the amplitude of the ABR is notorious-
ly variable in man.  Also, it is rare that both "before" and "after"
records are available from humans; consequently, abnormalities must
be defined on the basis of group data.  The ABR in the cat, however,
is more than forty times greater in amplitude, resulting in a marked

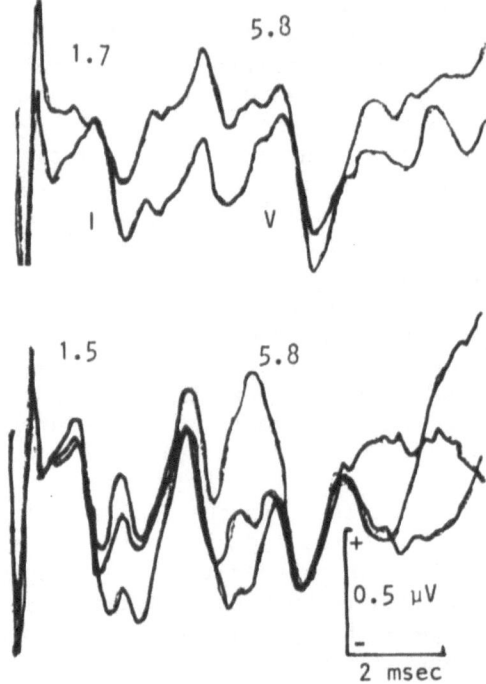

Fig. 8.  Auditory brain stem responses from monaural stimulation
of the right ear (upper) and left ear (lower) in a patient with a
tumor of the tectum of the midbrain.  Waves I and V are labeled.
Note that the latency of the components are normal as were central
conduction times (I-V < 4.4 msec).  The only finding vaguely suggestive of an abnormality is that the amplitude of Wave V is less
than I in two of the three responses from stimulating the left ear.
At the time of this recording the patient was confused (obstruction
of the aqueduct of Sylvius producing hydrocephalus), with a paralysis
of upward gaze.


improvement in signal/noise relationship and allowing the absolute
amplitude measures to be reliable.

    To demonstrate that the animal studies are relevant to the
clinical situation, we have encountered instances of lesions of the
inferior colliculus in man without abnormalities of the ABR.  Fig.
8 is from a patient who died with a tumor restricted to the tectum
of the midbrain (the inferior and superior colliculus) without
pressure or edema in the tegmentum of the brain stem.  The ABR was
normal throughout the two years the patient was observed.  This
result supports the animal studies in which lesions of the inferior
colliculus did not affect the ABR.  It is likely that the tegmentum
of the midbrain coupled with the pons provide the major generator

sites for the components designated as III and IV-V in man.  Furthermore attention should be paid to the vertex negative components in
man since certain lesions in the animal studies (lateral lemniscus)
had predominant effects on these troughs.

The ABR is an encouraging example of the clinical relevance of
evoked potential and neurophysiological research.  Its successful
application has been based on a relatively clear understanding of
peripheral and central auditory physiology and the ability to transfer this knowledge to the human condition.

## SUMMARY

The generation of auditory brain stem responses was examined
in anesthetized cats by using a field analysis of the potentials
evoked every 2 mm in the brain stem to click stimuli.  These field
maps were correlated with the peaks and troughs of the scalp recorded auditory brain stem responses.  The first three components
(P 0.8, N 1.0 and P 1.2) appear to be generated in the eighth nerve.
The remaining components, except for N4, are associated with large
amplitude fields in two or more separate sites along the classical
auditory brain stem pathway.  Acute and chronic electrolytic lesions
in portions of the auditory brain stem pathway in cats showed that
discrete lesions may effect more than one component of the auditory
brain stem responses.  However lesions in the inferior colliculus,
the dorsal cochlear nucleus and the dorsal acoustic striae may have
no effect on brain stem responses.  The lesions usually decreased
the amplitudes of the evoked potentials and had little or no effect
on latencies.  All of these results suggest that the generation of
auditory brain stem response cannot be attributed to a one-to-one
relationship between a particular component and a particular site
in the auditory pathway but rather reflect a complex interrelationship between the various structures.

## ACKNOWLEDGEMENTS

This research was supported by USPHS Grant NS11876.

## REFERENCES

Achor, J.  Field analysis of auditory brain stem responses.  Neuro-
    sci., Abstract, 1976, 2, 12.

Buchwald, J.S. and Huang, C.M.  Far field acoustic responses: Ori-
    gins in the cat.  Science, 1975, 189, 382-384.

Chiappa, K.H., Norwood, A.E. and Young, R.R.  Brain stem auditory
    evoked responses in clinical neurology:  Utility and clinico-
    pathological correlations.  Arch. Neurol., in press.

Davis, H.  Principles of electric response audiometry.  Ann. Otol.
    Rhinol. and Laryng., Suppl. 28, 1976, 85, 5-96.

Davis, H. and Hirsh, S.K.  Brain stem electric response audiometry
    (BSERA).  Acta. Otolaryngol., 1977, 83, 136-139.

Don, M. and Eggermont, J.J.  The analysis of the click evoked brain
    stem potentials in man using high pass noise masking.  J.
    Acoust. Soc. Amer., 1978, 63, 1084-1092.

Hecox, K. and Galambos, R.  Brain stem auditory evoked responses in
    human infants and adults.  Arch. Otolaryng., 1974, 99, 30-33.

Huang, C.M. and Buchwald, J.S.  Interpretation of the vertex short
    latency acoustic response:  A study of single neurons in the
    brain stem.  Brain Res., 1977, 137, 291-303.

Jewett, D.L.  Averaged volume conducted potentials to auditory
    stimuli in the cat.  Electroenceph. Clin. Neurophysiol., 1970,
    28, 609-618.

Lev, A. and Sohmer, H.  Sources of averaged neural responses record-
    ed in animal and human subjects during cochlear audiometry
    (electrocochleography).  Arch. Klin. Exp. Ohr. Nas. Kehlkof.,
    1970, 201, 79-90.

Mokotoff, B., Schulman-Galambos, C. and Galambos, R.  Brain stem
    auditory evoked responses in children.  Arch. Otolaryng., 1977,
    103, 38-43.

Robinson, K. and Rudge, P.  Abnormalities of the auditory evoked
    potentials in patients with multiple sclerosis.  Brain, 1977,
    100, 19-40.

Rowe, M.J.  Normal variability of the brain stem auditory evoked
    response in young and old adult subjects.  Electroenceph. Clin.
    Neurophysiol., 1978, 44, 459-470.

Schulman-Galambos, C. and Galambos, R.  Brain stem auditory evoked
    potentials in premature infants.  J. Speech Hear. Res., 1975,
    18, 456-465.

Sohmer, H. and Feinmesser, M.  Routine use of electrocochleography
    (cochlear audiometry) on human subjects.  Audiol., 1973, 12,
    167-173.

Squires, K., Chu, N.-S. and Starr, A.  Acute effects of alcohol on
    auditory brain stem potentials in humans.  Science, 1978, 201,
    174-176.

Starr, A.  Auditory brain stem responses in brain death.  Brain,
    1976, 99, 543-554.

Starr, A.  Clinical relevance of auditory brain stem evoked poten-
    tials in brain stem disorders in man.  In J.E. Desmedt (Ed.),
    Auditory Evoked Potentials in Man, Psychopharmacology Corre-
    lates of EPs, Prog. Clin. Neurophysiol., Vol. 2, Basel: Karger,
    1977.

Starr, A.  Sensory evoked potentials in clinical disorders of the
    nervous system.  Ann. Rev. Neurosci., 1978, 1, 103-127.

Starr, A. and Achor, J.  Auditory brain stem responses in neurologi-
    cal disease.  Arch. Neurol., 1975, 32, 761-768.

Starr, A., Amlie, R.N., Martin, W.H. and Sanders, S.  Development
    of auditory function in newborn infants revealed by auditory
    brain stem potentials.  Pediatr., 1977, 60, 831-839.

Starr, A. and Hamilton, A.  Correlation between confirmed sites of
    neurological lesions of far field auditory brain stem responses.
    Electroenceph. Clin. Neurophysiol., 1976, 41, 595-608.

Stockard, J.J. and Rossiter, V.S.  Clinical and pathologic correlates
    of brain stem auditory response abnormalities.  Neurol. (Min-
    neap.), 1977, 27, 316-325.

Stockard, J.J., Sharbrough, F.W. and Tinker, J.A.  Effects of hypo-
    thermia on the human brain stem auditory response.  Ann. Neurol.,
    1978, 3, 368-370.

Terkildsen, K., Huis in't Veld, F. and Osterhamel, P.  Auditory
    brain stem responses in the diagnosis of cerebellopontine angle
    tumors.  Scand. Audiol., 1977, 6, 43-47.

Thornton, A.R.D. and Hawkes, C.H.  Neurological applications of sur-
    face recorded electrocochleography.  J. Neurol., Neurosurg.
    Psych., 1976, 39, 586-591.

Yamada, O., Yagi, F., Yamane, H. and Suzuki, J.-I.  Clinical eval-
    uation of the auditory evoked brain stem response.  Auris Nasus
    Larynx., 1975, 2, 97.

COLOR EVOKED POTENTIALS:   CORTICAL AND SUBCORTICAL ELEMENTS

Carroll T. White and Roger W. Hintze

University of California Medical Center

San Diego, California 92103

In our work with responses to colored stimuli it was possible to identify specific components of the evoked waveforms as being related to three basic processes tentatively referred to as red, green and blue processes.  This was achieved by selectively sensitizing the eyes with light which was passed through a variety of limited spectrum filters while presenting flashes obtained with standard red, green and blue filters.

In the original report on this work (White et al., 1977) the results of using a number of background colors were presented, a method which made it possible to detect trends in the waveform that indicated the nature of the underlying processes.  The major results of that earlier work can be summarized by two sets of evoked waveforms, one representing red flashes against a blue-green background and the other being blue flashes against a yellow background.  Both are new data obtained from one of the subjects studied in the earlier work.

Fig. 1 shows the subject's responses to flashes of red light (Wratten filter #92) of constant intensity under increasing levels of blue-green lights.  The voltage values refer to the settings on a rheostat in series with the 60 watt tungsten bulb used to produce the background light.

The waveform for the in-dark condition (0 volts) is dominated by three positive peaks in the 100-200 msec time period.  The waveform for the highest level background exhibits only two positive peaks in that time range.  At intermediate background levels critical changes occurred.  As the background level was increased the second peak moved forward in time from its original 150 msec position and

431

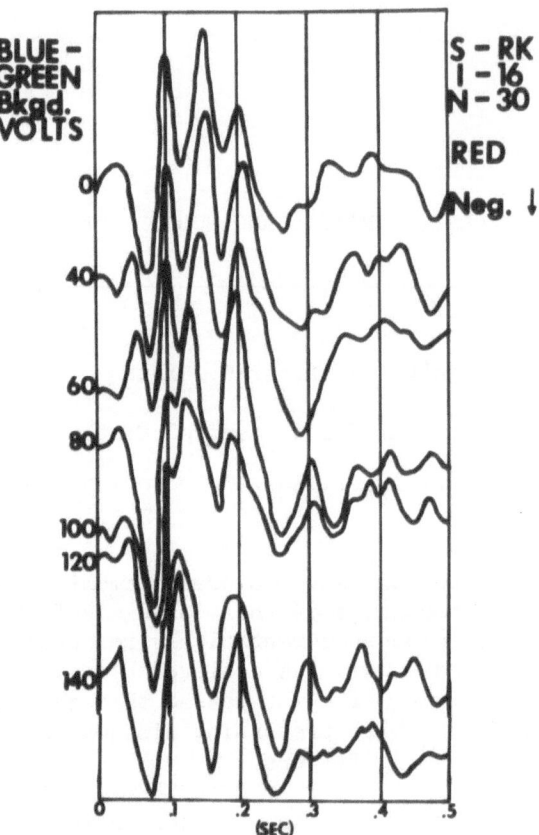

Fig. 1.  Responses of a subject to red flashes upon a blue-green background.  Montage:  Oz to linked earlobes.

merged with the first peak, having a final latency of about 120 msec. The first peak now appeared as a shoulder on the leading edge of the combined positive element.  With other backgrounds where higher intensities are possible (e.g., white or yellow) the second peak is much reduced in amplitude, finally appearing as a shoulder on the trailing edge of the first peak.

It is to be noted that the first peak did not change its latency as the background level was increased.  This is also true for the third peak (180-200 msec), which is such a dominant feature of the high background response.  On the basis of the responses obtained with the various background colors and the red flash stimuli, it was concluded that the first and third peaks (about 100 and 180 msec, respectively) are components related to the red color processes.

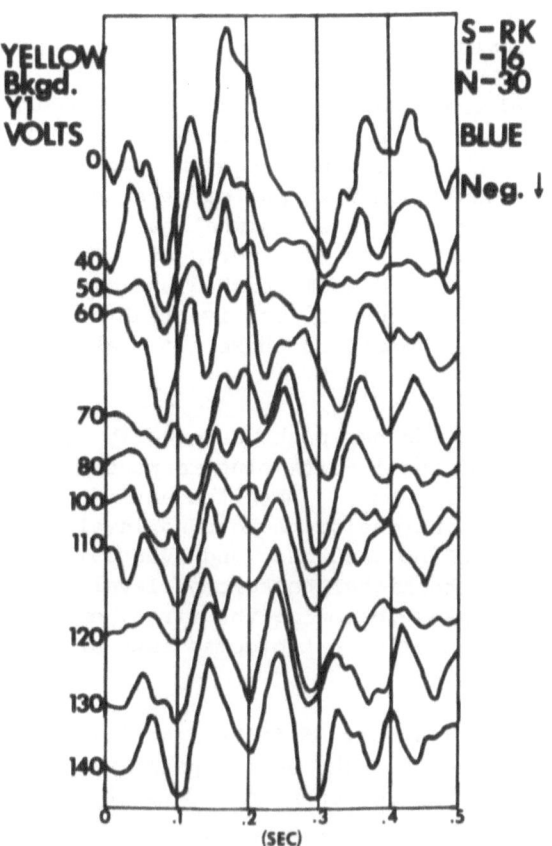

Fig. 2.   Responses of a subject to blue flashes upon a yellow background.   Montage:   Oz to linked earlobes.   This should be viewed obliquely in order to see the trends most clearly.

    In Fig. 2 responses are shown for blue flashes against a yellow background for various intensities.  The blue-yellow paradigm is ideal for helping to determine whether there are indeed sets of color specific components.  Because of the spectral characteristics of the three basic color processes, which have been determined by well established psychophysical techniques, stimulation by the blue flash will affect primarily the blue and the green.  The red processes will be affected to a slight degree, but for present purposes this can be ignored.  Likewise, the yellow background will affect only the green and red processes leaving the blue relatively unaffected.  It is to be noted that green would be affected by both

the stimulus flash and by the steady background light, a fact crucial
for the logic of this experimental design.

It is assumed that the in-dark waveform evoked by the blue
flash (top of Fig. 2) is made up of blue and green related elements. As the background is increased the amplitude of any green-
related elements should diminish and can thereby be identified.
An overview of Fig. 2 clearly shows what has occurred in the evoked waveform as the background was increased. The prominent positive
peak at 120 msec was markedly diminished and eventually completely
removed. This also is true for positive peaking at 200 msec. We
therefore tentatively identified these two peaks as components of
the green process.

What happened to another peak was equally dramatic. One of
the major features of the in-dark blue response was the marked positivity occurring at 180 msec. When the earlier (green?) component
disappeared with the increasing background level, the later peak
moved forward in time about 30 msec and eventually stabilized at
about 150 msec. At the higher background levels another peak
emerged at about 90 msec following the first, ending at about 240
msec. We concluded that these two components are related to the
blue process.

On the basis of a number of facts described in our earlier
paper it was concluded that the second positive peak in the red
evoked waveform (Fig. 1) represented the reaction of the green
process.

We have, therefore, isolated three pairs of components which
we tentatively relate to the red, green and blue color processes.
The red has the shortest latency, followed by the green, and then
the blue. Under light-adapted conditions and moderately high flash
intensities the peak latencies are around 90-100 msec for red, 120
msec for green and 140-150 msec for blue. The latencies of the
second peaks in the color pairs are 180, 200 and about 240 msec,
respectively.

The temporal characteristics of these tentative color components are in precise agreement with the results of earlier psychophysical studies by Pieron and his colleagues (1952) and the more
recent studies on reaction time to color stimuli (Mollon and Krauskopf, 1973). The spectral desensitization technique was earlier
used by Huber (1972).

The marked latency shifts shown by the green and blue components when the background was raised might be related to other data
indicating opponency between the basic color processes. Apparently
a very strong red response can delay the onset of the green process

by as much as 30 msec.  The same seems to be true for the green/blue
relationship with the green being capable of inhibiting the onset
of the blue process by that amount of time.

The above discussion of the color responses is based on our
work with color normal individuals.  When individuals with known
color deficiences were studied the results obtained were in general
agreement with our color-normal analysis, but there were marked individual differences shown among individuals with the same color
vision classification (White et al., 1977).

Some of the earliest work on color responses done in our laboratory dealt with binocular summation (Bartlett et al., 1963).  We
have recently finished an extensive parametric study on this topic
in which a number of individuals were presented a broad range of
stimulus/background conditions.  The usual individuality of our
subjects was found also in regard to this aspect of the VER, each
showing marked differences in terms of the degree of summation
shown for given conditions (White et al., 1978).

Under certain conditions the degree of summation shown by a
subject could be quite impressive, definitely out of line with the
results of psychophysical judgements dealing with binocular summation effects.  Two examples of marked summation are shown in Fig.
3.  They represent the reactions to two intensities of blue flashes
presented upon a rather high intensity yellow background.  This
stimulus background situation was overall the best for demonstrating the highest degree of summation for most of our group of
subjects.

Another finding which came out of this study was the fact that
some of our subjects' responses to left and right eye stimulation
were quite different.  This is illustrated in Fig. 4 (a).  The
stimulus was a relatively low intensity green flash (12 on the
Grass photostimulator) presented upon a relatively high level background.  Under these conditions the subject (myself) noticed that
he was having completely different color perceptions under the monocular conditions with one eye producing yellow and the other green.
It can be seen from the figure that when "green" was reported the
red component was missing.  When both the red and green components
were present in the evoked response a yellow flash was seen.


SUBCORTICAL ELEMENTS IN THE VER

In our earlier paper on color evoked potentials (White et al.,
1977) evidence was presented which indicated that the color specific
components around 100-150 msec were related to subcortical activity.  The strongest evidence was the fact that these response
components could be obtained even when there was no electrode in

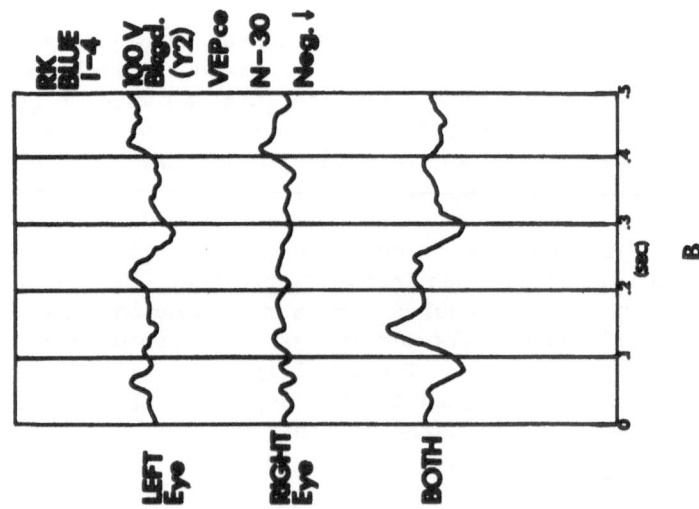

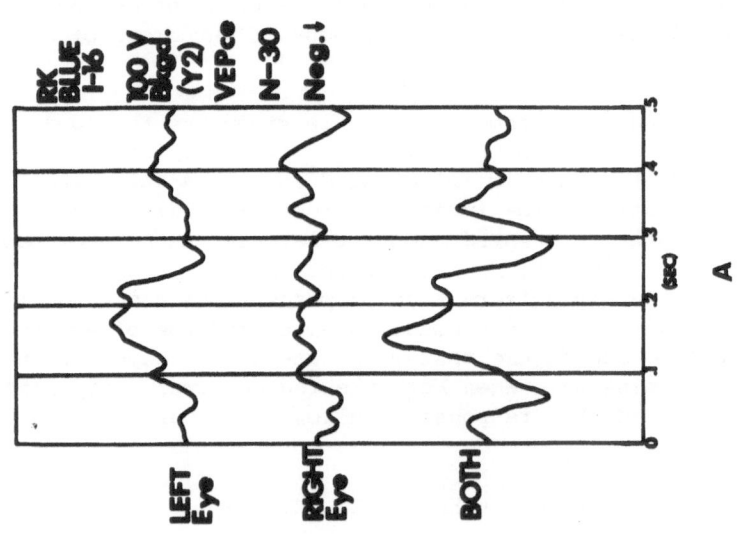

Fig. 3. Examples of binocular summation effects. Blue flashes upon a yellow background. Montage: Oz to cheekbones beneath the eye (VEP ce). (a) Flash intensity 116 (Grass photostimulator); (b) Flash intensity 14.

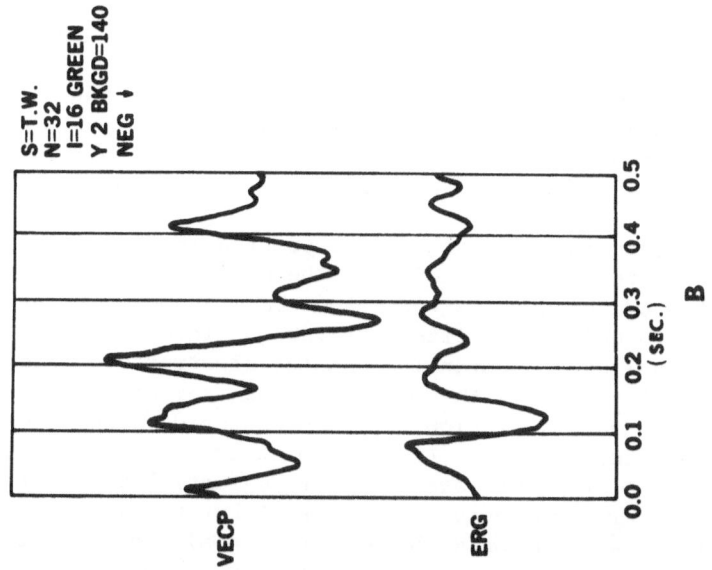

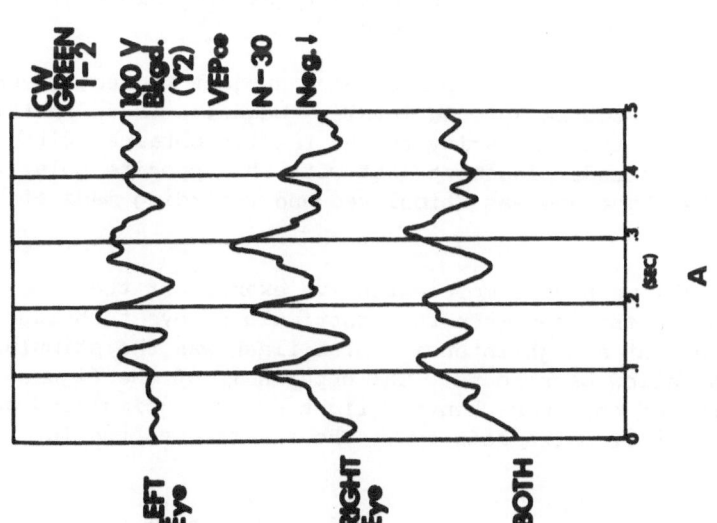

Fig. 4. (a) Example of differential monocular responses related to differences in color perception. Montage: Oz to cheekbones beneath the eyes. With right eye stimulation the subject saw a "yellow" flash; with the left a "green" flash. Note different responses around 100 msec. (b) Simultaneous recordings of VECP and "ERG". VECP montage: Oz to linked earlobes. "ERG" montage: Cheekbone beneath eye to linked mastoids. Right eye stimulated, recorded from left occluded eye.

place over the visual cortex. With the active electrode at the eye
and reference electrodes at the mastoids, for example, a red flash
will produce a sharp negative peak at 100 msec, precisely the time
at which a sharp positive peak would be obtained with an electrode
over the visual cortex with mastoids or earlobes as reference.
With the eye-mastoid montage the strong component at around 200 msec
does not appear, however, indicating that it is related to cortical
activity.

    Further evidence in this regard is presented in Fig. 4 (b),
which presents the results obtained when the cortex-mastoid and
eye-mastoid electrode placements were used simultaneously. It is
part of a series in which the effects of various levels of background on the visual evoked potential and the electroretinogram
(ERG) were being studied. As the background was raised the B-wave
(rod related) disappeared, leaving only the photopic (cone) elements of the light-adapted eye. At this point it was noted that
the early portions of the two waveforms were essentially mirror
images of one another (from about 40-160 msec) but became completely different from that time on with the strong positive activity
at 200 msec appearing only when using the cortex-mastoid montage.

    The presence of the scotopic B-wave limits the usefulness of
the ERG for studies such as this since only by light-adapting to
fairly high levels can one get photopic responses. It has been
found that responses evoked by flash stimuli can be obtained by
stimulating one eye and recording from one electrode placed on the
ridge of the cheekbone under the occluded eye. The B-wave does
not appear on the records so obtained. The components that do
appear are assumed to be related to activity at some higher level
in the visual system common to both eyes.

    Fig. 5 (a) presents the responses of a subject to red, green
and blue flashes at two background levels. Negative is up in this
figure to emphasize the similarity to the results obtained with
cortex-mastoid electrode placement (but with the opposite polarity).
In this case the right eye was stimulated and recording made at the
left eye.

    In Fig. 5 (b) we have a more extensive example of the type
of responses to be obtained when the nonstimulated eye technique
is used. Throughout a high intensity blue flash was the stimulus
with a varying yellow background. The upper half of the figure
shows the responses obtained when the right eye was stimulated and
recording was made from the left eye. The reverse is true for the
lower half.

    The results we see here support what we said earlier; the two
eyes appear to be different in their color sensitivity. In the

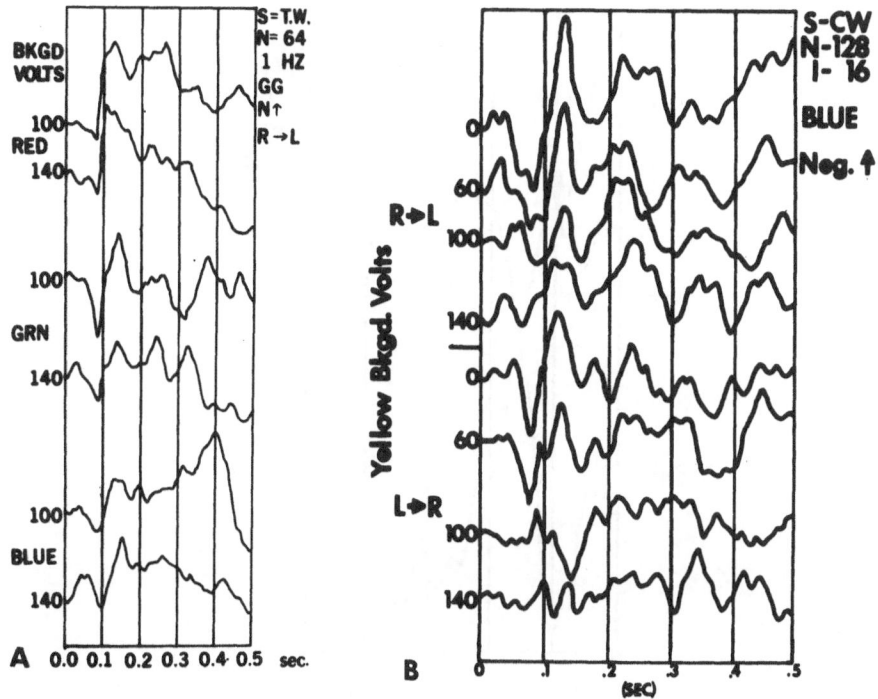

Fig. 5. (a)   Responses to red, green and blue flashes upon two
levels of yellow backgrounds (100 v and 150b).   Montage:   Cheekbone beneath eye to linked mastoids.   Right eye stimulated, recorded from left occluded eye.   (b)   Responses to blue flashes upon
yellow backgrounds.   Montage:   Cheekbones beneath eyes to linked
mastoids.   Upper records show right eye stimulated, recording from
left eye;   lower records show left eye stimulated and recording from
right eye.


lower half of the figure (L-R) a negative peak is prominent just
before 100 msec, while this is not the case in the R-L situation.
This finding has been consistent for this individual.   The difference is especially noticeable at the 100 volt background level.

     The findings here are consistent within themselves, but are
strikingly different from the records shown in Fig. 5 (a) wherein
similar stimulus/background conditions were used.   The very strong
peaking at 150 msec which has been identified as the first blue
component is not apparent as an outstanding feature.

     The responses in Fig. 6 seem to provide an answer, though not
now an explanation, to this problem.   Here is the same subject,
same flash intensity of the blue light, and with one of the yellow
background levels used in Fig. 7 (100 volts).   It can been seen

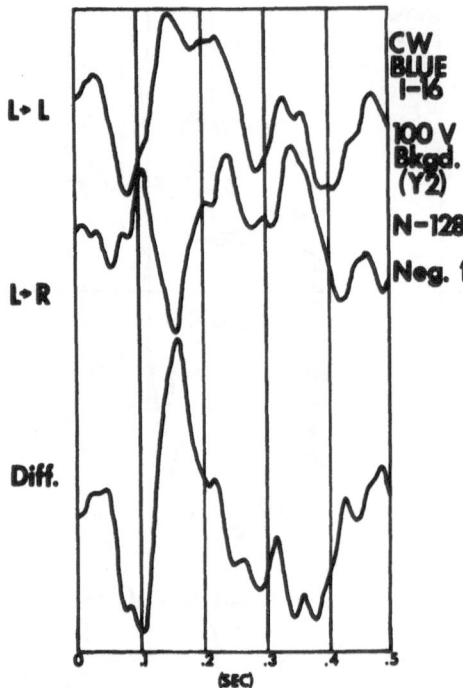

Fig. 6. Responses of subject CW to high intensity blue flashes
upon a 100v yellow background. Montage: Cheekbone beneath eyes to
linked mastoids. L - L: Left eye stimulated, recording from left
eye. L - R: Left eye stimulated, recording from right occluded eye.


that the morphology of the waveforms are similar for the L-R condition at that background level considering the expected day-to-day
variability.

The major difference to be seen in Fig. 6 is in the L-L condition, i.e., the left eye was stimulated and the recording was
made from beneath that eye. In this case there is a very strong
negative peak at 150 msec. The difference waveform is even more
emphatic; the strong negative peak at 150 msec does not carry across
to the unstimulated eye.

We would like to conclude our paper with a discussion of the
evoked waveforms shown in Fig. 7. In the first part [Fig. 7 (a)]
there is the comparison of the responses obtained in an eye to mastoid montage with the eye to midforehead montage. It is clear
that the prominent peak at 150 msec which has been so clearly related to the "blue" component of the VEP is also dependent on the
mastoid (or earlobe) electrode being used.

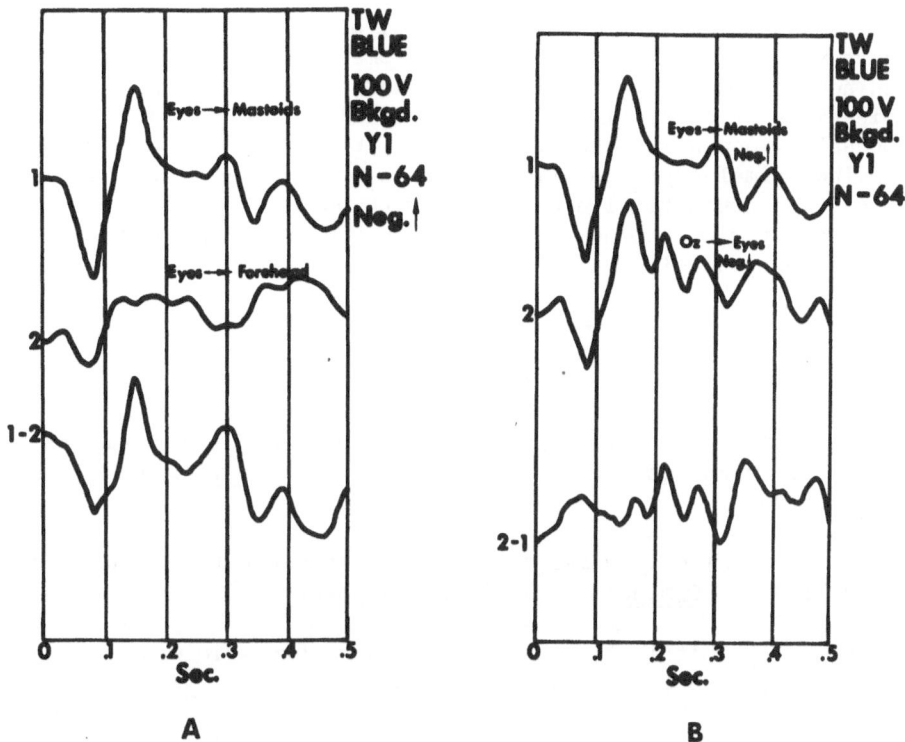

Fig. 7. (a) Responses of subject TW to blue flashes upon a 100v
yellow background. Upper response: eye to mastoid; center response:
eye to midforehead, a standard reference for the classic ERG; lower
waveform; the difference between these two waveforms. (b) Responses
of subject TW to blue flashes of 116 intensity upon a yellow background 100v. Upper waveform is eye-mastoid; middle record is cortex
to eye. Lower is the difference between the other two.

The second part of Fig. 7 (b) contrasts the eye-mastoid montage with the cortex to eye montage and the cortex to mastoid montage under this particular stimulus/background situation. Again
it is clear that the prominent peak at 150 msec is primarily dependent on an electrode being placed in the mastoid location while
the later components require the use of a cortical electrode.

SUMMARY

Previously published findings by our group regarding color
evoked potentials were replicated and examples from a recent study
on binocular summation of such potentials were presented. Our

earlier suggestion that certain elements of the evoked waveform represent visual processing activity at some subcortical level was
given added support by examples of evoked potentials obtained from
combinations of cortical and noncortical electrode placements.  The
strongest evidence was that the activity between about 40-160 msec
following stimulus presentation could be obtained with both the
cortical and noncortical electrodes (with opposite polarities),
while the activity around 200 msec and beyond was dependent on the
use of a cortical electrode.

REFERENCES

Bartlett, N.R., Eason, R.G. and White, C.T.  Binocular summation
    in the evoked cortical potential.  Percept. Psychophys., 1963,
    3, 75-76.

Huber, C.  Visual evoked responses during exposure to strong color-
    ed lights.  Ophthal. Res., 1972, 3, 55-62.

Krauskopf, J.  Contributions of the primary chromatic mechanisms
    to the generation of visual evoked potentials.  Vis. Res.,
    1973, 13, 2289-2298.

Mollon, J.D. and Krauskopf, J.  Reaction time as a measure of the
    temporal responses properties of individual color mechanisms.
    Vis. Res., 1973, 13, 27-40.

Pieron, H.  The Sensations: Their Functions, Processes and Mechan-
    isms, New Haven: Yale University Press, 1952.

White, C.T., Kataoka, R.W. and Martin, J.I.  Colour evoked poten-
    tials:  Development of a methodology for the analysis of the
    processes involved in colour vision.  In J.E. Desmedt (Ed.),
    Visual Evoked Potentials in Man:  New Developments, Oxford:
    Clarendon Press, 1977.

White, C.T., White, C.L. and Hintze, R.W.  The color evoked poten-
    tial:  Comparison of monocular and binocular effects.  Int. J.
    Neurosci., in press.

# ABSTRACTS

# INTERACTIONS BETWEEN TARGET AND MASKING STIMULI: PERCEPTUAL AND EVENT RELATED POTENTIAL EFFECTS

John L. Andreassi, Joseph A. Gallichio, Nancy E. Young
Baruch College, City University of New York

The purpose of this investigation was to determine the effects of target-mask contour interactions (backward masking paradigm) on perception and visual event related potentials (ERPs). Three experiments were conducted. In the first, masking stimuli closely bordered the target on 25%, 50%, 75% or 100% of its perimeter. Increased amounts of target-mask contour interaction resulted in progressively greater decreases in ERP amplitude (Oz recordings) to target stimuli. (In all experiments a positive ERP component which appeared at 200 msec after target presentations was used in data analyses.) Perceptual masking occurred with contour interactions of 50% and over.

A second experiment examined visual ERPs to the masking stimulus alone, target alone and to a target-mask condition which produced perceptual masking. The ERPs were recorded from Oz to Cz. Perceptual masking was accompanied by significant ERP attenuation at Oz only. The Cz response was similar under all conditions. Amplitude of response at Oz was significantly greater for the mask alone compared to the target alone condition.

A third experiment compared the target-mask condition at an effective interstimulus interval for masking (40 msec) with ISIs in which target and mask were perceived either as simultaneous (10 msec) or successive (100 msec) presentations. The most interesting finding was that target-mask conditions which did not produce masking (10 msec and 100 msec ISIs) were not accompanied by ERP amplitude attenuation. The effective masking condition (40 msec ISI) resulted in significantly attentuated ERP amplitudes. The ERP changes were specific to Oz recordings since Cz records showed no amplitude changes for the different conditions. The mask alone condition again produced a significantly larger response than target alone. This difference may have been due to the larger amount of perceived contour for the mask alone (sixteen sides) vs. target alone (four sides). The results suggest that cortical excitatory-inhibitory activity produced by target and mask stimuli is reflected in ERP recordings obtained from over the occipital cortex, but not at the vertex.

445

CEREBRAL ORGANIZATION OF EVENT RELATED POTENTIALS
ANALYZED BY MULTIDIMENSIONAL SCALING TECHNIQUES

Jackson Beatty
Department of Psychology
University of California, Los Angeles

One of the most important but difficult problems in the analysis of event related potentials (ERPs) is the determination of
interareal relationships from simultaneously obtained averaged
recordings.  One approach to this problem is suggested by the recent configurational analysis of the spontaneous EEG using multidimensional scaling reported by Beatty (Beatty, Neuroscience Letters,
8 (1978) 99-104).  The present paper reports the results of a
similar analysis of interareal relations for visual, auditory and
somatosensory ERPs using data originally described by Goff and
Allison.  From these data the latencies of ten reliably appearing
early or middle (less than 150 msec) components at eighteen sites,
were used to compute a half-matrix of the Euclidean distances between all possible electrode pairs for each stimulus type.  The
three resulting matrices represent the measured functional distances
between electrodes for which a two-dimensional configurational
solution was attempted using INDSCAL, a three-way multidimensional
scaling program.

INDSCAL was able to achieve a low error two-dimensional
solution with the following properties.  First, the obtained
dimensions might naturally be labelled anterior-posterior and left-
right.  Second, the grouping of recording sites in this functional
space indicates a clear division between frontal and posterior
cortex along the anterior-posterior dimension.  Third, the individual solutions for the three stimulus types indicate the anterior-
posterior dimension dominates the configuration for the visual ERP,
whereas the left-right dimension predominates for the somatosensory
ERP.  Finally, for all ERPs the orderly representation of occipital,
parietal, central and frontal zones, flanked on each side by
temporal cortex, may be reliably discerned.  Thus, it appears that
the configurational maps produced by multidimensional scaling
provide a means of representing functional units of the human
cerebral cortex in a comprehensible and meaningful fashion.

# ELECTROPHYSIOLOGICAL INDICATORS OF COGNITIVE DEFICITS IN CHRONIC ALCOHOLICS AND GERIATRIC SUBJECTS

H. Begleiter and B. Porjesz

Chronic alcohol abuse is known to produce information processing deficits. It has been postulated that these cognitive deficits are quite similar in alcoholic patients and in geriatric subjects. Therefore, we conducted a visual evoked potential (VEP) experiment designed to assess information processing deficits in chronic alcoholics, as compared to geriatrics and matched controls, using a P3 paradigm.

The experimental design required that the subject respond to rarely occurring (8.3%) target stimuli only, while withholding responses to frequently occurring (83.3%) non-target stimuli and rare (8.3%) "novel" stimuli. The target shape and non-target shape were alternated over four blocks (96 stimuli/block) in the first condition (Long Blocks) and were alternated four times as often (16 blocks) in the second condition (Short Blocks) containing 24 stimuli/block. Monopolar VEPs were recorded at Oz, Pz, Cz, Fz, F3 and F4, and peak-to-peak measurements (P1, N1, P2, N2, P3), as well as principal component factor analyses with varimax rotation, were performed on the data. This paper is limited to a discussion of the Pz electrode.

Our results indicate that the alcoholics manifested significantly depressed or absent P3s to target stimuli when compared to both the normal controls and the geriatric subjects. On the other hand, the geriatric subjects displayed significantly delayed latencies when compared to both the alcohol and control groups for all conditions. Therefore, our data does not support the view that CNS deficits in alcoholics are similar to those in geriatric subjects.

# GSR, AEP AND CNV IN DEPRESSED PATIENTS AND HEALTHY CONTROLS

J. Bolz, H. Giedke and H. Heimann
Psychiatric Clinic, University of Tübingen, West Germany

In eighteen patients with primary affective disorders and twenty-seven healthy, age matched controls, GSR (skin resistance level, number of spontaneous fluctuations, amplitude and habituation rate of orienting response, AEP and CNV (Fz, Cz) were measured in response to auditory stimuli. During the non-response condition, the resting subject heard pairs of tones (ISI 2 sec, III 7-12 sec), while in the response condition, he had to react upon the second stimulus by pressing a key.

Depressed patients develop AEP amplitudes (N1-P2 differences) which average 15% smaller and CNVs which are about 50% smaller than those of healthy controls.

|  |  | Patients | Controls |  |
| --- | --- | --- | --- | --- |
| AEP (N1-P2 µV) | Fz | 24.1+ 9.6 | 31.3+ 9.5 | p<0.01 |
|  | Cz | 22.8+10.4 | 31.7+16.2 | p<0.05 |
| CNV (µVsec) | Fz | 7.3+ 6.6 | 17.4+ 9.3 | p<0.001 |
|  | Cz | 10.4+ 7.7 | 19.2+10.5 | p<0.001 |

The last finding is at variance with the results of Small and Small (1971), in as far as these authors found smaller CNVs only when warning stimulus and imperative stimulus differed in modality and not when a single modality was used. A higher degree of inhibition in depressed patients, as measured in GSR, is confirmed in respect to number and mean amplitude of GSR orienting responses during response condition: depressed patients show less response and smaller response amplitudes. Our hypothesis that inhibition as measured in GSR is positively correlated with a reduction of AEP is only partially supported by the data: mean AEP amplitude is positively correlated with the number of spontaneous fluctuations and is negatively correlated with skin resistance level - but in the depressed group only. On the other hand, CNV (Fz) is negatively correlated with the number of spontaneous fluctuations and positively with skin resistance level - also in the depressed group only. Finally, mean GSR amplitudes during the response condition are positively correlated with CNV (Fz) in patients, as well as in healthy controls.

# SCALP-RECORDED VISUAL EVOKED SUBCORTICAL POTENTIALS IN MAN

Roger Q. Cracco and Joan B. Cracco
Brooklyn, New York

Short latency auditory and somatosensory subcortical evoked potentials (EP) have been recorded from the human scalp. Similar visual evoked potentials have not been described in man. In animals, however, short latency EP have been recorded from the optic nerve, tract, lateral geniculate body, optic radiation and visual cortex. We describe similar scalp-recorded visual EP in man.

EP to bright light flash stimulation were recorded from the scalp of fifteen adults. This response consisted of a series of potentials which were distributed widely over the scalp. The onset latency of the response recorded over anterior frontal regions was 9-17 msec, and the peak latency of the first potential was 11-21 msec. The oscillations (100-160 cps) persisted for up to 90 msec. The onset latency of the response recorded over central-parietal-occipital regions was 13-24 msec, and the peak latency of the first potential was 15-27 msec. These oscillations (80-180 cps) persisted for over 100 msec in some subjects.

These EPs were greater in amplitude at midline and parasagittal recording locations than in temporal leads. Over posterior head regions the first few waves were similar in amplitude in central, parietal and occipital leads and were lower in amplitude than subsequent ones. In some subjects the subsequent oscillations were similar in amplitude at central, parietal and occipital sites, while in others they were more prominent in occipital leads.

The source of these potentials recorded over anterior frontal regions is uncertain. Similar potentials have been recorded from the optic nerve and tract of animals and from the ERG of animals and man. However, under the conditions of sustained light adaptation used in this study, the optic nerve and tract potentials recorded in animals are maximal, but the ERG potentials are attenuated and are not consistently recorded in different preparations. This suggests that the oscillatory potentials recorded from anterior scalp regions in man may arise, at least in part, in anterior optic pathways including the optic nerve and tract.

The distribution of the oscillations recorded from posterior scalp regions is not consistent with an origin in the ERG. Their short onset latency and frequency are similar to the oscillatory potentials recorded from the lateral geniculate body, optic radiation and cortex of animals. It seems likely that these potentials arise in these structures.

# EFFICACY OF THE SCALP-RECORDED VISUALLY EVOKED POTENTIAL IN DEMONSTRATING MISROUTING OF OPTIC PROJECTIONS IN MAN

Donnell Creel, V. A. Hospital, Salt Lake City, Utah 84148
Frank E. O'Donnell, Jr., John Hopkins University, Baltimore
Richard A. King and Carl J. Witkop, Jr., University of Minnesota

Visual systems of albino mammals, including humans, are anomalous. Anomalies include: (1) reduced uncrossed optic projections, (2) disorganized lamination of lateral geniculate nuclei and (3) disorganization of projections to visual cortex. Abnormalities have been verified in nine species of mammals, including humans. Experiments with animals and humans have shown that visually evoked potentials (VEPs) recorded from surface electrodes reflect the disorganized retinogeniculostriate projections. The organization of uncrossed and crossed optic projections may be examined by comparing effects of binocular versus monocular stimulation while recording VEPs from both hemispheres.

Binocular versus monocular stimulation produces no significant alteration of the VEP in most normally pigmented humans. VEPs were recorded from sixty human total albinos and from ten human ocular albinos. Approximately 70 percent of human albinos and ocular albinos show significant alteration of VEPs following monocular stimulation, with one or more components of the VEP missing or significantly attenuated. Efficacy varies between luminance onset-offset, pattern onset-offset and pattern-reversal stimuli.

The asymmetric VEPs of monocularly illuminated human albinos reflect the disorganization of optic fibers similar to that reported for other albino mammals. The asymmetrical VEPs of human albinos are probably due to disorganization of cortical projections similar to the disorganization detailed for the Siamese cat. The missing VEP components are most likely the result of disorganized geniculostriate projections generating potentials in abnormally oriented areas of the visual cortex. The effect of misrouting of optic afferents found in albinos is similar to shifting the visual field midline ($0°$ meridian) up to $20°$. In the albino this shift is analogous to the effect of partial field stimulation in a normally pigmented subject. Changes in components of the VEP of monocularly stimulated human albinos are similar to those in the VEP of patients with homonymous hemianopsia or localized unilateral macular scotoma affecting the first $20°$ of the horizontal field. Scalp-recorded VEPs detect the abnormal cortical projections in patients with various types of albinism reflecting their lack of a normal neuronal substrate for cortical binocularity of vision.

450

# EVENT RELATED BRAIN POTENTIALS IN RESPONSE TO CONSCIOUS AND NON-CONSCIOUS STIMULI: HEMISPHERIC SPECIALIZATION AND THE EFFECTS OF ATTENTION

Richard J. Davidson
State University of New York at Purchase

Two experiments were performed on evoked brain potentials in response to consciously detected and non-conscious stimuli. The purpose of Experiment I was to determine whether selective attention influenced EPs to subthreshold stimuli. In the first experiment ten subjects were exposed to alternating stimuli in four classes: above threshold auditory (aa) and visual (av), below threshold auditory (ba) and visual (bv). Incremental thresholds were obtained for visual and auditory stimuli. Subjects received the following conditions: Attend Auditory (AA); Attend Visual (AV). EEG was recorded from O2, T4 and F4. The main hypothesis tested in the present data is that the amplitude of the EP in response to unconscious stimuli will be enhanced during attention to the modality of the target stimulus. The results confirmed the prediction for visual stimuli; in the seven subjects showing an EP in response to bv stimuli, N1 at F4 was significantly higher during AV versus AA. Although we recorded from only right hemisphere leads in Experiment I, in pilot work the T3 EP to suprathreshold stimuli was larger than the T4 EP, with the opposite obtained in response to subthreshold stimuli. Experiment II was designed to: a) further explore this finding; b) develop more rigorous psychophysical methods for characterizing conscious and unconscious stimuli. Six right-handed subjects were exposed to a two-interval forced choice detection paradigm. Two standard tones separated by a 1 sec interval were presented binaurally. Subjects were required to detect in which interval a 40 msec amplitude increment occurred. The amplitude of the increment was varied to maintain 75% correct detection. Subjects also rated their degree of confidence in their response. EEG was recorded from T3, T4, F3 and F4. For each subject, EPs were obtained in response to correctly detected stimuli and misses with the constraint that the mean amplitude increment be equivalent for both sets. The results revealed significant differences in the N2-P3 component between hits versus misses for T3 and F3 but not for T4 and F4. The T3 response to hits was larger than that for T4; in addition, the difference between hits versus misses was greater in T3 versus T4. Five of six subjects showed a difference of greater than 2 μV between hits versus misses in T3 with only one of six showing a comparable difference in T4 (p=.039). These findings suggest that identical stimuli, which are detected versus missed, evoked different brain responses and specifically indicate that the left hemisphere shows an enhanced responsiveness to conscious stimuli compared to the right.

CLINICAL USE OF THE ABR IN AN INFANT INTENSIVE CARE UNIT

P. A. Despland, University of California, San Diego and
R. Galambos, University Hospital of Lausanne, Switzerland

The auditory brain stem response (ABR) yields information on both the neurological and the audiological status of infants, children and adults. We have developed a procedure for extracting each type of information for separate study and have applied it to over 100 premature infants (28 to 42 weeks gestational age) in an intensive care unit. The procedure is based on these well known facts: (1) the interval between waves I and V is constant at a given age; (2) the threshold lies close to that stimulus intensity where wave V is smallest in amplitude and longest in latency.

Using click stimuli at rates of 37 or 70 per second, we have identified four infants with neurological disorder, eleven with audiological disorder and two with both. The I-V interval and the response threshold were considered to be normal in 91. For the audiological cases, the clinical history was analyzed in an effort to identify the risk factors for hearing loss and estimate their importance.

Nine such factors were identified, and the combination of perinatal hypoxia and postnatal acidosis appeared most frequently.

THE EVOKED POTENTIAL AS A MEASURE OF BRAIN DYSFUNCTION:
AGING, DOWN'S SYNDROME, ALCOHOLISM, AMYOTROPHIC
LATERAL SCLEROSIS AND RENAL DISEASE

R. E. Dustman, E. C. Beck and E. G. Lewis
Veterans Administration Hospital
Salt Lake City, Utah 84148

In an attempt to develop the evoked potential (EP) technique
into a useful procedure for evaluating brain dysfunction, we have
recorded EPs from several hundred normal subjects whose ages ranged
from the first through the eighth decade.  These data reveal striking age related changes which must be taken into account when evaluating patient populations.

EPs recorded from 66 Down's syndrome (DS) individuals aged
5-62 years were significantly larger than those of normals.  While
the EPs of normals clearly habituated over time, those of the DS
group did not.  The EPs of the DS group did not show age related
trends similar to those observed in the EPs of normal subjects.
These findings support the concept that deficits in central inhibition characterize the DS brain.

To determine if alcoholism promotes CNS aging, twenty young
alcoholics, young normals and normal oldsters were compared with
respect to EPs, WAIS subtests and a battery of neuropsychological
tests.  Despite a nearly forty year age difference between the
young alcoholics and the oldsters, the EPs and test performances
of the two groups exhibited a surprising number of similarities.

Amyotrophic lateral sclerosis (ALS) is a chronic, progressive
degenerative disease which selectively destroys the motor system
from cortex to anterior horn cells.  Somatosensory EP waves of ALS
patients were delayed and of smaller amplitude than those of
normals.  We speculate that these changes in somatosensory EP waves
reflect alterations of motor or pyramidal feedback acting on the
somatosensory system.

The short term effects of hemodialysis on the CNS were assessed with EP and neuropsychological test measures which were
obtained 1, 24, 42 and 66 hours following dialysis.  A highly
consistent relationship between time since dialysis and EP
latency was found.  Latencies were shortest at 24 hours following
dialysis and longest at 66 hours.  Performance on two tests of
visual-motor speed and accuracy paralleled the EP latency findings:
performance was best 24 hours following dialysis.  The results
indicate that there are consistent changes in the CNS as time since
dialysis lengthens.

# A NEW TEST OF BRAIN FUNCTION:
## BRAIN STEM TRANSMISSION TIME (BTT)

M. Fabiani, H. Sohmer, C. Tait, M. Gafni, R. Kinarti

Department of Physiology, Hebrew University-Hadassah
Medical School, Jerusalem, Israel

For several years auditory nerve and brain stem responses (BSR) have been used routinely in auditory diagnosis to give objective information regarding both hearing threshold and site of lesion. Recently the value of BSR in neurological diagnosis, lesion localization and psychopathology has been demonstrated. One of the characteristic electrophysiologic response deviations observed is prolonged response latency of later waves which is best quantified by measuring the time interval between the latency of the first response wave (N) and a certain late brain stem response wave. This measure has been called brain stem transmission time (BTT). The purpose of this study was to describe BTT as a recorder in normal subjects under various conditions. BTT was recorded in normal subjects in several age groups from neonates to late childhood-adulthood and under several stimulus conditions.

BTT is the time interval between the peak of compound auditory nerve response (wave 1) (the input to the brain stem) and the trough of the earlobe positive wave generated in the region of the inferior colliculus (output) BTT is longest in neonates and approaches adult values at the age of three years. BTT is relatively independent of click intensity, conductive (middle ear lesion) hearing loss, click rate (except for high click rates) and click frequency (filtered clicks).

This finding that for a given age group, BTT is generally independent of most stimulus conditions, makes it a useful, functional test of brain stem activity in audiology, neurology and psychopathology.

EQUIVOCATION IN PREDICTION VERSUS NO-PREDICTION SCHEDULES:
EFFECTS ON ERSP MEASURES

B. Fenelon and B. Frost

University of Newcastle, Australia

The classical CNV paradigm involves a static S1-S2 relationship which is an inadequate analog of real-life learning situations
in which anticipations and expectancies are developed.  The P300
component may more plausibly be associated with imperative events
and antecedent psychological factors.

Six experiments were performed in a series on the same subjects
(N=14 adults, half strongly dextral, half strongly sinistral).
Three paradigms were employed: 1) prediction-response to accuracy
of prediction; 2) prediction-response to accuracy of stimulus sequence; 3) no prediction-response to accuracy of stimulus sequence.
Four experiments involved analysis or synthesis of simple geo-
metrical figures; the other two involved presentation of alphabetic
series.  The differential motor response of the subject followed S3.

Preliminary ANOVA results (for sites iP4, iP3 only) indicate
that S2-S3 negativity (CNV) varies greatly between schedules.  For
certain conditions in interaction there are significant handedness
groups differences, and these groups also differ in interhemispheric
response.

The difference between hemispheres in post-S1 positivity (P300)
(right hemisphere amplitude greater than left) is higher when the
sequence of stimulation is incorrect than when it is correct.  Post-
S3 positivity (P300) is significantly small in the alphabetic
schedule compared with the other paradigms.  Overall, the amplitudes
of this component for correct versus incorrect outcome sequences,
interact with the nature of the schedule.

These preliminary results show that the magnitude of ERSP components is much affected by stimulus-organism-response factors,
singly and in interaction, which are omitted from many experimental designs.

# THE UTILITY OF ERPs IN DETERMINING AGE-RELATED DIFFERENCES

Judith M. Ford and Adolf Pfefferbaum
Langley Porter Neuropsychiatric Institute,
University of California, San Francisco, Ca. 94143

ERPs provide unique information about age related neural and cognitive deficits. ERPs are better than behavioral techniques alone because they can: (1) be recorded to both unattended and attended stimuli; (2) be recorded from subjects performing no task; (3) supplement reaction time (RT) measures for estimating timing of different mental events. We describe three experiments in which ERPs were used in these ways to compare young (20-29 years) to old (74-89 years), non-senile, extraordinarily healthy women.

To determine if elderly subjects can ignore irrelevant auditory stimuli and detect target stimuli, we used a technique devised by Hillyard et al. (1973). The results for N1 reflected that both groups could attenuate irrelevant stimuli, while the results for P3 indicated that, although elderly subjects could identify targets, they were slower than were young subjects.

To demonstrate age related neural differences without demanding task involvement we recorded ERPs to four tone intensities from passive subjects. The amplitude of N1 increased with intensity for young and old subjects. The amplitude of P2 increased with intensity for young but decreased for old subjects. The amplitudes of an early peak (P1) and a late sustained potential were more negative in young than in old subjects.

To estimate separately the speed of some mental processes, we used both RT and the latency of P3 to the target in a Sternberg task. On each trial, subjects received a memory set of 1-4 digits followed by a target digit. Subjects pressed one of two buttons indicating whether the target was a member of the memory set. RT P3 latency to the target were increasing linear functions of the number of items in the set. Some of the slopes and intercepts of these functions, the mental processes they may reflect and the time taken to complete the processes for old and young are listed in the table below.

| | RT Intercept | P3 Latency Slope | P3 Latency Intercept | RT-P3 Latency Intercept |
|---|---|---|---|---|
| Hypothetical mental processes | Encoding + Motor | Memory Scanning | Encoding | Motor |
| Time to complete the process: | | | | |
| Old | 1028 ms | 27 msec/digit | 448 msec | 582 msec |
| Young | 720 ms | 29 msec/digit | 369 msec | 350 msec |

APPLICATION OF ERPs IN THE STUDY OF DRUG USE AND ABUSE IN MAN:
A CLOSE LOOK WITH MORE SENSITIVE TASKS
AND MEASUREMENT TECHNIQUES

Ronald I. Herning, Ph.D. and Reese T. Jones, M.D.
Langley Porter Institute, Department of Psychiatry
University of California, San Francisco
San Francisco, California 94143

Components of the sensory evoked response later than 75 msec are
limited to processes other than pure sensory stimulus reception.
Although there is some disagreement as to the exact nature of this
process(es), as well as which component(s) appears to reflect which
process(es), there is no doubt that these latter components involve
an evaluation of the stimulus at some level, and can be dependably
altered by slight psychological manipulations.  The components in
75 to 250 msec range are also altered by a variety of psychoactive
drugs.  Most often these midrange components are decreased by de-
pressants and increased by stimulants.  However, the effects of few
drugs have been studied on components later than 250 msec in paradigms
designed to maximize these components.

Drugs are often abused for their psychoactive properties.  Are
these altered perceptual states detectable and quantifiable by ERP
methods on other than the sedation continuum?  Do abused drugs have
some common effect on the ERP?  To answer these questions, we have
studied the effects of single doses of alcohol, hexobarbital, THC
(marijuana), nicotine and morphine on the auditory ERPs of normal,
healthy adults performing the oddball task.  For all drugs except
alcohol, the ERPs were recorded at times of maximal drug effects.
All drugs produced a decrease in P300 of the auditory response to
the rare tone.  Table 1 lists the percentage decrease from pre or
control for each of the drugs.  These and possibly other psychoactive drugs alter or reduce the cortical processing of rare occurring stimuli.

Table 1

| Drug | Dose | Test Time After Dose | % Decrease at $P_z$ |
|------|------|----------------------|---------------------|
| Ethanol | 1 ml/kg Oral | 2.5 hr | 9% |
| Morphine | .14 mg/kg I.M. | 45 min | 18% |
| Hexobarbital | 500 mg Oral | 3 hr | 20% |
| Nicotine | One "Camel" | At end of smoking | 27% |
| THC | 10 mg THC Smoked | 15 min | 30% |

# AUDITORY EVOKED POTENTIALS AND PSYCHOPHYSICAL PARAMETERS
## IN CIRCADIAN STUDIES

G. A. Kerkhof and J. H. Werner
Department of Physiology and Department of Psychology
University of Leiden, Leiden, The Netherlands

In the past few years there has been increasing evidence of a close relationship between detection behavior and the averaged evoked potential (AEP) and the importance of nonsensory, as well as sensory, factors has also been established (Hirsh, S.K., Psychon. Sci., 1971, 22, 173-175). The relationship between these nonsensory factors and the P3 component has been studied chiefly within the context of the Theory of Signal Detectability (Hillyard, S.A. et al., Science, 1971, 172, 1357-1360). With respect to circadian variation in auditory psychophysical performance and related AEPs, the results are not unequivocal (Conroy, R.T.W.L. and Mills, J.M., Human Circadian Rhythms. J. and A. Churchill: London, 1970). The main objective of the present study is to clarify this problem.

In three diurnal studies (10.00 and 19.30 h) we employed yes/no ratings and 2AFC procedures. The subject had to judge whether or not a burst of white noise contained a weak sinusoidal signal. No evidence was found for diurnal fluctuations of perceptual sensitivity, response bias, P3 amplitude or the relationships between the two detection parameters and P3. We also conducted an around-the-clock experiment involving a rating task at four different times of the day (04.00, 10.00, 16.00 and 20.00 h). The AEPs were analyzed by principal components analysis. For some components slight but significant effects were found. In current data analysis, particular attention is given to the relationship between single EPs and detection behavior by the use of multivariate analysis procedures; latency characteristics of the single EPs as well as alternative detection parameters, are under investigation. Our present approach is directed at characterization of detection and performance in terms of perceptual sensitivity and response bias on the basis of single EPs. This should enable us to establish short-term changes in neurophysiological correlates of detection behavior.

# EFFECTS OF METHYLPHENIDATE ON HYPERACTIVE CHILDREN'S EVOKED RESPONSES DURING PASSIVE AND ACTIVE ATTENTION

R. Klorman, L. F. Salzman, H. L. Pass,
A. D. Borgstedt and K. B. Dainer
University of Rochester

This study was aimed at assessing the effects of methylphenidate on hyperactives' evoked responses (ERP) and performance in the Continuous Performance Test (CPT). Eighteen hyperactive boys were removed from methylphenidate treatment for 6-51 days and were tested in two different sessions in which they received methylphenidate (0.3 mg/kg) and placebo in multiple blind fashion and counterbalanced order. In addition, seventeen normal boys were tested without drugs. For both samples vertex-derived evoked potentials were recorded to the fifty go- and the fifty preceding no-go stimuli of the CPT. When the task was administered without a requirement to respond, there were no electrophysiologic differences between hyperactive and normal children.

In the active CPT, normal children made fewer errors of omission ($F(1/31)=18.06$, $p < .001$) and commission ($F(1/31)=21.27$, $p < .001$) and displayed faster reaction times ($F(1/31)=6.33$, $p < .025$) than hyperactives tested under placebo. In addition, the late positive component (LPC; P320) of the evoked responses evoked by both go- and no-go stimuli was smaller in placebo treated hyperactives than in normals ($F(1/31)=5.47$, $p < .05$). Methylphenidate increased the amplitude of hyperactives' LPC ($F(1/13) =4.88$, $p < .05$) and ameliorated their performance, especially commission errors ($F(1/13)=5.55$, $p < .05$) and reaction times ($F(1/13)=4.69$, $p < .05$). These results confirmed previous findings of normalization by methylphenidate of hyperactives' performance and electrophysiologic activity during active attention.

EVOKED POTENTIALS IN SENILE DEMENTIA

S. Laurian, J.-M. Gaillard, G. Gruber, H. Heimann,
A. Lobrinus, J. Reigner, J. Wertheimer
Clinic of Psychiatry, University of Lausanne, Switzerland

In order to evaluate the modifications of brain evoked responses
n senile dementia we performed two studies.

In the first one, visual evoked responses (VER) to flashes were
ecorded at occipital (Oz) and vertex (Cz) leads in twelve patients
uffering from severe senile dementia and twelve young normal adults.
hereas the occipital responses were rather similar in the two groups,
ertex responses were of lower amplitude in patients than in con-
rols and sometimes were hardly discernible. Therefore, the vertex
esponses to flashes seemed to be impaired in senile dementia.

In order to further elucidate this finding and to obtain a con-
rol group matched for age, we performed a second study on ten pa-
ients suffering from simple senile dementia (SD; mean age = 83.4
ears), seven patients suffering from Alzheimer's disease or senile
ementia evolving towards an Alzheimer condition (AD; mean age =
3.5 years). The experimental procedure was similar to that used in
he precedent study; in addition, we investigated the responses to
uditory stimuli (AER). The analysis of the results revealed that
n SD, the vertex VERs presented a quite standard configuration, but
ith longer latencies and greater interindividual variability than
n controls. In AD the vertex VERs were not discernible, the N1-P2
omponent being replaced, on the grain mean (obtained by averaging
ll responses of all patients), by a positive wave of low amplitude.
n the other hand, the vertex AERs were present in all subjects,
he latencies being longer in patients than in controls. Therefore,
n AD the vertex VER is missing, while the vertex AER is preserved.
part from its clinical implications, this finding puts into question
he generally admitted opinion of the nonspecificity of the vertex
esponse.

ELECTROPHYSIOLOGICAL AND BIOCHEMICAL STUDIES
IN AUTISTIC CHILDREN TREATED WITH VITAMIN B6

G. Lelord, J. P. Muh, J. Martineau, B. Garreau and S. Roux
School of Medicine, 37032 Tours, France

Previous studies have indicated that certain autistic children
are favorably influenced by vitamin B6 (Rimland B., Callaway, E.
and Dreyfus P., Am. J. Psychiat., 1978, 135, 472-475). Our recent
laboratory study of forty-four autistic children disclosed fifteen
who were improved by large doses of B6. In addition, many of these
children showed a large decrease in the excretion of urinary
homovanillic acid during the B6 treatment.

A study of event related potentials (ERP) in some of these
children has been carried out before and during the treatment with
B6. Thirteen autistic children (average age, 9.5 years) and eleven
normal children (10 years) were recorded. Following a classical
conditioning paradigm, sound (1 KHz, 25 dB, 4 msec) was used as the
conditional stimulus and light (1 200 Lux, 0.1 msec) as the uncon-
ditional stimulus. Interstimulus interval was 800 msec. Evoked
potentials (EP) were recorded from the vertex and from the occiput
and measured in three windows: 0-100 msec (early EP), 100-400 msec
(medium EP), 400-800 msec (late EP).

Before treatment, early EP were larger (p<.05), and medium EP
smaller (p<.001), at the vertex in autistic children. Late negative
EP percentage was higher (p<.05) in normal children. B6 treatment
reduced early EP (p<.02), enhanced medium EP (p<.01) and increased
negative EP percentage (p<.05) in autistic children. The reduction
in homovanillic acid excretion was observed only in the autistic
children and not in the normal children. Thus, a tendency to normalization of electrophysiological as well as biochemical data was
observed in autistic children under vitamin B6 treatment.

Supported by CNRS, E.R.A. 697, INSERM ATP 78-97; DGRST, DNP 28-78.

# VISUAL EVENT RELATED POTENTIALS OF PILOTS AND NAVIGATORS

G. W. Lewis

Navy Personnel Research and Development Center
San Diego, California 92152

Recent research suggests relationships between hemisphere
lateral asymmetry, habituation and occupational performance. This
center is evaluating these hypotheses on several Navy occupational
groups. The present study is based on analyses of VERP data and
information processing task performance of a group of 58 aviators
from a Navy fighter squadron (28 pilots, 30 navigators). Eight
channels of VERP data (F3, F4, C3, C4, P3, P4, O1, O2) were acquired by a NOVA 2 computer acquisition system installed in a mobile
laboratory parked inside the squadron hangar. Technical problems
encountered in this operational environment will be discussed. A
simple recognition information processing task was performed by
each subject prior to VERP acquisition. The pilot group consisted
of thirteen instructors and fifteen students. Amplitude variates
($\mu$Vrms) at C3 (F=6.53, dF=1,56,p<.02) and F3 (F=5.28, dF=1,55,p<.05)
discriminated pilots from navigators. Seventy-one percent of aviators were correctly classified ($X^2$=8.35,p<.01). C3 amplitude was
less than C4 within the navigator group (t=3.10, dF=58,p<.01), but
not within the pilot group. Total hemisphere asymmetry (F=5.94,
dF=1,56, p<.018), site (F=186.88,dF=3,168, p<.001) and hemisphere
asymmetry-by-site interaction (F=3.41,dF=3,168, p<.019) were significant for all subjects. VERP habituation was assessed by comparing
VERPs of the first fifty flashes with the second fifty flashes.
Habituation was statistically significant (F=5.98,dF=1,27,p<.021)
for instructors, but not students. No reaction time differences
in information processing were found between the groups. The pilots
and navigators were placed in a high or low group based on performance ratings; P4 was greater than P3 amplitude for the high group
pilots, P3 was greater than P4 amplitude for the lows. P3 was
greater than P4 amplitude for the high group navigators, while P4
was greater than P3 amplitude for the lows. Asymmetry (R-L) standard deviations (SDs) were greater for both low pilot and navigator
groups than for the high groups. The SDs were greater in the
parietal-occipital areas than in frontal-central areas for the
low groups. Other Navy groups have shown similar VERP-performance
relationships, low performers having greater VERP SDs than high
performers (e.g. trainees on a sonar simulator).

# EFFECTS OF SLOW CORTICAL POTENTIALS ON REACTION TIME

W. Lutzenberger, T. Elbert, B. Rockstroh, N. Birbaumer
University of Tübingen

The relationship between slow cortical potentials (SCP) and response latency was investigated by inducing different shifts of SCP: visual feedback of SCP was provided by means of a little sketched rocket moving across a television screen into one of two goals during intervals of six seconds each; subjects were asked to direct the rocket into one of the goals depending on one of two signal tones which were presented in randomized order.

In the present experiment consisting of two identical sessions, series of reaction time trials alternated with series of feedback trials; during reaction time trials subjects heard the same signal tones as during the feedback trials and were additionally asked to escape an aversive noise following the signal tones by pressing a microswitch with their dominant (right) hand. Two groups of ten subjects each were investigated, one group receiving feedback of C4-recording of SCP, the other group receiving a C3-feedback.

Results demonstrate that subjects achieve significant instrumental control of SCP. During feedback intervals negative shifts were more pronounced in the right hemisphere (C4) than in the left (C3). The better control of SCP was achieved under conditions of C4-feedback. This result can be explained by the hypothesis that our feedback - spatial representation - was processed in the right hemisphere. In reaction time trials both groups showed pronounced differences in SCP between required negativity and required positivity. After feedback training, response latency was significantly shorter in trials with required negativity. An analysis of covariance for response latency with C3- or C4-scores respectively as covariate provided significant regression constants in both groups only for C4 (right hemisphere). This does not support a motor hypothesis which would suggest that differences in SCP recorded from sensorimotor areas (interpreted as motor potentials) are responsible for differences in response speed. Interpreting SCP as sign of (readiness for) information processing would also suggest that differences in response speed - as observed in the present reaction time task - may be due to differences in SCP but not necessarily due to differences recorded from the primary motor areas of the right hand.

# EFFECT OF SOUND PRESSURE DIRECTION AND FREQUENCY SPECTRUM OF CLICKS ON BRAIN STEM RESPONSES IN CHILDREN

Edward M. Ornitz

Both immaturity and high frequency hearing loss increase differences in brain stem responses to rarefaction and condensation clicks. Recent reports suggest abnormal brain stem responses to combined rarefaction and condensation clicks in autistic and other developmentally disabled children. Because of these developments, a parametric study of the influence of both the direction of sound pressure and the frequency spectrum of click evoked acoustic stimuli on brain stem responses in children seem advisable. Brain stem responses to four types of acoustic stimuli were collected from nine normal and six autistic children. The stimuli were either rarefaction or condensation clicks with peak acoustic energies of either 3150 Hz or 5000 Hz. All clicks were monaurally delivered at a rate of 10/sec at 68 dB (HL). Responses were recorded from a vertex to ipsilateral mastoid derivation. The peak latencies of vertex positive waves I, II, III, IV and V and brain stem transmission time were measured in response to each of the four types of clicks separately. Significant interactions between the influence of the direction of sound pressure and the peak acoustic energy of the stimulus occurred. Rarefaction (R) clicks induced a significantly earlier wave IV response than did condensation (C) clicks, regardless of peak acoustic energy, while wave I and wave II latencies were significantly earlier in response to R than to C clicks only at the higher peak acoustic energy. The C-R difference was significantly greater in response to the 5000 Hz than to the 3150 Hz clicks for wave II. Five thousand Hz clicks induced a significantly later wave II response than did 3150 Hz clicks for C clicks and a significantly earlier wave II response for R clicks. There were no such differences in respect to the other peaks when responses to C and R clicks were computed separately. On the other hand, when the responses to C and R clicks were algebraically combined in the computer (as is common practice), these differences were not seen while the latency of wave IV was significantly later in response to 5000 Hz clicks than to 3150 Hz clicks. The latter finding was not reflected in differences associated with separate computations of responses to R and C clicks. These results suggest that the practice of combining brain stem responses to R and C clicks may be misleading in some applications and that it is necessary to know the acoustic characteristics (frequency spectrum) of the click stimulus. On the other hand, brain stem transmission time was relatively unaffected by sound pressure direction or acoustic frequency spectrum. These results were utilized in a comparison of brain stem evoked response parameters in normal and autistic children. Recently reported latency differences and differences in brain stem transmission time were not confirmed.

# RELATIONS BETWEEN CONTINGENT NEGATIVE VARIATION
# AND BEHAVIOR UNDER PSYCHOACTIVE DRUGS IN MAN

J. Paty, M. Gioux, G. Boulard, Ph. Brenot, Ph. Deliac, B. Claverie,
J. M. A. Faure
Department of Experimental Medicine and Physiopathology
University of Bordeaux, France

We have tested the reliability of the contingent negative
variation (CNV) as an index for behavioral evaluation under psychoactive drugs in fifteen voluntary subjects.  Statistical analysis
was performed of the relevant relationships between electrophysiological parameters [amplitudes of the pre-imperative negativity (N)
and of the post-imperative positivity (P)] and reaction time (RT).

Five conditions were studied: (1) Standard (S1-L2), paired
stimulations of a conditioning sound (S1) and an imperative light
(L2) with motor response; (2) Disagreeable (S1-E2, with an electric
shock as an imperative stimulus; (3) Uncertainty (S1-?) with a
randomized suppression of the imperative stimulus and a separate
averaging of complete and incomplete sequences; (4) Positive
Reinforcement (S1-L2-RT) by indicating RT; (5) Negative Reinforcement
(S1-L2-E3) with an electric shock when RT was too long.

In five patients CNVs were studied during three sessions before
and after administration of chlorpromazine (CP) 10 mg, morphine (Mo)
1 cg or placebo (Pl) (intravenous injection).

In ten patients CNV were recorded during three sessions, after
oral administration of a benzodiazepine (lorazepam - Lo; diazepam -
Di) or placebo (Pl).  Placebo effect was seen only after intravenous
injection (low increase of amplitude and greater dispersion of RT).
CP and Mo modified the CNV in all the situations.  There were
increased N and P amplitudes of CNV and increased RT with CP.  Under
Mo, RT was unchanged while CNV decreased, then disappeared with
reversal after 45 minutes.  CNV and RT changes after Di and Lo were
selective, only seen in reinforcing conditions (increased N, decreased P waves of CNV and increased RT as compared to the standard
conditions).

These data suggest that there is no linear relation between CNV
amplitudes and RT.  Further CNV studies for the evaluation of psychoactive drugs must be referred to individual psychometric tests.

EVOKED POTENTIAL ABNORMALITY AND DISABILITY
IN BRAIN DAMAGED PATIENTS: A REPLICATION STUDY
AND PRELIMINARY FINDINGS IN RELATION TO OUTCOME

M. Rappaport, K. Hall, K. Hopkins, T. Belleza,
S. Berrol and R. Hamilton
University of California, San Francisco

Evoked potentials were obtained in a clinical setting from
brain damaged patients (with head injury and other types of CNS
damage) using auditory, visual and somatosensory stimuli.  Brain
stem and cortical responses were judged for degree of evoked potential abnormality (EPA).

Correlations between EPAs and initial disability ratings for
brain damaged patients (N=92) were positive and significant.  Findings in this study replicate those previously reported.  In addition,
the EPA rating procedure was tested and found to have significant
inter-rater reliabilities.  It is concluded that EPA ratings can be
used to aid in the assessment of the clinical condition and degree
of overall brain dysfunction in brain damaged patients at all levels
of consciousness.

In a selected sample of head injury patients (N=30) a significant relationship was found between extremes of EPA score and even-
tual outcomes.  These are preliminary findings and require replication.

Evoked potentials representing cortical activity were found to
be the most informative in reflecting overall brain functional status.
The major components of these EPs have been shown by others to be
related to basic cognitive functions such as habituation and attention.  It is felt that the degree to which these higher level brain
functions are preserved indicate a patient's potential for positive
outcome.

The need for further refinement in EP testing procedures and
in the method of utilizing combined EP and other pertinent clinical
data to improve prediction of outcome is indicated by cases with
paradoxical outcomes.

ELECTROCORTICAL MANIFESTATIONS OF COMPLEMENTARY
HEMISPHERIC SPECIALIZATION IN AN EXPECTANCY TASK

Charles S. Rebert, Roland C. Lowe and Jean M. Hatchel
SRI International
Menlo Park, California

Subjects were tested in a cued reaction time (RT) task wherein
warning stimuli (WS) were briefly presented as five letter words or
dot patterns randomly intermixed across trials. After 2 sec, an
imperative stimulus (IS) of the same category as the WS appeared,
and the subjects pressed a key with the left or right hand. The
right key was pressed if the IS word was a synonym of the WS word
or if the IS dot pattern was the same as the WS pattern, and the
left was pressed for antonyms or different patterns. It was predicted that CNVs would be larger over the left than right hemisphere on word trials and vice-versa on pattern trials in accordance
with speculations concerning hemispheric specialization. The CNV
was lateralized as expected, most prominently on pattern trials.
In addition, a negative transient potential and a late negative
post-imperative slow wave were similarly lateralized. P300 waves
were very large, and largest to the IS when the IS differed from
the WS, but P300 exhibited no lateralization. The results indicate
that it is possible to induce CNV differences in the hemispheres
without employing overt verbalizations by subjects in response to
the IS, so avoiding associated artifacts and enhancing the clinical
usefulness of CNV asymmetry. The lateralized anticipation may be
construed as a differential attentional set. Lateralization of the
negative component of the response to the IS is compatible with such
an interpretation as that component appears to reflect attention to
stimulus parameters that define an input channel. Attentional channels, then, may be defined in terms of specialized hemispheric/cog-
nitive functions. The substrate of cognitive set onto which a
stimulus impinges may strongly influence the extent to which EPs
evoked by the stimulus are lateralized. Thus, the failure to assess
"prior state" in EP asymmetry studies may account for much of the
confusion in that literature.

# THE EFFECTS OF OPTICAL BLUR AND GRATING ADAPTATION ON AMPLITUDE AND PHASE OF EVOKED POTENTIALS

Ingo Rentschler and Donatella Spinelli
Laboratory of Neurophysiology, CNR, Pisa, Italy

Optical image degradation and preadaptation of the eye to high contrast gratings (Blakemore and Campbell, 1969) both may reduce the visibility of low contrast gratings. We showed how these effects are correlated to reductions of EP amplitude. Significant temporal EP phase shifts have been observed only as a result of grating adaptation.

We used the EP recording technique of Campbell and Maffei (1970). The EP amplitude measured as a function of spatial frequency reveals significant effects of blur only at frequencies above 5 Hz. The EP phase linearly increases with log spatial frequency and closely correlates with the latency of neuromagnetic responses (Williamson et al., 1978) and Breitmeyer's (1975) psychophysical reaction time data. The phase, however, is not significantly affected by blurring the retinal image. Briefly, the accuracy of meridional EP refractometry is better than $\pm$ 0.5 D only if EP amplitudes are considered and the eye is stimulated at higher spatial frequencies (Rentschler and Spinelli, 1978).

Grating preadaptation of the eye causes a loss of EP amplitude and induces EP phase shifts as well. These effects show interocular transfer, as it is known, from psychophysical studies. We observed a decrease in latency when preadapting the ipsilateral eye and an increase in latency when adapting the contralateral eye. No subjective counterpart of such effect is known. The interocular transfer of grating adaptation might be used as an EP technique for testing binocular function in children.

# OPERANT EVOKED POTENTIAL CONDITIONING IN ANIMAL AND MAN

M. Roger, G. Sanfourche and G. Galand
E.R.A., C.N.R.S. no. 07.0624 (Neurophysiologie de la Vision).

With the operant conditioning technique, we trained ninety human subjects to modify their visual EP configuration. For half of them, training induced stable modifications restricted only to the reinforced wave. These modifications disappeared with extinction. Such results led us to some fundamental questions: (i) Is it possible to rule out any peripheral mechanism, i.e., are we dealing with true CNS activity conditioning? (ii) Which pathways and/or structures can account for these modifications? Some answers came from animal studies. We were able to train curarized rats to change their visual cortical EP waveform. Modifications exhibited the same characteristics as for man; they were strictly restricted to the wave submitted to reinforcement, susceptible to polarity reversal and disappeared with extinction. According to Graybiel (The Neurosciences, Third Study Program, 1974, M.I.T. Press), we recorded the responses of some structures along the "lemniscal line" and the "lemniscal adjunct" system. We could not find at the LGN level the waveform modifications evoked at the trained cortical site. We also recorded the EP activity of the NPT (nucleus posterior thalami) where Disterhoft and Stuart (J. Neurophysiol., 1976, 39, 266) found the earliest neural responses to a conditioning paradigm. This nucleus exhibited the same waveform alterations as those emitted in the cortical trained site. Moreover, successful training of the visual evoked activity of NPT itself showed us that this center must play an important role in operant conditioning of neural events. But further investigations are necessary to determine whether the observed modifications of NPT activity have a real subcortical origin or if they are a simple reflection of cortical activity.

# VISUAL EVOKED POTENTIALS DURING STIMULUS
## DISCRIMINATION LEARNING

Frank Rösler
University of Kiel, West Germany

During stimulus discrimination, learning the relevancy of
stimulus attributes changes with increasing practice.  At the beginning all the stimulus attributes will be seen as equally important,
and they will be processed with an equal amount of attention.  At
later stages of the acquisition phase, the subject can concentrate
solely on those attributes which have been shown to be relevant and
ignore all the others.  The present experiment was designed to determine whether these hypothesized changes in attentional set are
reflected in amplitude changes of the vertex evoked potential.
Method: Two-element visual stimuli, each composed of a circle
(varying in size) and a triangle (varying in shape), were paired
with different responses.  In one group of subjects only the dimension circle-size was relevant for the correct stimulus-response
identification, while triangle-shape was irrelevant.  In another
group the opposite held.  The two attributes of each stimulus were
presented separately in time.  Thus, evoked potentials picked up
from Cz to A2 could be averaged separately for different stages of
the acquisition phase and separately for the relevant and the irrelevant stimulus attributes.  The experiment was run with a total of
thirty-one subjects.  Results: While percentage of correct stimulus-
response associations increased linearly over blocks, systematic
amplitude changes could be observed in two positive peaks (P160 and
P330) of the AEPs.  First, the amplitudes of both components decreased continuously with increasing learning progress.  Second,
with increasing practice the amplitudes to the irrelevant attributes
became significantly smaller than those to the relevant attributes.
Third, the point at which the amplitudes to relevant and irrelevant
attributes diverged was different for the two components.  It was
earlier for the P330 and later for the P160.  The fact that the
amplitudes of the two positive peaks showed different trends with
increasing practice suggests that they reflect functionally distinct
processes of attentional set.

# THE UTILIZATION OF EVOKED POTENTIALS IN PSYCHOPHARMACOLOGY AND PHARMACOPSYCHIATRY

B. Saletu
Department of Pharmacopsychiatry and Psychiatry
University of Vienna, Austria

Quantitative evaluation of drug-induced alterations of latencies and amplitudes of human evoked potentials (EP) of normal volunteers resulted in characteristical "pharmaco-EP profiles" for the major classes of psychotropic drugs. Anxiolytics produce EP profiles characterized by a latency increase in early peaks and a decrease in late peaks of the secondary components, as well as by an attenuation of the amplitudes in general. In contrast, neuroleptics induce a latency increase in all peaks which, together with an amplitude attenuation, is especially prominent in the late portion of the EPs. This was also observed in chronic schizophrenic patients. Interestingly, therapy responsive patients showed different changes than therapy resistant ones: while the former revealed a marked latency increase during neuroleptic therapy, the latter showed only minor alterations or even changes in the opposite direction. There were no significant inter-group differences. Neuroleptic treatment of psychotic children resulted in an increase of both latencies and amplitudes, which was correlated with clinical improvement and represented a ("normalization") shift towards the EP patterns observed in age and sex matched normal children. Stimulatory drugs produced in normals a latency decrease in the early as well as in the late part of the EP. Contrarily, in hyperkinetic children an increase in latency was observed with d-amphetamine (as was observed with the neuroleptic thioridazine), which seems to be the neurophysiological correlate of the well known "paradoxical" clinical response of these children patients to amphetamine. Therapy responsive children showed more latency increase and amplitude augmentation than therapy resistant ones. Some pre-treatment VEP values were correlated with clinical outcome. EP profiles of antidepressants depend largely on their chemical structures: while MAO-inhibitors induce alterations similar to those of stimulants, tricyclic antidepressants produce a latency decrease in early and a latency increase in late EP components. The amplitudes are generally attenuated. The neotropic drug Hydergine was found to increase SEP amplitudes. Based on these pharmaco-EP profiles, new compounds were successfully classified: while halazepan and clorazepate and the anti-androgene cypoterone acetate induced changes typical for anxiolytics, the androgene mesterolone produced alterations similar to thymoleptic drugs.

# DISCRIMINATE FUNCTION MODELS OF ERP DATA
## IN HYPERACTIVE CHILDREN

James H. Satterfield, M.D.

Data will be presented that illustrate several problems in using event related potential data to discriminate between hyperactive and normal children (ages 6 to 12 years). Since some ERP amplitudes change twofold in this age range and since these changes differ between normal and hyperactive children (interaction with age), careful attention to this interaction is a necessary first step. Spuriously high (95%) correct classification can occur if too many variables are used to construct the model. With a reduction of the number of variables to only eight, a discriminate function developed on the same set of cases (as in the problem with 95 variables) correctly classified 90% of the training set and 76% of an unknown set.

The percent of cases correctly classified is dependent upon the chance way in which the split is carried out for the simulated replication. This was demonstrated by pooling all hyperactive and all normal cases and then randomly selecting one-half of each of two groups. Half of the cases in each group were combined and used as a training set, with the remaining cases used as an unknown set. All cases were then repooled and the above procedure repeated twenty times. Twenty discriminate functions were developed from the twenty training sets thus selected, and those functions were tested against twenty unknown sets. The mean correct classification for the twenty sets of training cases was 82% (SD = 7.8). The mean correct classification for the twenty unknown sets was 81% (SD = 8).

Major conclusions: (1) The success of the classification of twenty random split halves found here suggests potential usefulness of discriminate function models of ERP data as an aid in diagnosis. (2) The percent of cases correctly classified in split half replication studies using discriminate function models varies considerably, depending upon the particular (chance) split utilized. (3) The mean performance on a series of split half simulated replications is a better estimate of the ability of such models to separate groups than is any individual simulated replication. (4) When looking for ERP abnormalities in children, group interactions with age must be considered.

# AUDITORY EVOKED POTENTIALS AS PROBES OF LATERALIZED INFORMATION PROCESSING IN ADULTS AND INFANTS

D. W. Shucard and J. L. Shucard
Brain Sciences Laboratories
Department of Behavioral Sciences
National Jewish Hospital and Research Center
Denver, Colorado

Recently, Shucard, Shucard and Thomas (1977) reported a study in which cerebral specialization of function was assessed using auditory evoked potentials (AEPs) to pairs of task-irrelevant tones to probe activated brain sites involved in ongoing information processing. Other investigations have been conducted in our laboratory to elaborate on the original findings and to study the phenomenon in infants.

The original findings have been replicated in a new adult sample. In exploring the relationship between monopolar and bipolar placements, a negative relationship was found between AEP peak amplitudes obtained from temporal scalp placements references to $C_z$ ($T_4-C_z$, $T_3-C_z$) versus temporal placements referenced to linked ears. For example, when $T_3-C_z$ showed a higher amplitude response relative to $T_4-C_z$ during verbal information processing, and $T_3$-linked ears showed a lower amplitude response relative to $T_4$-linked ears during the same task. These findings indicate that reliable predictions can be made about evoked activity at the temporal sites whether a $C_z$ or linked ears reference is used.

Using our "two-tone probe technique" to study the development of cerebral specialization of function in awake, three-month old infants, we found significant sex dependent differences in left versus right hemisphere AEP amplitudes. While listening to complex auditory stimuli such as language and music, seven out of eight male infants showed a higher amplitude right hemisphere AEP as compared to the left for $N_{300}$, whereas, seven out of eight females showed a higher left hemisphere response relative to the right for the same peak. Similar results were obtained as well for $P_{200}$ and $P_{400}$ AEP peak amplitudes. No such relationships were found when the tones were presented alone without the verbal and musical stimuli. These findings support previously reported behavioral studies of developmental sex differences in analytical and spatial information processing which may be related to the influence of sex hormones on the developing brain.

The auditory probe technique might prove clinically useful for early detection of disabilities which are thought to be related to disturbances in cerebral organization. (Supported in part by NICHD Grant HD 11747.)

# AUDITORY EVOKED POTENTIALS INDICATE ATTENTIVE DYSFUNCTIONS IN HYPERKINETIC ADOLESCENTS

John S. Stamm and David L. Loiselle
Department of Psychology
SUNY, Stony Brook, N.Y. 11794

From the files of a children's clinic, thirteen 12 to 13 year-old boys were selected who had childhood diagnoses for hyperkinesis (HK), IQ above 84 and no neurological or psychiatric disorders. The controls (CG) were fifteen age-matched normal boys. The selective attention (SA) task consisted of dichotic series of 180 tone pips (50 msec, 75db SPL) of 800 Hz to one, and 1500 Hz to the other ear, with random interstimulus intervals (mean of 793 msec). Approximately 20 signals (840 Hz or 1560 Hz) were randomly interspersed. Subjects were instructed to count signals to one ear (Attend). Four series were given, counterbalanced for the attended ear and frequency. Averaged EPs (vertex to mastoid) to the pips were computed to the attend (AT) and non-attend (NA) channels. N100 amplitudes (baseline to peak) showed no significant group differences for NA. N100 was significantly higher under AT than NA conditions for the CG, but not for the HK group. Mean amplitude enhancements were 43% for CG and 13% for HK. P300 to the attend signals was found for every boy, with means of 9.51 μV for the CG and 6.74 μV for the HK (insignificant difference). Correlations between P300 and N100 AT were .48 for CG and .20 for HK. P300 to nonsignal pips were unremarkable.

Two behavioral tasks were button-press responses to the signals for the SA and for a 10 minute vigilance task which consisted of binaural 1500 Hz pips (40 per min) with 64 signals of 1560 Hz. On both tasks the HK made significantly fewer correct responses and more errors of commission than the CG. Also, on the vigilance task, reaction times to correct responses were significantly longer and more variable for the HK group. For SA, correlations between correct responses and N100 AT enhancements were -.03 for CG (mean 81% correct) and .57 for HK (mean 42% correct). Dichotic listening to sixty pairs of real syllables (pa, da, etc.) resulted in mean correct responses of 63.7% for CG and 54.7% for HK, and insignificant right-ear advantages for each group (means of 7.73 and 6.77). For lateral preferences, the incidence of consistent right hand-eye preferences was 67% for CG and 23% for HK, while crossed preferences were, respectively, 20% and 77%.

These findings demonstrate the applicability of the SA paradigm for EP measures of attentive dysfunctions in HK children. Their deficient N100 enhancements reflect deficits in selective attention, while their normal P300 waves would indicate adequate detection of the relevant signals. (Supported by a grant from The Grant Foundation.)

# DIMINISHED CNV REBOUND AND PERSEVERATIVE ATTENTION SET IN OLDER SUBJECTS

J. J. Tecce

Tufts University School of Medicine
Boston, Massachusetts,  U.S.A.

There are two CNV effects of potential value in clinical work - the CNV distraction effect which is exaggerated in schizophrenics and psychosurgery patients, and the CNV rebound effect which is absent in psychosurgery patients.  The present study assessed these effects in two age groups.  Twenty-one young subjects (ages 18-28) and thirty-one healthy older subjects (ages 56-85) were tested in two CNV paradigms.  The first was a control condition where a light flash (first stimulus of S1) was followed in 1.5 secs by a continuous tone (second stimulus or S2) which was terminated by an operant key press (control trials).  The second condition involved a random presentation of two types of trials: no-letters trials which were identical to control trials, and letters trials which were similar to control trials, except that three successive visual letters were presented within the S1-S2 interval for recall after the key press to S2.  A control condition preceded and followed the mixed condition.  Both young and older subjects showed a slowing of reaction time ($p < .001$) and a reduction in amplitude of CNV ($p < .01$) recorded at Fz, Cz and Pz in letters trials compared to control trials (CNV distraction effect).  For the young group, amplitude of CNV reached supranormal elevations (above control values) ($p < .01$) in the no-letters trials at each recording site (CNV rebound effect). The older group showed CNV rebound effects at Cz and Pz ($p < .01$) but not at Fz.  CNV rebound appears to reflect a switching of attention process between the divided-attention set of attending to letters and tone in letters trials and the unified attention set of attending to tone in no-letters trials.  Consequently, the absence of normal CNV rebound in frontal brain areas of the elderly may indicate some type of loss of resiliency of brain functioning that becomes expressed in a perseverative attention set.

# LATE COMPONENTS OF THE AUDITORY EVOKED RESPONSE IN SCHIZOPHRENICS

M. Timsit-Berthier and A. Gerono
Laboratory of Clinical Neurophysiology
University of Liege, Belgium

This study was carried out using ten normal controls and twenty patients selected from forty-five recorded patients (ten acute and ten chronic schizophrenics). All were matched for age, sex and educational level, and patient groups were matched for medication dosage level. They were exposed to a 15 min sequence of frequent/ infrequent auditory stimuli (85% of 60 dB – 320 Hz vs 15% of 60 dB – 1000 Hz with interstimulus intensity (ISI) : 5 sec), and were told to count infrequent stimuli. All the controls counted correctly, but only ten of the twenty patients were able to execute the task. Averaged evoked potentials (AEP) were recorded for the frequent and infrequent stimuli from Cz and Pz and one ocular site.

The most interesting findings were the following:

1. _Nosological effect_: The late positive component (LPC) amplitude (peak of maximum positivity between 300-500 msec) was larger for controls than for schizophrenics, but there was no difference between acute and chronic schizophrenics. Since some patients did not perform the task we could not distinguish the effect of the psychotic process from that of the subject option.

2) _Behavioral effect_: As could be expected, the most striking differences were seen between the LPC of controls and schizophrenics who counted poorly (Cz and Pz – $p < 0.001$). In this last group, there was no significant difference between the AEPs evoked by frequent and infrequent stimuli. This finding demonstrated that the attitude of the patient toward the experiment played a major role.

However, there were also differences between controls and schizophrenics who counted well. The latter displayed clear LPC but no significant difference between frequent and infrequent stimuli. These patient-control differences were seen in P3a and SW components, particularly in the development of N210 and the occurrence of an additional negative peak N3 (mean latency: 380 msec) which overlapped the early positivity process.

Thus, patients may have different electrophysiological potentials even when they perform a task as well as the normal subjects. These data raised the problem of whether we are faced with a different strategy or with a different brain reactivity.

HAAR TRANSFORMS OF EVENT-RELATED POTENTIALS:
TOWARD AN OPTIMAL RE-EXPRESSION OF THE DATA

Jacques J. Vidal and Eric D. Helfenbein
University of California, Los Angeles

Linear transform methods, routinely used to reduce ongoing EEG
data, have been applied sporadically to event related potentials
as a way to re-express the data with fewer variables (i.e. to reduce
dimensionality).

The most popular transforms with fixed basis function, Fourier
and Walsh-Hadamard, are pure frequency representations that span the
whole epoch and blur the information contained in the physiologically
significant time sequence of ERP components. The Haar transform es-
capes this loss by using basis functions that occupy separate time
windows. At each successive level (i.e., order) the windows become
narrower (by one half).

A comparative study is presented that shows the efficiency of
the transform in encoding visual ERP information. Discriminant
analyses (stepwise) applied to both raw and transformed data demonstrated simultaneously an increase in discrimination performance
and a reduction of dimensionality.

The Haar re-expression lies halfway between time and frequency analysis. It is sensitive both to local and global features
of the signal with the high-order terms becoming progressively more
local. The ability to capture local components is a major asset for
ERP analysis. In addition, the Haar functions take the form of
single "alterations", a waveform characteristic that mimics ERP components fairly well.

Finally, it seems that further improvements could be obtained
if the constraints imposed by orthogonality and basis functions
fixed in time were relaxed. Such a waveform directed data transformation is certainly realizable but still remains to be implemented
and tested. It would bring the long sought after capability for
automatic component separation.

477

DEVELOPMENTAL CHANGES IN ERP PRECEDING MOVEMENT:
RELATION TO VARIABILITY AND IQ

Charles Warren and Rathe Karrer
Illinois Institute for Developmental Disabilities and
University of Illinois, Chicago

Waveforms preceding right thumb flexion vary with development
and mental retardation (Karrer et al., in press).  We have replicated these waveforms in children, preadolescents and in normal and
mentally retarded young adults.  EEG during thumb flexion (button
press) was recorded DC between Oz, Cz, C3, C4, Fz and linked ears.
Activity occurring 920 msec pre-EMG to 320 msec post-EMG was classified by form using explicit criteria.

The frequency of waveforms at Cz confirmed developmental changes
in their distribution.  The retarded's distribution of waveforms
was different from the normal's.  Positive components at 600 and
150 msec prior to movement characterize the child's waveform.  Young
adults had typical negative-going waveforms.  Retarded had uniphasic
positive-going waveforms.  Preadolescents exhibited all waveform
types.  We also confirm the relation of positivity to a measure of
movement extraneous to the task (discarded eye movement artifact).
In all children positivity at C4 is directly related to the amount
of extraneous movement (r = +.49), and this is strongest in children
showing the typical "child's" waveform (r = +.85).  This relation
resides at different leads depending on waveform in children, preadolescents and MR, but not in adults.  Waveforms did not differ
on number of trials averaged, trials excluded due to eye movements
or in trial-to-trial variability, nor were they a function of background EEG.  Variability for all waveforms increased over the epoch
to a maximum at the response.  Between groups there was a variability
increase with decreasing age and mental retardation.  However, within
groups there was no relation of IQ to variability.

Children showing a waveform characteristic of the adult had
higher IQ (X=113) than those showing the typical "child's" waveform
(X=101) though there was no age difference.  For "adult" waveforms,
the less the positivity the greater the IQ for adults (Fz:r = -.83),
children (Fz,Cz:r -.90,-.78) and retarded (Oz:r = -.79 p<.1).  This
positivity that relates to IQ occurs between 600 msec and response
depending on group and lead.

These data support the concept that different waveforms preceding movement occur as a function of age and mental status.  The
positivity that characterizes the waveform of the physically and
mentally immune is functionally related to IQ and to the inhibition
of movement irrelevant to performance.

Supported by NICHD grant HD08265.

EVOKED POTENTIALS IN THE DIFFERENTIAL DIAGNOSIS OF SENSORY AND
NEUROLOGIC IMPAIRMENT IN CHILDREN

Ira P. Weiss and Ann B. Barnet
EEG Research Laboratory, Children's Hospital National Medical Center
Washington D.C. 20010

A combination test consisting of cortical auditory evoked
potentials (EPs), brain stem auditory EPs and visual EPs to flash
has been found to be very useful in assisting in the differential
diagnosis of sensory and neurologic impairment in children.  Data
on clinical referrals for such testing over a one year period at
C.H.N.M.C. were analyzed.  Among children who had normal brain
stem EP thresholds, those referred with a suspicion of hearing loss
had cortical auditory EP amplitudes approximately 50% lower than
children with no auditory symptoms.  No differences in BEP latencies
were found between the two groups.

EP latency did, however, differentiate between children with
and without a history of neurologic deficits.  Children with known
neurologic deficits had longer brain stem and cortical auditory EP
latencies than children with no neurologic symptoms whether or not
they presented with symptoms of an auditory deficit.

An evoked potential index (EPI) was devised to quantify the
"abnormality" of an EP.  The EPI was found to differentiate normal
children from those suffering from the effects of severe malnourish-
ment (marasmus).  Although the EPIs of the children improved during
the course of treatment, they were still deviant at the time of dis-
charge and at follow-up tests a year or more later.  These abnormalities may reflect a long lasting effect of malnutrition on brain
function (Barnet et al., Science, 1978, 201, 450-452).

In addition to the above findings, six case studies taken from
patients seen in this laboratory in the past six months are discussed.
The patients presented with symptoms of auditory and visual deficits.
EP test results helped confirm a variety of final diagnoses including brain stem encephalopathy, hemianopsia, cortical blindness,
peripheral hearing loss and "cortical deafness".  The patients
ranged in age from six months to five years.  The utility of EPs in
these differential diagnoses was dependent upon careful individual-
ized design of the test parameters and procedures for each patient.
Benefits of EP testing were maximized when the test was designed to
allow the patient to serve as his own control.  Analysis of EP
results was often assisted by comparing BEPs and AEPs, results from
left ear or eye and those from the right or results from two test
sessions.

# CONTRIBUTOR INDEX

# AUTHOR INDEX

Acheson, E.D. 381
Achor, L.J. 16, 427, 429
Adachi, T. 134
Adam, N. 117
Aine, C. 396
Ajax, E.T. 281
Alamanea, Y. 167
Albee, W. 118
Albin, S. 199
Aldridge, V.J. 267
Aleev, L.S. 13
Allen, A. 14
Allison, T. 13, 14, 54, 249,
   300, 301, 362, 446
Alm, M. 233
Altair, D. 411
Amabile, G. 342
Amadeo, M. 234, 282, 344, 362
Amlie, R.N. 429
Anders, T.R. 342
April, R.S. 134
Arden, G.B. 28
Armington, J.C. 13, 28, 301
Asselman, P. 13, 380
Axford, J.G. 28
Barber, C. 28
Baren, M. 103
Baribeau-Braun, J. 15, 412
Barkley, R.A. 165
Barnet, A.B. 410, 479
Barrett, G. 68, 151, 213
Bartlett, F. 233, 442
Bartlett, N.R. 442
Basar, E. 28
Beauchamp, M. 15, 16, 102

Beaumont, J.G. 232
Beck, E.C. 231, 411
Becker, D.P. 14
Becker, P.E. 120
Bedrosian, E. 81
Begleiter, H. 118, 411
Behrman, J. 15
Beidler, L.M. 300, 301
Benson, P.J. 249, 250, 264, 281
Bernardi, G. 342
Biersdorf, W.R. 282
Bigum, H.B. 411
Black, J.L. 15, 381
Blake, R. 182
Blakemore, C. 28, 182, 468
Blumhardt, L.D. 151, 213
Borenstein, S. 101
Bosley, T.M. 14
Botwinik, J. 394
Bragdon, H.R. 41, 67, 68
Braley, B.W. 166, 234
Braren, M. 282, 316
Breitmeyer, 468
Brent, G. 394
Brizzee, K. 395
Brown, D. 233
Brown, J.W. 41
Brown, W.S. 41, 42, 134, 281
Bruner, J.S. 199
Brunko, E. 100, 102, 264
Buchsbaum, M.S. 53, 54, 81,
   117, 165, 361
Buchthal, F. 13
Buchwald, J.S. 15, 411, 412,
   427, 428

489